OXFORD MEDICAL PUBLICATIONS

Duchenne Muscular Dystrophy

OXFORD MONOGRAPHS ON MEDICAL GENETICS

General Editors:

ARNO G. MOTULSKY
PETER S. HARPER
MARTIN BOBROW
CHARLES SCRIVER

Former Editors:

J. A. FRASER ROBERTS
C. O. CARTER

OXFORD MONOGRAPHS ON MEDICAL GENETICS No 15

Duchenne Muscular Dystrophy

ALAN E. H. EMERY

MD, DSc, PhD, FRCP, MFCM, FLS, FRS(E)

*Emeritus Professor of Human Genetics,
and University Fellow, Edinburgh
Visiting Fellow, Green College, Oxford*

OXFORD   NEW YORK   TOKYO
OXFORD UNIVERSITY PRESS
1987

Oxford University Press, Walton Street, Oxford OX2 6DP

Oxford New York Toronto
Delhi Bombay Calcutta Madras Karachi
Petaling Jaya Singapore Hong Kong Tokyo
Nairobi Dar es Salaam Cape Town
Melbourne Auckland
and associated companies in
Beirut Berlin Ibadan Nicosia

Oxford is a trade mark of Oxford University Press

Published in the United States
by Oxford University Press, New York

British Library Cataloguing in Publication Data
Emery, Alan E. H.
Duchenne muscular dystrophy. — (Oxford
monographs on medical genetics; no. 15)
— (Oxford medical publication)
1. Muscular dystrophy — Diagnosis
2. Muscular dystrophy — Treatment
I. Title
616.7'48   RC935.M7
ISBN 0-19-261556-4

Library of Congress Cataloging in Publication Data
Emery, Alan E. H.
Duchenne muscular dystrophy.
(Oxford monographs on medical genetics; no. 15)
(Oxford medical publications)
Bibliography: p.
1. Duchenne muscular dystrophy.   I. Title.
II. Series.   III. Series: Oxford medical publications.
RJ482.D78E44   1987   616.7'48   86–28427
ISBN 0-19-261556-4

Set by Colset Private Limited, Singapore
Printed in Great Britain by Butler & Tanner Ltd
Frome, Somerset

To

Kyle Grace

memories of whose ever-cheerful

disposition was a continual

source of encouragement

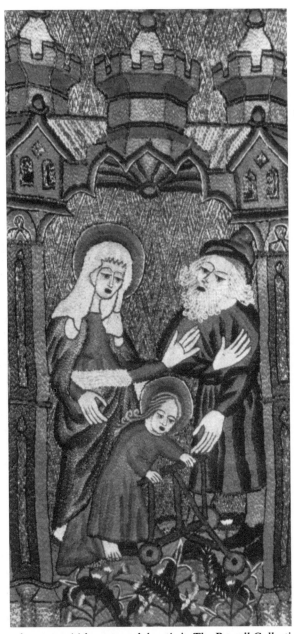

Detail of an orphrey on a 14th century dalmatic in The Burrell Collection, Glasgow. (Reproduced with permission.)

Foreword

JOHN WALTON

Warden, Green College, Oxford;
former Professor of Neurology, University of Newcastle upon Tyne;
Chairman, Muscular Dystrophy Group of Great Britain and
Northern Ireland

World-wide interest in diseases of muscle has burgeoned within the last 30 years. All of those working in the field accept that the Duchenne type of muscular dystrophy, the commonest of the inherited myopathies and the most devastating in its effects upon the affected individual and his family, presents to both doctors and scientists a formidable research challenge. Ever since I myself began, some 35 years ago, to work in this field with the late Professor Nattrass, until his death Honorary Life President of the Muscular Dystrophy Group of Great Britain, the tragic consequences of this disease have been at one and the same time a spur and also a reproach to research workers in myology. But at a time when it seems at last that markers have been identified which lie within the Duchenne gene on the X chromosome, and when full characterization and sequencing of the gene can only be regarded as imminent despite its evident complexity, the practical consequences of these exciting discoveries are already beginning to be felt in relation to carrier detection and antenatal diagnosis. Research is now beginning to give genuine hope to patients with the condition, to their families, and to those who care for them.

It is therefore timely that a book devoted to this subject should be published, to bring the knowledge accumulated in the last century, since the disease was first clearly delineated by Duchenne de Boulogne, into modern perspective.

The contributions which Professor Alan Emery has made to our understanding of neuromuscular disease over the last three decades are well known, especially in the field of genetics. It is therefore entirely appropriate that he should have chosen to devote his very considerable talents to undertaking a detailed and scholarly survey of the literature, enlivened by the fruits of his personal experience, in order to set down in print a succinct but nevertheless current review of present knowledge of this disease. This monograph represents a very considerable achievement. It reviews critically and in my view dispassionately the substantial volume of published work on Duchenne

dystrophy and related diseases, beginning with a fascinating historical introduction before going on to discuss the clinical features, diagnostic methods,
differential diagnosis, the non-muscular manifestations of the disorder and
subsequently its biochemistry, pathogenesis, genetics, and molecular pathology. Very properly, the last few chapters deal with prevention, genetic counselling, and management, and there are several useful appendices, one of
which lists the Muscular Dystrophy Associations which have been established
to aid in research and in patient care and welfare in many countries throughout the world.

So-called 'single disease monographs' can never be expected to be best-
sellers, but everyone with an interest in muscular dystrophy from whatever
standpoint should read this book and I hope that many will wish to possess it
as it presents an invaluable 'state of the art' review of where we stand at a time
when explosive and exciting new knowledge is emerging. Neurologists,
paediatricians, geneticists, biochemists, pathologists, nurses, physio-
therapists, occupational therapists, social workers, teachers, and many other
members of the caring community are all likely to find something within this
book to interest and stimulate or fuel their concern for the unfortunate
sufferers from this disease. In writing it, I believe that Professor Emery has
done his profession and society a considerable service.

Oxford, September 1986

Preface

Duchenne muscular dystrophy is one of the most serious and common genetic disorders. Although it has generated a considerable amount of research over the last few decades, no effective treatment has yet been found and the cause remains unknown. An attempt has been made in this book to present a broad picture of the disease encompassing the various clinical features as well as some of the findings in the basic sciences. It is hoped that it might therefore be of interest to all those involved in the field who are not necessarily experts.

Writing the book was undertaken during the tenure of a Leverhulme Emeritus Fellowship and a Senior Visiting Research Fellowship at Green College, Oxford, the latter being funded by the Nuffield Provincial Hospitals Trust. I am most grateful to the Warden, Sir John Walton, and the Fellows of Green College, as well as Professor John Edwards, for providing excellent facilities.

I am also grateful to the following for permission to reproduce certain illustrations and published data:
Frontispiece (Burrell Collection), Figs 1.1 and 1.3 (Professor R. Krstić and Springer-Verlag, publishers), Fig. 1.2 (Dr M. J. Cullen), Fig. 2.1 (Professor P. E. Becker), Fig. 2.3 (Musei Vaticani), Fig. 2.4 (National Galleries of Scotland, Edinburgh), Figs 2.5 and 2.9 (*Founders of Neurology*, edited by W. Haymaker, 1953, courtesy of Charles C. Thomas, publishers, Springfield, Illinois), Fig. 2.7 (Dr Macdonald Critchley), Fig. 3.3 (Dr Sarah Bundey), Figs 3.7 and 13.6 (Professor V. Dubowitz and W. B. Saunders Company Limited, publishers), Fig. 4.6 (NI Medical, Redditch, Worcestershire, England), Fig. 4.9 (the Editor of the *British Medical Journal*), Fig. 4.16 (Dr J. Trevor Hughes and Lloyd-Luke, publishers), Figs 3.1, 5.1, 5.2, and 8.1 (Churchill Livingstone, publishers), Fig. 6.2 (Editor of the *Journal of Medical Genetics*), Fig. 6.3 (Dr J. K. Perloff and the editor of the *American Journal of Medicine*), Fig. 6.5 (Sir John Walton), Fig. 7.1 (Dr S. P. Frostick), Table 8.4 (Dr F. Schanne and the American Association for the Advancement of Science), Fig.10.3 (Mr G. Spowart and the editor of *Lancet*), Fig. 10.6 (Dr Kay Davies), Fig. 11.9 (John Wiley and Sons Limited, publishers), Fig. 13.2 (Ms Sylvia Hyde), Figs 13.5 and 13.7 (Dr G. M. Cochrane and the Mary Marlborough Lodge), Fig. 13.8 (Mr G. R. Houghton), Fig. 13.11 (Dr M. Brooke and the editor of *Muscle and Nerve*), Fig. 13.12 (Dr Mayana Zatz).

I should also like to thank Dr A. Cuthbertson for generously allowing me to consult his unpublished dissertation, Dr R. Pennington for helpful advice, Miss J. Ferguson, Librarian of the Royal College of Physicians, Edinburgh; Mrs D. Magee of the Ashmolean Museum, Oxford; and Mr G. Davenport, Librarian of the Royal College of Physicians, London. Finally I should particularly like to thank Dr Sarah Bundey for reading the entire script and making several useful suggestions, and Mrs Isobel Black for her excellent secretarial assistance.

Edinburgh/Oxford   A. E. H. E
April 1986

Contents

1 Introduction

Duchenne muscular dystrophy is the second most common genetic disorder in Man and has been recognized as a distinct entity for over a hundred years. In the last thirty years or so it has generated a great deal of interest among research workers and in their bibliograpy of what they considered to be the more important publications on the subject, Herrmann and Spiegler (1985) list no less than 789 references. Yet despite all the interest, the cause still remains elusive. This may in part be due to the fact that the tissue which is predominantly affected, namely skeletal muscle, is complex as must also be the genetic repertoire responsible for its normal development and functioning.

There are 434 different muscles in the human body which in the adult contribute to over 40 per cent of the total body weight. Much has been written on the development and morphology of muscle, and an excellent review is given by Landon (1982), but here only some general principles need be emphasized. The essential element of muscle is the *muscle fibre* (myofibre) which has been defined as '. . . a multinucleated cell that contains a large number of myofibrils embedded in a matrix of undifferentiated protoplasm, all enclosed within a fine sheath, the sarcolemma' (Adams 1975, p. 15). Muscle fibres are grouped together into fascicles and a network of collagen fibres surrounds each fascicle (perimysium), and extends between individual muscle fibres (endomysium). Each muscle fibre, which vary in length from one muscle to another, is bounded by the plasma membrane (*plasmalemma*) and an outer basement membrane (*basal lamina*). The latter along with the endomysium constitute the *sarcolemma* though this term is sometimes also used when referring to the plasma and basement membranes together (Fig. 1.1). Each multinucleated muscle fibre is formed during development by the fusion of several dividing mononucleated myoblasts derived from the myotomes. After fusion the nuclei of the fibre do not divide again and lie in the cytoplasm (*sarcoplasm*) along with the contractile elements. Small mononucleated *satellite cells* are situated between the plasma and basement membranes of the muscle fibre. These cells contain many ribosomes and are particularly frequent in diseased muscle, though how this occurs is unknown (Mauro 1979). They are believed to be a persistent population of myoblastic stem cells which retain the ability to divide and are a source of additional muscle fibre nuclei during growth and regenerative repair (Fig. 1.2). A muscle fibre contains many *myofibrils* which are the contractile elements of muscle and display alternating dark (A) and light (I) bands, and through the

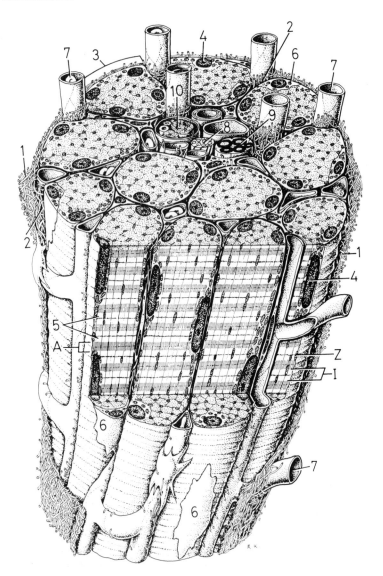

Fig. 1.1. Diagrammatic representation of a small fascicle of muscle fibres. (1, perimysium; 2, endomysium; 3, muscle fibre (myofibre); 4, nucleus; 5, contractile myofibrils; 6, satellite cells; 7, capillaries.) (Fom Krstić (1978) reproduced with kind permission of the author and publishers.)

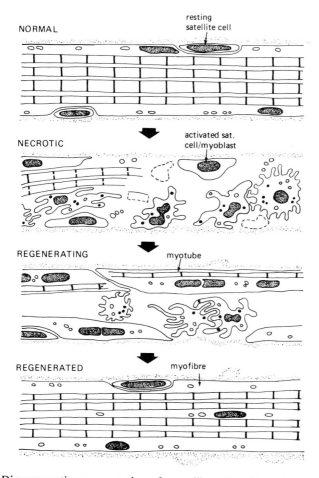

Fig. 1.2. Diagrammatic representation of a satellite cell and its role in muscle fibre regeneration. (Reproduced by kind permission of Dr M. J. Cullen.)

centre of the latter is the dense Z-line (band or disc) (*see* Fig. 1.1). The myofibrils are themselves composed of thick and thin *myofilaments*. During contraction and relaxation of the muscle, thin filaments slide between the thick filaments. In addition to nuclei and myofibrils, the sarcoplasm of a muscle fibre contains mitochondria, glycogen granules, lipid bodies, ribosomes, the transverse system of tubules (*T-system*), and the *sarcoplasmic reticulum*. The latter is equivalent to the endoplasmic reticulum of cells in other tissues and forms a network of tubules which run between the myofibrils. The T-system consists of transversely arranged, fine, interconnecting, tubular extensions of the plasma membrane. A single T-tubule and two dilated ends of the sarcoplasmic reticulum form so-called *'triads'* which are concerned with the excitation and contraction of muscle fibres. A nerve impulse, via the neuromuscular junction, produces depolarization of the muscle cell surface membrane which then spreads inwards along the T-system to the triads. This results, by a mechanism which is still not clear (Beam *et al.* 1986), in the rapid release of calcium from the sarcoplasmic reticulum into the sarcoplasm, which in turn then results in the interaction between thick and thin filaments producing muscle contraction (Fig. 1.3).

This account, although brief and sketchy, emphasizes the complex nature of skeletal muscle. But as this is not the only tissue affected in Duchenne muscular dystrophy, an obsession with changes in skeletal muscle could obscure ideas of the fundamental nature of the basic defect. Furthermore, in attempting to maintain an open mind about tissue expression, it might also be helpful to remember that there is no absolute certainty that *all* cases of the disease will have the same identical biochemical defect. The biochemical literature is replete with many examples of this, as for instance in episodic rhabdomyolysis and myoglobinuria (Kark and Becker 1981; Rowland 1984). Furthermore, even if the gene product were the same in all cases, it seems very unlikely that the precise molecular defect will be identical in all cases.

No doubt the Duchenne gene (or more likely 'gene cluster') will soon be isolated, cloned, and sequenced. It will then be possible to devise rational approaches to treatment. Such information will doubtless throw light not only on the pathogenesis of the disease, but also help to answer more fundamental questions including differential gene expression in different groups of muscles. Once the cause of Duchenne muscular dystrophy is known, a great deal more about normal muscle biochemistry and physiology will be understood.

Any attempt to mention all the reported findings in this disease would be in danger of turning into a mere catalogue because so many appear to be unrelated and often contradictory. Futhermore, on present knowledge it is difficult to find a satisfactory explanation for all the various observations which have been reported. During the process of selecting and emphasizing certain findings for the sake of clarity, it is inevitable that the resultant picture may be oversimplified, somewhat idiosyncratic, and probably inconsistent. The only defence is that voiced by Miguel de Unamuno in Erwin Schrödinger's book *What is life?* (1944) which Watson and Crick and many others found so illuminating:

If a man never contradicts himself, the reason must be that he virtually never says anything at all.

The references have been selected because they are of historical interest, or present helpful and detailed reviews, or are considered to be particularly seminal in regard to pathogenesis. Apart from Herrmann and Spiegler's bib-

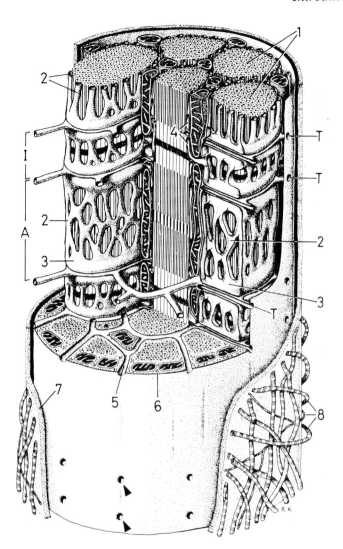

Fig. 1.3. Diagrammatic representation of a single muscle fibre. (1, myofibril; 2 and 3, sarcoplasmic reticulum; T and 5, transverse tubular system; 4, triads; 6, plasma membrane; 7, basement membrane; 8, endomysium.) (From Krstić (1978) reproduced with kind permission of the author and publishers.)

liography (1985), the Muscular Dystrophy Association of America publishes monthly abstracts from the world literature on clinical and basic science research into muscular dystrophy and related disorders. This is *the* single, most helpful literature source available to research workers in the field.

Finally, there have been several monographs in recent years which present detailed reviews of the muscular dystrophies and related disorders in general, such as Swash and Schwartz (1981), Dubowitz (1987), and Walton (1987), as well as several which deal with specific aspects of the disease, especially muscle pathology (Mastaglia and Walton 1982; Schröder 1982; Kakulas and Adams 1985; Dubowitz 1985). The comprehensive text of Engel and Banker (1986) covers the anatomy, biochemistry, and physiology of normal muscle as well as detailed reviews of various neuromuscular disorders.

This book, which is partly based on cases and families studies by the author, is not intended for the expert in any particular field, but rather for those with more catholic interests who are involved in this distressing and perplexing disease, which Gowers himself (1879b) referred to as being '. . . one of the most interesting and at the same time most sad'.

2 History of the disease

Early beginnings

Muscular dystrophy has no doubt afflicted Man from earliest times. Since the ancient Egyptians in their wall paintings often depicted physical abnormalities with some care, so that they can often be identified as diseases we now recognize, such as paralytic poliomyelitis and congenital dwarfism, it is just possible that they might have portrayed muscular dystrophy. In fact it has been suggested (Pöch and Becker 1955) that this might be so in a relief painting on the wall of a tomb in ancient Egypt, dating from the 18th Dynasty of the New Kingdom, that is, about 1500 BC (Fig. 2.1). The subject depicted

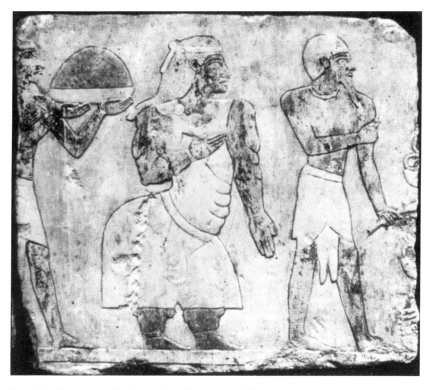

Fig. 2.1. Egyptian relief painting from the 18th Dynasty. (Reproduced by kind permission of Professor P. E. Becker.)

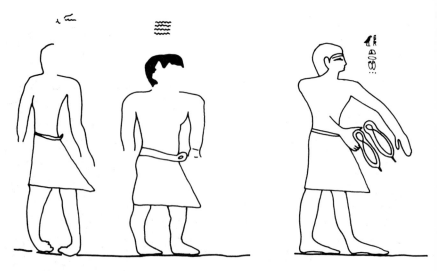

Fig. 2.2. Drawings from a tomb at Beni Hasan (*circa* 2800–2500 BC.)

on the wall of the Temple of Hatshepsut is the Queen of Punt who shows lumbar lordosis and who, it has even been suggested, may also have some calf enlargement. However in comparison with the adjoining figure she seems generally fatter, and perhaps what is shown is no more than generalized obesity, which is also the opinion of an expert Egyptologist (Riad 1955). However on the wall of a tomb (No. 17 in Newberry 1893) at Beni Hasan, dating from the Middle Kingdom (*circa* 2800–2500 BC), there are depicted two figures of interest (Fig. 2.2). The first has bilateral club foot. In the middle, however, is a boy with what could just possibly be muscular dystrophy. He has lost the normal arch of his feet, which is usually clear in Egyptian wall paintings as seen in the figure to the right. Also, his calves seem somewhat enlarged, and he may have some degree of (pseudo) hypertrophy of certain upper limb muscles. On the other hand as the hieroglyph above his head implies he may have been a dwarf.

The *Transfiguration* was Raphael's last great work, and was unfinished when he died on Good Friday, 1520, at the untimely age of 37. Vasari, in his *Lives of the Artists*, considers the boy in the painting to be 'possessed by a devil', an idea which may have prompted subsequent observers to suggest that it could illustrate a case of epilepsy. However, Duchenne himself, after whom the commonest form of muscular dystrophy is named, when visiting the National Hospital for Nervous Diseases in London where a reproduction of the painting hung, commented at the time that the boy depicted by the artist could be cited as an example of pseudohypertrophic muscular dystrophy (Fig. 2.3).

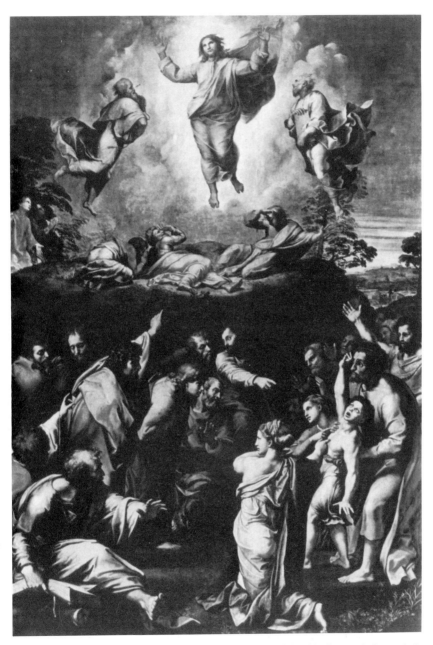

Fig. 2.3. Raphael's the *Transfiguration*. (Reproduced by kind permission of the *Musei Vaticani.*)

However, such observations can only be speculative. The first clinical descriptions of dystrophy, at least in the English language, do not appear until the 19th century.

Charles Bell was born in Fountainbridge in Edinburgh in 1774, where he studied medicine and subsequently worked as a surgeon–anatomist, often illustrating his works with his own carefully executed drawings. At the age of thirty he moved to London where he spent most of his working life, and was a Founder of the Middlesex Medical School. He returned to Edinburgh to the Chair of Surgery in 1835, and died in 1842 from angina. He is best remembered for being the first to describe paralysis of the facial nerve (Bell's palsy) and, with the French experimental physiologist, François Magendie, for discovering the distinct functions of the posterior (sensory) and anterior (motor) nerve roots of the spinal cord (Fig. 2.4).

Among his numerous publications is his *The nervous system of the human body* first published in 1830 and which subsequently ran to several editions.

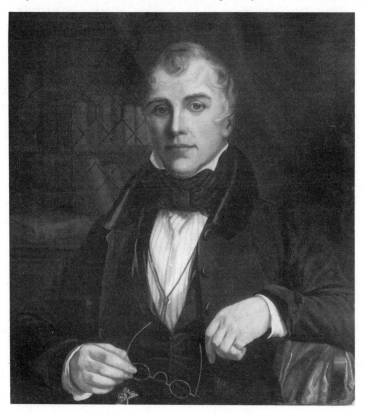

Fig. 2.4. Sir Charles Bell. (Reproduced by kind permission of the National Galleries of Scotland, Edinburgh.)

In it he describes (Case 89) a young man of eighteen with wasting and weakness of the quadriceps muscles which began some 8 years previously and which

... disabled him from rising; and it is now curious to observe how he will twist and jerk his body to throw himself upright from his seat. I use this expression, for it is a very different motion from that of rising from the chair.   (Bell 1830, p. CLXIII)

There was no sensory loss. Without muscle pathology the diagnosis cannot be certain, but the description would certainly be compatible with muscular dystrophy.

Gowers (1879), whose seminal contributions to the subject will be dealt with in more detail later, refers to the possibility of the disease having been described in 1838 by Coste and Gioja from Naples. Unfortunately it has not been possible to trace the original report in the *Ann. dell' Osped. degl. Incur. di Napoli* for 1838 but this was abstracted in Schmidt's *Jahrbücher* (Schmidt 1838). It concerns two brothers who, about the age of ten, developed progressive muscle wasting and weakness associated with marked enlargement of certain muscle groups, including the calf muscles (? pseudohypertrophy) with subsequent development of widespread contractures by the age of 18. Again, since there was no muscle pathology the diagnosis must remain speculative. However, in 1847 a Mr Partridge presented a case to the pathological Society of London (reported in the *London Medical Gazette* Vol. 5, p. 944) of a boy who, from about the age of nine, had developed progressive muscle wasting and weakness, had enlarged calves and muscle contractures and who died after an attack of measles at age 14. Examination of muscle tissue at autopsy revealed widespread fatty degeneration. In the same year, 1847, Dr W.J. Little, a physician at the London Hospital, studied two affected brothers aged 12 and 14 which he reported in detail in 1853 in a book entitled *On the nature and treatment of the deformities of the human frame*. Both brothers presented a similar picture. Onset was in early childhood with a tendency to walk on the toes and a peculiar gait with the '. . . head and body having been inclined backwards'. There was progressive muscle wasting and weakness affecting the neck, trunk, and upper and lower extremities associated with enlargement of the calf muscles and contractures 'behind the heels'. Sensation was normal. Both boys were unable to walk by the age of 11. The elder died at 14 and at autopsy, examination of the gastrocnemius and soleus muscles (and some other muscles as well) revealed that the muscle tissue had been largely replaced by fat ('adipose degeneration'). The brain and spinal cord appeared normal. These findings would certainly be consistent with the diagnosis of the severe form of muscular dystrophy which predominantly affects boys. However, the fullest and earliest description of this disorder must be credited to Dr Edward Meryon of St. Thomas's Hospital, London.

Unfortunately, not very much is known about Meryon. He was born in

1809 and studied medicine in Paris and University College, London. He qualified as a Member of the Royal College of Surgeons in 1831, proceeding to an MD degree in 1844. His chief appointments were at St. Thomas's Hospital and the Hospital for Nervous Diseases where it is just possible he may have been acquainted with the young William Gowers. He was apparently a man of wide learning and published several books relating to the nervous system. He also embarked on a *History of medicine* but unfortunately did not get beyond a first volume. In Feiling's *History of the Maida Vale Hospital* the only reference to him reads: 'Edward Meryon although not really distinguished in medicine, was clearly a well-known figure in London society at the time' (Feiling 1958, p. 5). He died at his home in Mayfair in 1880, at the age of 71.

In a communication addressed to the Royal Medical and Chirurgical Society in December 1851 and which was published in the Transactions of the Society the following year, Meryon described eight affected boys in three families. Interestingly, one of the two affected brothers in the second family is the case on which Partridge had earlier reported his autopsy findings in 1847. Meryon was particularly impressed by the familial nature of the condition and its predilection for males, and in his book *Practical and pathological researches on the various forms of paralysis* published in 1864, he details a family in which there were four affected cousins with the disorder having been transmitted through three sisters. Secondly, he subjected muscle tissue to microscopic examination and reported that . . .

the striped elementary primitive fibres were found to be completely destroyed, the sarcous element being diffused, and in many places converted into oil globules and granular matter, whilst the sarcolemma and tunic of the elementary fibre was broken down and destroyed   (Meryon 1852, p. 76)

He therefore used the term 'granular degeneration' for the microscopic changes he observed. Thirdly, he observed that

. . . the relative proportion of the grey matter to the white in the cord, and the ganglionic cells of the former, and the tubular structure of the latter, as well as of the nerves and the white substance within the neurolemma, wherever examined by the microscope, all bore evidence of the healthy condition of the nervous system   (Meryon 1852, p. 78)

Thus, he concluded that this was a familial disease which primarily affected muscle tissue and was not a disease of the nervous system. Meryon's clear delineation of the disorder and his understanding of its nature were very significant contributions. It is therefore unfortunate that he has not always been given the credit he deserves and that his work is completely overshadowed by that of Duchenne.

Duchenne de Boulogne

Guillaume Benjamin Amand Duchenne, Duchenne de Boulogne as he signed himself in order not to be confused with Duchesne of Paris, was born in the town of Boulogne-sur-Mer on 17 September 1806 (Fig. 2.5). He studied medicine in Paris where his teachers included Cruveilhier, Dupuytren, and Laennec. He then returned to Boulogne with the intention of being a family doctor (Guilly 1936). However, this proved a very unhappy time, for his young wife died of puerperal sepsis 14 days after giving birth to their son Emile in 1833, and for several years afterwards he remained depressed and lost interest in his work. In 1839 he remarried, this time to a widow, but this does not seem to have been a happy marriage. Then in 1842, at the age of 36, he returned to Paris where he spent the rest of his life. Cuthbertson (1977) suggests there may have been three factors instrumental in his return to Paris and to neurology: his growing interest in the possible therapeutic effects of electricity, his own family history of a 'nervous' disease, and his disastrous second marriage. Whatever the reasons he quickly settled in Paris where he became a sort of itinerant physician mainly at the Salpêtrière. He never held an official hospital or academic appointment and was therefore completely free to pursue his obsessional interests in the electrical stimulation of muscle, muscle function, and neuromuscular diseases. He studied the mechanisms of facial expression, a subject which had also interested Charles Bell some years previously. His painstaking observations led to clear descriptions of several

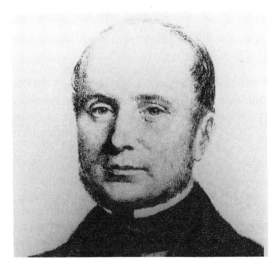

Fig. 2.5. Duchenne de Boulogne. (Reproduced from *The founders of neurology*, edited by Webb Haymaker 1953. Courtesy of Charles C. Thomas, Publishers, Springfield, Illinois.)

disorders, his name now being most closely associated with progressive muscular atrophy (with Aran) and progressive bulbar palsy (both part of the motor neurone disease complex), and of course pseudohypertrophic muscular dystrophy. He devised a strength gauge or dynamometer and a special needle-harpoon for muscle biopsy. His numerous publications have been translated, edited, and condensed for the New Sydenham Society by Poore (1883). The last five years of his life saw him famous but tragic: his wife died in 1870 and his son shortly afterwards from typhoid fever. He suffered a cerebral haemorrhage in August 1875, and Potain and Charcot never left him during the last weeks of his illness, taking it in turns to sleep by his bed. He died on 17 September 1875 on his 69th birthday. On 30 October the Paris correspondent of the *Lancet* (see Appendix A), commenting on Duchenne's life and work, wrote that despite many adverse circumstances

. . . his reputation has come out clear and bright as an honest, hard-working, acute, and ingenious observer, an original discoverer, a skilful professional man, and a kind-hearted, benevolent gentleman.

Despite his abounding interest in research, it seems he never lost a bedside manner.

Duchenne's interest in muscular dystrophy was first aroused in 1858 when his attention was drawn to a case, details of which he published in 1861 in the second edition of his book *De l'électrisation localisée* (Duchenne 1861). Later, in 1868, he reviewed in considerable detail his original case plus 12 further cases, two of whom were young girls, and referred to a further 15 cases in the German literature (Duchenne 1868). By 1870 he had seen some 40 cases of the disease, not counting those he saw when he visited the London hospitals around this time (Fig. 2.6).

Duchenne defined the disease as being characterized by: progressive weakness of movement, first affecting the lower limbs and then later the upper limbs; a gradual increase in the size of many affected muscles; an increase in interstitial connective tissue in affected muscles with the production of abundant fibrous and adipose tissue in the later stages. The onset was in childhood or early adolescence, was more prevalent in boys than girls, and could affect several children in the same family. Though Meryon had studied the histology of affected muscles, his observations had been limited to material obtained at autopsy. Duchenne on the other hand, used his needle-harpoon (*enporte-pièce histologique*) to obtain biopsy specimens in life. In fact, using this technique, he was able to study material from the same patient at different stages of the disease. His observations led him to conclude that the fundamental anatomical lesion was hyperplasia of the interstitial connective tissue which therefore prompted him to use the term *paralysie myosclérosique* as an alternative to *paralysie musculaire pseudohypertrophique*. Previously, a pathological diagnosis could only be made at autopsy–so-called

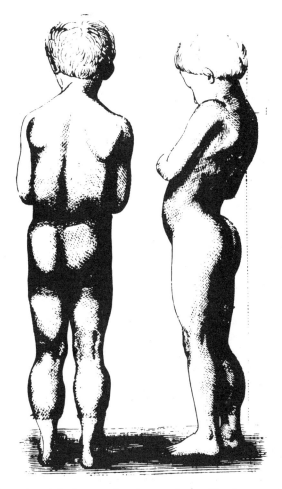

Fig. 2.6. Duchenne's original case, showing marked calf enlargement and lumbar lordosis. (From *Arch. Gén. Méd.* Vol. 11, p. 8 (1868).)

diagnosis of Morgagni. But Duchenne's technique meant such a diagnosis could be made in life. He believed, correctly, that unlike progressive (spinal) muscular atrophy of childhood the disease was not caused by a lesion in the spinal cord. In this matter it is rather disappointing that Duchenne felt he should dismiss Meryon's contributions when he says that the latter confused the disease with progressive muscular atrophy, and therefore thought it had a neurogenic basis, which as we have seen he did not, and Duchenne goes further by giving the date of Meryon's address to the Royal Medical and Chirurgical Society as 1866 when in fact it was some 15 years earlier in 1851.

Duchenne carefully weighed the available evidence regarding the possible aetiology of the disorder, particularly with regard to possible neurological or vasomotor factors, but had to conclude, just as we would today '. . . la pathogénie de la paralysie pseudo-hypertrophique est très obscure; elle doit être réservée . . .'.

William R. Gowers

Considerable interest now began to be shown in the disease and numerous case reports appeared in the French, English, German, American, Australian, and Danish literature (Dubowitz 1978). However, the next physician to enter the stage who made a significant contribution to the subject was William R. Gowers. Gowers was born in 1845 and spent all his life in London. He had a brilliant undergraduate career at University College Hospital where he was awarded medals in almost every subject of the medical curriculum and graduated with first class honours. He later became Professor of Medicine at University College, as well as being a physician at the National Hospital for Nervous Diseases. He was a man of immense intellect and wide interests. He was a knowledgeable botanist and an authority on mosses, an accomplished artist (he exhibited at the Royal Academy), and an obsessional shorthand writer. He introduced into medicine a number of new terms such as 'knee jerk', 'fibrositis', and 'abiotrophy'. He described several clinical signs including the nasal smile in myasthenia gravis, as well as the so-called Gowers' manoeuvre. He also invented a haemocytometer which was widely used for many years. It is understandable that in his day he was therefore widely admired and respected. He remained, however, a reserved and very private individual with few intimate friends. He died in 1915 at the age of 70 (Critchley 1949) (Fig. 2.7).

Gowers' interest in muscular dystrophy was kindled when working as a premedical student apprentice to a Dr Thomas Simpson in Coggeshall, Essex. Here he came across a family with four brothers afflicted with a '. . . strange disorder of locomotion with wasting of some muscles and enlargement of others'. Later he learned that the disease had been described in 1852 by Meryon and in 1879 he delivered a series of lectures on the disorder at the National Hospital which were published in *Lancet* (Gowers 1879a) and subsequently made into a monograph (Gowers 1879b). The latter was based on information from 220 cases, which included 24 he had seen himself, 20 seen by colleagues, and the remainder from the literature. In deference to Duchenne he referred to the disease as 'pseudohypertrophic muscular paralysis', and in his monograph he attempted to give as complete a picture of the disease as possible with detailed discussions of the clinical features, pathology, prognosis, and possible treatment. As with all of Gowers' writings,

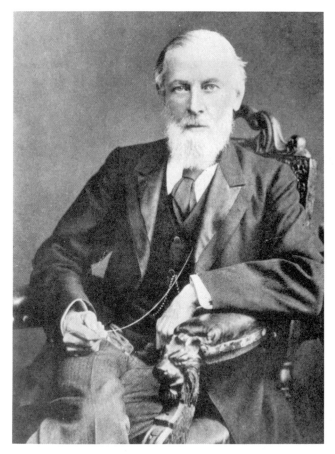

Fig. 2.7. Sir William Gowers. (Reproduced by kind permission of Dr Macdonald Critchley.)

clarity, thoughtfullness and good prose are evident. This is illustrated in the graphic opening paragraph:

The disease is one of the most interesting and at the same time most sad, of all those with which we have to deal: interesting on account of its peculiar features and mysterious nature; sad on account of our powerlessness to influence its course, except in a very slight degree, and on account of the conditions in which it occurs. It is a disease of early life and of early growth. Manifesting itself commonly at the transition from infancy to childhood, it develops with the child's development, grows with his growth–so that every increase in stature means an increase in weakness, and each year takes him a step further on the road to a helpless infirmity, and in most cases to an early and inevitable death.

The interest in the book lies mainly in the detailed presentation of the clinical features of the disease, and describes what is nowadays usually referred to as Gowers' manoeuvre or Gowers' sign (Fig. 2.8). Weakness of the hip and knee extensors causes difficulty in rising from the floor or a chair. As a result, when getting up patients

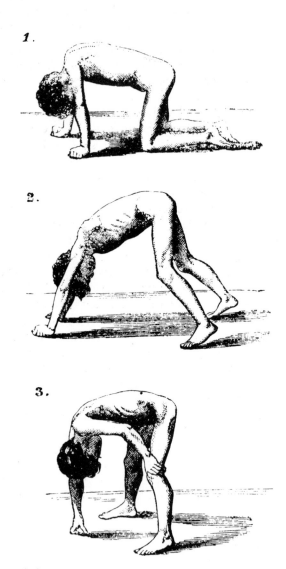

Fig. 2.8. Gowers' sign or manoeuvre. (From W. R. Gowers' *Pseudo-hypertrophic muscular paralysis*, 1879.)

. . . first put the hands on the ground (1), then stretch out the legs behind them far apart, and, the chief weight of the trunk resting on the hands, by keeping the toes on the ground and pushing the body backwards, they manage to get the knees extended so that the trunk is supported by the hands and feet, all placed as widely apart as possible (2). Next the hands are moved alternately along the ground backwards so as to bring a larger portion of the weight of the trunk over the legs. Then one hand is placed upon the knee (3), and a push with this and with the other hand on the ground is sufficient to enable the extensors of the hip to bring the trunk into the upright posture.

Gowers recognized that this had also been noted by Duchenne: 'If he bent forward he could only recover his position by catching hold of the furniture, or by supporting his hands on his thighs' (Poore 1883, p. 184). At first Gowers thought the action of putting the hands on the knees, then grasping the thighs higher and higher ('climbing up his thighs') so as to extend the hips and push up the trunk was pathognomonic for the disease. However, he later realized that it could also be seen in other diseases in which the same muscle groups were affected.

Gowers also emphasized that the disease was primarily a disease of muscle and that the spinal cord was unaffected. Further, he was impressed by the predilection for males and was clearly convinced of the hereditary nature of the disorder. Of the total of 220 cases only 30 were females and these were usually less severely affected. Although isolated cases were common, he was impressed by the frequency with which other relatives could be affected (of the 220 cases, 102 were isolated and 118 were grouped in 39 families). Perhaps his most revealing observation was that '. . . the disease is almost never to be heard of on the side of the father; when antecedent cases have occurred they have almost invariably been on the side of the mother'. Gowers also observed that a woman could have affected sons by different husbands, but found no instance in which members of the father's family suffered from the disease. He concluded that limitation to males and inheritance only through the mother was the same as haemophilia. This pattern of inheritance was already recognized at the time, and sometimes referred to as Nasse's law (Nasse 1820), although in fact it had been appreciated since the days of the Talmud some 1500 years earlier. The Jews excused from circumcision the sons of all the sisters of a mother who had a son with the 'bleeding disease'. The sons of the father's sibs were not so excused. The genetic basis for this mode of inheritance was appreciated through the rediscovery of Mendelism in 1900 and its cytological basis (X-linkage) recognized a few years later (reviewed in McKusick 1964).

Wilhelm Heinrich Erb

By this stage in the story it was now quite clear that the disease primarily affected skeletal muscle and was hereditary. However, it was also clear that not all cases presented with exactly the same clinical features: females were occasionally affected and sometimes the disease in males would pursue a more benign course with survival into at least the third decade (for example, Gowers' cases 23, 35, and 36). This raised the possibility that perhaps after all there was more than one disease, an idea first pursued by Erb.

Wilhelm Heinrich Erb (Fig. 2.9) was born in 1840 in Bavaria and studied medicine at Heidelberg, Erlangen, and Munich. His subsequent professional life was spent almost entirely in Heidelberg. Erb was without doubt one of the greatest clinical neurologists of all time. But he was also a great clinical teacher–the archetype of the time: severe, cultured, and always impeccably dressed. He died of a heart attack when he was 81; it is said whilst listening to Beethoven's *Eroica*.

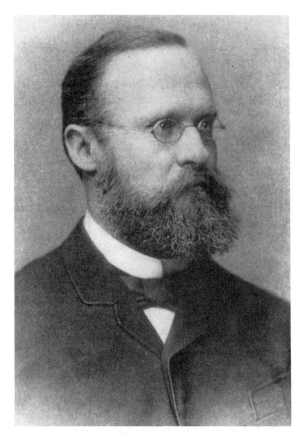

Fig. 2.9. Wilhelm Heinrich Erb. (Reproduced from *The founders of neurology*, edited by Webb Haymaker, 1953. Courtesy of Charles C. Thomas, publishers, Springfield, Illinois.)

Erb was greatly influenced by the studies of Duchenne, both with regard to the possible diagnostic and therapeutic uses of electricity in neurology, as well as his work on muscle disease. His pathological studies convinced him that the disease was due to a degeneration of muscle tissue and coined the term 'Dystrophia muscularis progressiva' or progressive muscular dystrophy, a term which has been used ever since (Erb 1884). Many of the cases he studied were clearly different from cases described by Duchenne and he was well aware of this. In fact he is credited with being the first to attempt to classify this group of diseases (Erb 1891). The details of his classification would now be questioned, but the idea that this was not one disease but a heterogeneous group of disorders was certainly true.

More recent developments

Over the next few decades, as physicians began to study their patients in increasing detail, attempts began to be made to categorize different types and to classify them according to various clinical criteria, such as distribution of muscle weakness, age at onset and progression, and later was added the mode of inheritance. Although there were a few who continued for a while to believe that muscular dystrophy was essentially one disease (for example, Milhorat and Wolff 1943), this view was gradually abandoned. However, there is a serious problem in considering heterogeneity within a group of disorders such as the muscular dystrophies. Differences between disease entities may be more apparent than real: variations within a spectrum and not necessarily a reflection of true genetic differences. This is constantly to be borne in mind when attempting to resolve apparent heterogeneity. The sentiments of Francis Bacon in 1620 are therefore apt:

The steady and acute mind can fix its contemplations and dwell and fasten on the subtlest distinctions: the lofty and discursive mind recognises and puts together the finest and most general resemblances. Both kinds however easily err in excess, by catching the one at gradations the other at shadows.

Those who contributed most significantly to our present ideas on classifying the muscular dystrophies include Bell (1943), Tyler and Wintrobe (1950), Levison (1951), Stevenson (1953), Becker (1953, 1964), Lamy and de Grouchy (1954), Walton and Nattrass (1954), and Morton and Chung (1959). How heterogeneity within this group of diseases was gradually resolved makes a fascinating byway in the history of medicine. However, there would be little value here in summarizing the detailed findings of these earlier studies, which in any event have been critically reviewed by Walton and Nattrass (1954). More recent classifications have been proposed by Emery and Walton (1967), Becker (1972), and by Walton and Gardner-Medwin (1981). One favoured by the author (Emery 1983) is reproduced in Table 2.1.

Table 2.1   *Clinical and genetical classification of the muscular dystrophies*

---

1. *X-linked dystrophies*
   (*a*) Proximal
       (*i*) Duchenne
       (*ii*) Becker
       (*iii*) Others (Mabry, Emery–Dreifuss)
   (*b*) Scapuloperoneal (?)
   (*c*) Quadriceps
       (*i*) Quadriceps myopathy (?)
2. *Autosomal recessive dystrophies*
   (*a*) Proximal
       (*i*) Congenital forms
           rapidly progressive
           slowly progressive (numerous variants)
       (*ii*) Childhood form(s)
       (*iii*) Adult forms
           scapulohumeral
           pelvifemoral (?)
   (*b*) Quadriceps
       (*i*) Quadriceps myopathy (?)
3. *Autosomal dominant dystrophies*
   (*a*) Facioscapulohumeral
       (*i*) Usual form
       (*ii*) With Coats' disease
   (*b*) Scapuloperoneal
   (*c*) Proximal
       (*i*) Dominant limb girdle dystrophy
       (*ii*) Hereditary myopathy limited to females (Henson)
       (*iii*) Hereditary myopathy limited to males (De Coster)
   (*d*) Distal
       (*i*) Childhood form
       (*ii*) Adult form
   (*e*) Ocular
       (*i*) Ocular form
       (*ii*) Oculopharyngeal forms (AD, AR)

At this point perhaps it would be appropriate to consider which disorders are included under the heading 'muscular dystrophies'. Unfortunately a precise definition is not possible because the basic biochemical defect is not yet known. However, for practical purposes a useful definition is *a group of inherited disorders which are characterized by a progressive muscle wasting and weakness, in which the muscle histology has certain distinctive features (muscle fibre necrosis, phagocytosis, etc.) and where there is no clinical or laboratory evidence of central or peripheral nervous system involvement or myotonia*. Excluded are, therefore, the myotonic syndromes and the various congenital myopathies. However, such a definition encompasses disorders which vary considerably in their onset, severity and distribution of muscle involvement. At one extreme there is the rapidly progressive form of congenital muscular dystrophy which is present at birth with generalized muscle involvement and leads to death within a few months. At the other extreme there is ocular muscular dystrophy where onset is in adult life, the disease is often limited to the extraocular muscles and may be no more than a minor inconvenience. Because of these uncertainties it is perhaps best to retain an open mind about aetiology and consider each type of dystrophy separately. Here we shall concentrate on that form of dystrophy which is associated with the name of Duchenne. Until fairly recently eponyms were retained for several other forms of dystrophy such as the scapulohumeral (Erb), pelvifemoral (Leyden–Möbius), and the facioscapulohumeral (Landouzy–Dejerine) forms. But this habit has now been largely abandoned in favour of a clinical-genetical nomenclature. However, there remains one important exception; the retention of Becker's name for the X-linked form of the disease which clinically resembles Duchenne muscular dystrophy but is more benign, affected individuals often surviving into middle age.

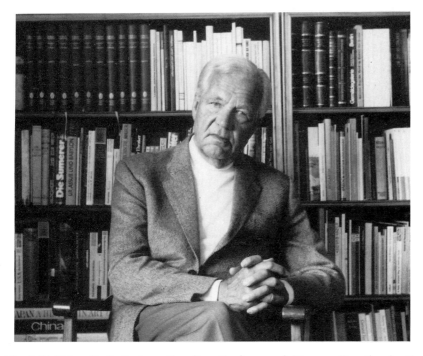

Fig. 2.10 Peter Emil Becker. Emeritus Professor of Human Genetics in the University of Göttingen.

Becker was, until his retirement in 1975, Professor of Human Genetics at the University of Göttingen, a position he had held since 1957 (Fig. 2.10). Although by training a neurologist and psychiatrist, most of his work has centred on human genetics. The dystrophy which bears his name was first brought to his attention by Dr Franz Kiener, a psychologist in Regensburg, who sought Becker's advice on the disease which affected several of his own relatives. Together, they studied the family in detail (Becker and Kiener 1955) and a few years later Becker reported two further families with the same disease (Becker 1962). Patients with the disease had been observed previously by others, but it was Becker who showed that it was clearly a separate clinical and genetic entity.

From this brief historical introduction to the subject, it will be evident that the earliest contributions were made by clinical neurologists and neuropathologists who defined the disease in terms of its clinical presentation and muscle pathology. Later geneticists added to our understanding of this group of diseases. Finally, in the very recent past, molecular biologists have entered the lists with some exciting consequences.

3 Clinical features

In the preclinical stage of Duchenne muscular dystrophy, before there are any signs of the disease, muscle histology is abnormal. Furthermore, significant histological and histochemical abnormalities have now been detected in muscle tissue from fetuses at risk for Duchenne muscular dystrophy as early as the second trimester of pregnancy (see Chapter 4). The disease is therefore already manifest in the fetus. Postnatally, however, the onset of clinical signs and symptoms is insidious and parents may be unaware that anything is wrong for some time.

Onset

Occasionally mothers volunteer that their affected son seemed 'floppy' at birth and in infancy. However, this is never as pronounced or as frequent as in the congenital forms of muscular dystrophy (Fig. 3.1) or infantile spinal muscular atrophy (Werdnig–Hoffmann disease).

The term amyotonia congenita (myatonia congenita, Oppenheim disease)

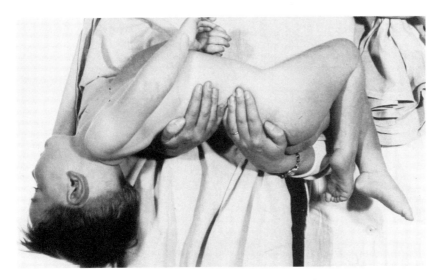

Fig. 3.1. A 3-year-old boy with a relatively non-progressive form of congenital muscular dystrophy. He has generalized hypotonia with retarded motor development and can still not sit without support. (From Emery (1983) with permission.)

has been applied to the syndrome of generalized muscular hypotonia, feebleness of voluntary movements, and depressed or absent tendon reflexes which is present at birth or is manifest shortly after birth. In one careful follow-up study (Walton 1956) of all infants affected in this way, over 60 per cent proved to have Werdnig–Hoffmann disease, 20 per cent a myopathy of one form or another, and the remainder had a variety of conditions including cerebral palsy and mental handicap. Three of the 109 cases in the study went on to develop Duchenne muscular dystrophy. However, in many cases of amyotonia, no cause is found, and these have been referred to as 'benign congenital hypotonia' because most of them resolve completely in childhood (Dubowitz 1978). However, this diagnosis should be accepted with some caution because refinements in muscle histochemistry and biochemistry in recent years have revealed several specific myopathies which can present in this way (Brooke *et al.* 1979).

'Failure to thrive' may, in some cases, be associated with the subsequent development of Duchenne muscular dystrophy (Call and Ziter 1985) as may also speech delay (Katlan and Elias 1986), and most boys show a delay in motor development in early childhood (Dubowitz 1963a; Gardner-Medwin *et al.* 1978). Any male infant who fails to thrive or where there is delay in motor, mental, or speech development for no apparent reason should have his serum creatine kinase level determined (p. 43) in order to exclude the possibility of Duchenne muscular dystrophy.

Often mothers notice that there is a delay in learning to walk. Of 114 cases in which this information was reliably documented, in 64 (56 per cent) walking was delayed until at least 18 months (Table 3.1) and roughly a quarter did

Table 3.1 *Distribution of age in learning to walk in 114 affected boys*

Age (months)	No.	Cumulative %
8–9	1	0.9
10–11	3	3.5
12–13	10	12.3
14–15	20	29.8
16–17	16	43.8
18–19	26	66.6
20–21	6	71.9
22–23	3	74.5
24–25	21	92.9
26–27	1	93.8
28–29	0	93.8
30–31	3	96.4
32–33	0	96.4
34–35	0	96.4
36	4	99.9

Table 3.2 *Percentile distribution of age at apparent onset in 144 affected boys*

Percentile	Age (years)
25	<2
50	2.4
60	2.8
70	3.4
75	3.7
80	4.1
90	5.1
95	6.1
99	7.8

not walk until they were at least 2 years old. In normal children, by comparison, the average age in learning to walk is about 13 months, and 97 per cent are walking by 18 months (Neligan and Prudham 1969).

Approximate percentiles for age at apparent onset in 144 cases are given in Table 3.2. In this and other age related events based on cases studied by the author, percentiles were obtained by fitting the best curve to the data. It will be seen that in 90 per cent of cases onset is before school age (about 5 years). These data, however, should be accepted with a little caution because age at onset is notoriously difficult to assess with any accuracy, although parents can usually give a good idea as to when they first noticed that something seemed to be wrong with their son.

It is often stated that if the parents have already had an affected son, the onset of the disorder in a second affected son is noted to be earlier because

Table 3.3 *Age (years) at onset in affected brothers*

Case no.	1st born	2nd born	3rd born
11	2	7	–
90	5	3	–
100	$2\frac{1}{2}$	5	–
111	$2\frac{1}{2}$	4	–
121	$1\frac{3}{4}$	$1\frac{1}{2}$	–
528	$1\frac{1}{2}$	6	–
587	4	$2\frac{1}{2}$	–
593	$7\frac{1}{2}$	$7\frac{1}{2}$	–
1761	$4\frac{1}{2}$	$4\frac{1}{2}$	$4\frac{1}{2}$
2009	3	$1\frac{1}{2}$	–

they are conscious of the possibility. But this is by no means always true as shown in Table 3.3 where age at onset is given for affected brothers in cases where this information was personally recorded *at the time the diagnosis was confirmed* in each case.

On close questioning in almost all cases, the affected child *was never able to run properly*. Other complaints at the time of onset included waddling gait, walking unsteadily with a tendency to fall easily, walking on toes, and difficulty in climbing stairs. In a few instances weakness was first noticed after the child had sustained a fracture following a fall. Sometimes the parents noted a tendency to 'throw out his leg' when walking, for the 'feet to turn in', or their attention was even drawn to enlargement of the calf muscles (Fig. 3.2).

However, although most cases in the present series presented in early childhood, there were five cases (which were all isolated cases) where onset was apparently delayed until the age of 8 or 9. This exceptionally late onset raises the possibility that these cases might not in fact be Duchenne muscular dystrophy but the more benign Becker type of muscular dystrophy in which age at onset is often somewhat later. However, the subsequent clinical course in all but case 144 would be compatible with the diagnosis of Duchenne muscular dystrophy (Table 3.4)

Muscle pseudohypertrophy

The most obvious feature in the early stages of the disease is enlargement of the calf muscles which are often said to feel 'firm' or 'woody'. Of 89 cases where the size of the calves was noted at some time in the course of the disease, in at least 85 (96 per cent) they seemed much larger than normal. However, such enlargement may also involve the masseters, deltoids, serrati anterior, and quadriceps, and occasionally other muscles as well. Macroglossia is not uncommon. Muscle enlargement, at least in part, is due to an excess of adipose and connective tissue, and therefore the term 'pseudohypertrophy' is widely used. But true (work) hypertrophy may also play a

Table 3.4 *Cases with delayed onset*

Case no.	Age (years)			Comments
	Onset	Chairbound	Death	
144	8	–	–	Now age 10 and moderately affected
124	8	11	20	–
1741	8	12	–	Parents not good witnesses
2197	9	11	–	Severely mentally retarded (IQ < 50)
112	9	12	21	–

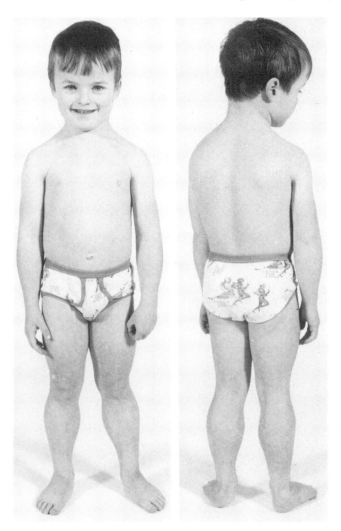

Fig. 3.2. A 4-year-old boy with Duchenne muscular dystrophy. Note the enlarged calves.

role as a compensation for weakness in other muscles (Bertorini and Igarashi 1985). However, in Duchenne muscular dystrophy it is difficult to imagine this as being an important factor because in some cases such muscle enlargement can be extensive (Fig. 3.3). Interestingly, if in an affected boy a limb becomes affected by poliomyelitis then there is no pseudohypertrophy in that limb and therefore, presumably, it depends on an intact nerve supply (Tyler 1950). Pseudohypertrophy is not pathognomonic for Duchenne muscular

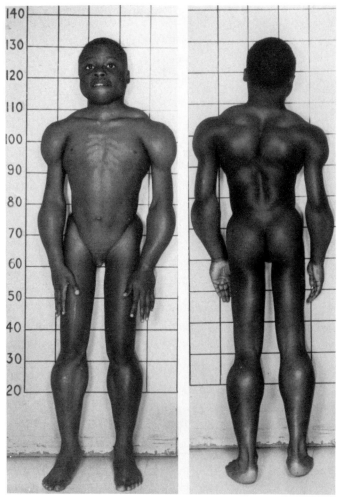

Fig. 3.3. Extensive muscle enlargement (pseudohypertrophy) in a case of Duchenne muscular dystrophy. (Reproduced by kind permission of Dr Sarah Bundey.)

dystrophy since it can also occur in some other forms of dystrophy and even occasionally in spinal muscular atrophy.

Distribution of muscle weakness

Muscle involvement is always bilateral and symmetrical. In general, in the early stages of the disease, the lower limbs are affected more than the upper limbs, and the proximal muscles more than the distal muscles. At this stage certain muscles are predominantly affected. These include the latissimus dorsi, sterno-costal head of the pectoralis major, brachioradialis, biceps, triceps, iliopsoas, glutei, and quadriceps muscles. The involvement is highly selective. For example, the quadriceps are more affected than the hamstrings, triceps more than biceps, wrist extensors more than flexors, neck flexors more than extensors, dorsiflexors of the feet more than the plantar flexors. Even within a single muscle there is differential involvement. For example, the sterno-costal head of the pectoralis major muscle is more affected than the clavicular head, but in contrast the clavicular head of the sternomastoid muscle is more affected than the sternal head. This differential muscle involvement, which has been elaborated upon by Bonsett (1969), becomes less clear as the disease progresses so that ultimately such patterns are no longer obvious. Later slight facial weakness often develops and the intercostal muscles also become affected, but sphincter control, chewing, and swallowing are never affected.

Early signs

This pattern of muscle involvement results in several well defined physical features associated with the disease. Weakness of the gluteus medius and minimus muscles (which abduct the hip and hold the pelvic bone down to the greater trochanter of the femur) results in the pelvis tilting down toward the unsupported side when an affected child raises his leg from the ground. To compensate for this he inclines toward the supporting leg. As he moves forward this action is continually repeated and results in the broad-based, waddling gait which is so characteristic of Duchenne muscular dystrophy. But, as Professor Dubowitz has pointed out, 'not everything that waddles is muscular dystrophy' for other conditions can also produce this type of gait (for example, spinal muscular atrophy). Weakness of the gluteus maximus muscle (which powerfully extends the hip) results in a tendency for the pelvis to tilt forward and in order to compensate for this a lumbar lordosis develops. In order to maintain his balance, and possibly because of an imbalance between the dorsiflexors and plantar flexors, he also tends to walk on his toes. However, the mechanical effects of muscle weakness on the gait in this disorder are complex and have been analysed in considerable detail by Sutherland and colleagues (1981).

Weakness of the knee and hip extensors results in the classical Gowers' manoeuvre: the child climbs up his thighs in order to extend the hips and push up the trunk (Fig. 2.8 and 3.4). However, it may be impossible to elicit this sign before the age of 4 or 5. Even before this age I have found that an affected child is unable to rise from a sitting position on the floor if he is asked to *keep his arms folded* (which prevents him from pushing on his thighs or on the floor) whereas a normal child can accomplish this quite easily.

In the early stages of the disease it may also be difficult to elicit weakness of

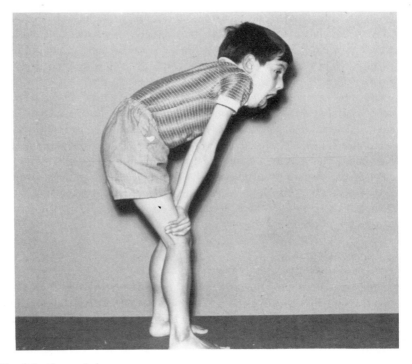

Fig. 3.4. Gowers' sign or manoeuvre.

the pectoral girdle musculature by formal testing. However, if the child is grasped around the chest from behind and an attempt made to lift him there is a tendency to 'slide-through' the examiner's arms. Also, by placing the examiner's hands inside the upper arms a normal child can be held up with comparative ease, but not an affected child. Both these signs are positive by the age of 4 and sometimes earlier. As the disease progresses, winging of the scapulae becomes apparent.

The affected muscles are not tender (which could suggest myositis) and there is no voluntary or percussion myotonia. As the muscles become weaker and wasted, the corresponding tendon reflexes become depressed, though good ankle jerks are retained for a long time and are the last of the tendon reflexes to disappear. The plantar responses are always flexor and there is no sensory loss.

In the early stages of the disease, apart from the obvious difficulties of trying to keep up with his peers, affected boys usually make few complaints apart from occasionally cramp and perhaps stiffness, particularly in the calf muscles. However, when such symptoms are severe this raises the possibility of some other myopathy (such as McArdle's syndrome or carnitine palmityl-transferase deficiency) or perhaps myositis. More than a third of affected boys show some degree of intellectual impairment and some are severely mentally retarded. This aspect of the disease will be dealt with later (p. 99).

Progression

The weakness is progressive but nevertheless often shows periods of apparent arrest. It is because of this fluctuation that the assessment of the efficacy of any suggested therapy has to be evaluated with considerable care.

As the disease progresses the lumbar lordosis becomes more exaggerated and the waddling gait increases. Shortening of the heel cords (Achilles tendon) becomes more marked and an equinovarus deformity develops, though this is more obvious when the boy becomes confined to a wheelchair.

Although, initially, an affected boy may find he only needs a wheelchair at certain times (for example when going outside) after a few weeks he will inevitably become permanently confined to a wheelchair. The age at which this occurs is more precise and much better documented than the age at onset (Table 3.5). In the present series, with very few exceptions which have been exculded, no attempts had been made to prolong ambulation by various orthopaedic measures and therefore the data relate to the natural progress of the disease.

Of the 120 affected boys in which the age at becoming confined to a wheelchair was reliably known, in 95 per cent of cases this occurred by the age of 12. Age at becoming confined to a wheelchair was not significantly correlated with age at onset but was significantly correlated with age at death

Table 3.5 *Percentile distribution of age at becoming confined to a wheelchair in 120 affected boys*

Percentile	Age (years)
10	6.7
20	7.4
30	7.8
40	8.2
50	8.5
60	8.9
70	9.3
75	9.6
80	10.0
90	11.0
95	11.9
99	13.2

Table 3.6 *Age at death related to age at becoming confined to a wheelchair*

	$\leqslant 7$	8	9	10 or more
		Age (years) confined to a wheelchair		
No.	9	18	15	13
Mean	15.65	16.52	17.44	18.15
s.d.	3.36	2.29	2.65	3.00
No.		27		28
Mean		16.23		17.77
s.d.		2.66		2.79

($N = 55$, $r = 0.33$, $P < 0.02$). The difference in mean age at death in boys who became chairbound by 8 years of age ($N = 27$, mean 16.23, s.d. 2.66) compared with those who became chairbound after 8 years of age ($N = 28$, mean 17.77, s.d. 2.79) is statistically significant ($P < 0.05$). It would seem that age at death after 15 increases roughly by one year for each year that a boy remains ambulant after the age of 7 up to the age of 10 or more (Table 3.6). In general terms, the earlier a boy becomes confined to a wheelchair, the poorer the prognosis.

Assessment of motor ability

It is often valuable to be able to chart the course of the disease in patients. A number of systems have been devised for doing this which depend on assessing either muscle strength or functional ability:
1. *Muscle strength*
   MRC grading (0–5)
   Ergometry
2. *Functional ability*
   Swinyard grade (1–8)
   Vignos grade (1–10)
   Hammersmith motor ability score (0–40)
   'CIDD' grade for upper limbs (1–6)

Details of the various grading systems are given in the Appendices B–F and will be discussed in more detail later. Since there is inevitably a subjective element in such methods, in order to make comparisons either between different patients or with the same patient over a period of time, they are best carried out by the same person. For many years I have assessed the Swinyard and Vignos grades of most patients examined (186 observations on 110 patients), and the results are given in Figs 3.5 and 3.6.

Both grades correlate well with the progress of the disease. However, there

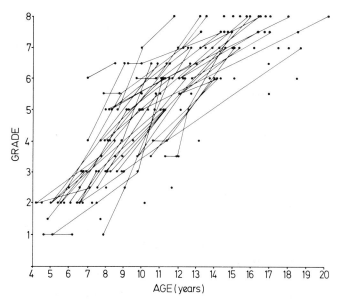

Fig. 3.5. Swinyard grade and age in boys with Duchenne muscular dystrophy. Points are joined for assessments on the same individual.

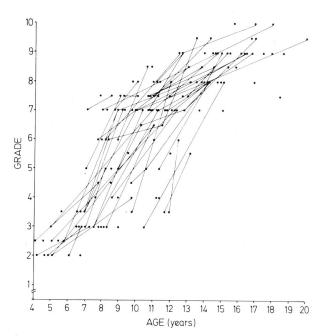

Fig. 3.6. Vignos grade and age in boys with Duchenne muscular dystrophy. Points are joined for assessments on the same individual.

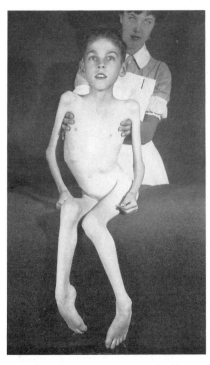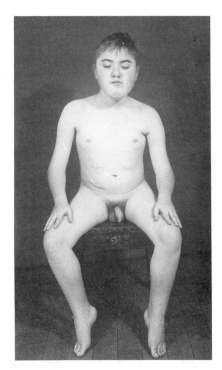

Fig. 3.7. A 13-year-old boy (*left*), and a 12-year-old boy (*right*) with Duchenne muscular dystrophy. (Reproduced by kind permission of Professor V. Dubowitz and W. B. Saunders Company, Publishers.)

is clearly considerable variation between different boys of the same age, and this has been well documented by others (Allsop and Ziter 1981; Cohen *et al.* 1982; Brooke *et al.* 1983). But apart from variations in motor ability between boys of the same age, affected boys also differ in their general appearance. Some retain their subcutaneous fat and muscle bulk whereas others become thin and atrophic. This is graphically demonstrated in the two boys of similar age shown in Fig. 3.7. The reason for this is not clear but there is a tendency for affected brothers to follow a similar pattern. In most cases sexual development is normal though puberty is delayed in a proportion of cases.

Later stages

As the disease progresses and muscle weakness becomes more profound, contractures increasingly develop, particularly flexion contractures of the elbows, knees and hips. Later, movements of the shoulders and wrists also become limited. Talipes equinovarus deformity becomes marked with the talus bone protruding prominently under the skin on the dorsum of the foot. Unless adequate support is provided in the wheelchair a severe kyphoscoliosis develops. These various deformities have been well illustrated by Rideau (1979). Thoracic deformity poses the most serious problem as it restricts adequate pulmonary airflow on the compressed side (Fig. 3.8).

The respiratory problems are also aggravated by weakness of the intercostal muscles. About halfway through the course of the disease a gradual deterioration begins in pulmonary function with reduced maximal inspiratory and expiratory pressures. By the later stages there is a significant reduction in total lung capacity and an increase in residual volume. Oxygen tension (P_{O_2}) and carbon dioxide tension (P_{CO_2}) are usually normal and an increase in P_{CO_2} in a patient without respiratory infection indicates a bad prognosis (Inkley *et al.* 1974). However, differences in pulmonary function in the upright and supine positions are small, indicating that diaphragmatic function is relatively preserved. This may account for why respiratory failure develops late in the course of the disease and chronic alveolar hypoventilation

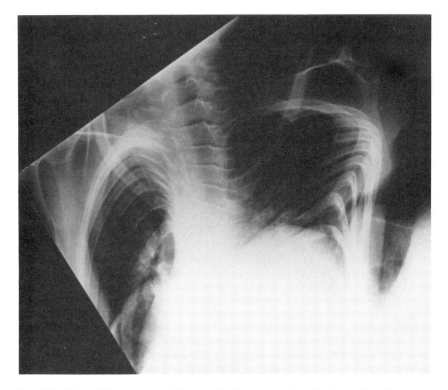

Fig. 3.8. Chest X-ray of an 18-year-old boy severely affected with Duchenne muscular dystrophy showing gross thoracic deformity.

appears to be rare. The effects of respiratory function are somewhat different in other forms of dystrophy (Newsom-Davis 1980).

Cardiac muscle is also affected, as will be discussed later, but it is very rare for a boy to succumb to heart failure though occasional cases of sudden death may be attributable to cardiac involvement. In the present series of patients, 14 cases came to autopsy and the primary cause of death was given as pneumonia (11), 'respiratory failure' (1), diphtheria at age 8 (1), and acute cardiac arrhythmia (1).

That age at death might be in some way related to socio-economic factors is not borne out in the present study; when information on social class was available there was no apparent relationship with age at death (Table 3.7).

Table 3.7 *Age at death in Duchenne muscular dystrophy and social class of parents*

	Social class					
Age (years) at death	5	4	3	2	1	*Total*
<10	–	–	1	–	–	*1*
10–14	1	1	4	2	–	*8*
15–19	4	15	11	5	1	*36*
20–24	2	–	1	–	–	*3*
Total	*7*	*16*	*17*	*7*	*1*	*48*

$$(\chi^2 = 10.92; P > 0.05)$$

Table 3.8 *Percentile distribution of age at death in 129 affected boys*

Percentile	Age (years)
10	12.0
20	13.4
30	14.3
40	15.0
50	15.5
60	16.2
70	17.0
75	17.6
80	18.1
90	19.5
95	20.5
99	23.5

Age at death was not significantly correlated with age at onset but, as we have seen, it was correlated with age at becoming confined to a wheelchair. The percentile distribution of age at death is given in Table 3.8. In 90 per cent of cases this occurred before the age of 20.

These figures, however, could be biased towards earlier deaths since they exclude affected individuals who are still alive. However this seems unlikely to be important because in cases where year and age at death were well documented there was no significant difference between mean age at death in those who died between 1934 and 1963 compared with those who died between 1964 and 1973 (Table 3.9).

Gardner-Medwin in a detailed study of the natural history of the disease in the north-east of England (Gardner-Medwin 1982a) has suggested that recently boys with Duchenne muscular dystrophy might be surviving longer, perhaps because of some improvement in treatment. The present data do indicate a slight increase in mean age at death over the years. However, the mean age at death in the last 10 years ($N = 28$, mean 16.83, s.d. 2.53) does not differ significantly from the mean in the preceding 40 years ($N = 45$, mean 16.49, s.d. 3.03), although it is just significantly different ($0.02 < P < 0.05$) from the mean calculated from data given by Gowers in 1879 ($N = 25$, mean 15.36, s.d. 2.46) for cases that would now be categorized as Duchenne muscular dystrophy but excluding two of his cases who died accidentally in early childhood. But then some of Gowers' cases died of intercurrent infections, such as acute gastroenteritis and scarlet fever, which are uncommon causes of mortality in childhood in Britain nowadays. It would seem that if there has been any improvement in survival over the last 100 years this has been slight.

There is considerable variation in age at death, some boys succumbing as early as 8, while others survive into their mid-twenties. In the literature one case has been recorded as having fathered in his twenties a son and a carrier daughter (Thompson 1978), and another confirmed case survived, despite considerable physical handicap, to the age of 34 when he died an accidental death (Johnson *et al.* 1985). But such cases are very much the exception.

The ages at which the three main events marking the disease occurred

Table 3.9 *Age at death and year at death recorded in 73 affected boys over the 50-year period 1934 to 1983 inclusive, compared with data from Gowers (1879b)*

	1934–1963	1964–1973	1974–1983	Gowers (1879b)
No.	13	32	28	25
Mean	16.27	16.63	16.83	15.36
s.d.	4.09	2.60	2.53	2.46

Table 3.10 *Ages at which the three main events marking Duchenne muscular dystrophy occur*

Region	Onset			Chairbound			Death				Reference
	No.	Mean	s.d.	No.	Mean	s.d.	No.	Mean	s.d.	Range	
Brazil	58	3.32	1.79	55	9.55	1.79	24	17.05	3.56	12–27	Zatz (1986)
Canada	–	–	–	49	9.94	1.57	59	16.56	2.25	12–21	Murphy (1985)
France	100	3.15	1.68	?	10.16	1.76	?	17.72	3.76	10–25	Rideau (1979)
Germany	41	3.07	2.24	42	9.36	2.62	40	14.71	3.76	8–23	Becker (1962)
Japan	105	3.7	1.9	128	10.8	1.9	65	18.0	2.9	–	Sugita (1985)
Poland	483	2.3	1.46	234	10.1	1.90	58	18.1	3.31	–	Hausmanowa-Petrusewicz *et al.* (1986)
Switzerland	88	2.89	1.29	83	9.81	1.50	47	17.79	3.22	11–29	Moser (1986)
UK											
England (N)	144	2.6	–	86	9.5	–	–	18.7	–	13–28	Gardner-Medwin (1982)
England (S)	64	3.07	1.75	56	9.05	2.02	7	15.57	2.82	11–18	Dubowitz (1978); (cases studied in 1960)
Scotland	144	3.26	1.74	120	9.39	1.69	129	16.27	3.12	8–25	Present series
USA											
Utah	46	3.76	2.15	–	–	–	25	17.68	3.34	13–25	Stephens & Tyler (1951)

(onset, confined to a wheelchair, and death) in the present series are compared with those in other studies (Table 3.10). There is reasonable agreement between the various studies which are drawn from different populations, but all show considerable variation in these three main events.

The considerable variation in the disease is also illustrated in Table 3.11 from which it can be seen that some boys may become chairbound, or even die from the disease, before the apparent onset in other boys.

Disorders in affected boys other than muscular dystrophy

Apart from mental handicap and problems directly relating to muscle weakness, most boys have very few other health problems. The only other

Table 3.11 *Numbers of boys with Duchenne muscular dystrophy with different ages at onset, becoming confined to a wheelchair, and death (author's series)*

Age	Onset	Chairbound	Death
<2	24	–	–
2	46	–	–
3	27	–	–
4	23	–	–
5	14	–	–
6	2	2	–
7	3	15	–
8	3	27	2
9	2	31	2
10	–	19	1
11	–	14	2
12	–	6	6
13	–	4	7
14	–	2	19
15	–	–	10
16	–	–	25
17	–	–	15
18	–	–	11
19	–	–	12
20	–	–	7
21	–	–	6
22	–	–	–
23	–	–	2
24	–	–	1
25	–	–	1
Total	*144*	*120*	*129*

disorders recorded in the present series were recurrent urinary infections (2), left hydronephrosis with associated impaired renal function (1), unspecified congenital heart disease (1), undescended testes (1), and insulin dependent diabetes mellitus (1); in the last case the same disease also affected the boy's father.

Summary and conclusions

Onset of the disease is insidious but an important hallmark in the very early stages is an inability to run properly. In over half the cases walking is delayed until at least 18 months of age. Manifestations of the disease are apparent in most cases before 5, but some remain apparently healthy until 8 or even 9 years of age. Pseudohypertrophy of the calf muscles is present in almost all cases and in some instances many other muscles are also affected. Wasting and weakness predominantly affects the proximal limb girdle musculature but early on muscle involvement is highly selective. A waddling gait, Gowers' sign, and 'sliding-through' the examiner's arms are useful diagnostic signs. However, even before Gowers' sign can be elicited, affected boys are unable to rise from a sitting position on the floor if asked to keep their arms folded. The age at becoming confined to a wheelchair (which is usually by the age of 12) is a prognostic sign in that age at death after 15 increases roughly by one year for each year that a boy remains ambulant after the age of 7 up to the age of 10 or more. Ninety per cent of boys die before the age of 20, usually from respiratory problems. However, as with the other main events in the natural history of the disorder, there is considerable variation from one individual to another. Apart from problems relating directly or indirectly to dystrophy, most affected boys have very few other health problems.

4 Confirmation of the diagnosis

It is unlikely that an experienced physician would have any difficulty in suspecting Duchenne muscular dystrophy in an otherwise healthy schoolboy who presents with a waddling gait, pseudohypertrophic calves, and a positive Gowers' sign. However, the diagnosis may not be so obvious in the very young or in those cases where onset is delayed until late childhood. Also, because of the uniformly poor prognosis and the parents' need for reliable genetic counselling, it is essential that the diagnosis be firmly established as soon as possible. This depends on the serum level of creatine kinase, electromyography, and muscle pathology (Swash and Schwartz, 1981).

Serum creatine kinase

The enzyme creatine kinase (E.C.2.7.3.2) catalyses the reversible transfer of a phosphate group from creatine phosphate to adenosine diphosphate (ADP) forming creatine and adenosine triphosphate (ATP):

$$\text{Creatine phosphate} + \text{ADP} \rightleftharpoons \text{Creatine} + \text{ATP}$$

The International Union of Biochemistry suggested the systematic name ATP: creatine phosphotransferase with creatine kinase as the acceptable trivial name.

Over the years a number of methods have been developed for measuring the activity of the enzyme, each depending on one of three approaches. First, creatine is incubated with ATP in the reaction mixture and the formation of creatine phosphate (as inorganic phosphate) is determined (Kuby *et al.* 1954). Secondly, the amount of ADP produced in the reaction is determined by a series of coupled reactions, in the original method pyruvate kinase and lactate dehydrogenase systems being used (Tanzer and Gilvarg 1959). Thirdly, the preferred faster reaction may be utilized whereby creatine phosphate is incubated with ADP and the formation of creatine (or ATP) is determined (Ennor and Rosenberg 1954). We have favoured a modification of this last method (Rosalki 1967) where the amount of ATP generated is estimated by coupling the reaction with hexokinase and glucose-6-phosphate dehydrogenase (G6PD), the formation of reduced nicotinamide-adenine dinucleotide phosphate (NADPH) being finally determined:

$$\text{Creatine phosphate} + \text{ADP} \longrightarrow \text{Creatine} + \text{ATP}$$

$$\text{ATP} + \text{glucose} \xrightarrow{\text{Hexokinase}} \text{Glucose-6-phosphate} + \text{ADP}$$

$$\text{Glucose-6-phosphate} + \text{NADP} \xrightarrow{\text{G-6-PD}} \text{6-Phosphogluconate} + \text{NADPH}$$

A thiol compound (e.g. cysteine) is incorporated in the reaction mixture to enhance enzyme activity. The amount of activity in serum is expressed in International Units (iu) as the amount of enzyme which catalyses the transformation of 1 micromole of creatine phosphate/min/1000 ml of serum at 30 °C. Since there is very little enzyme in erythrocytes, assays on serum are not affected by haemolysis which is an important practical consideration.

In healthy infants in the immediate newborn period, the level of activity of serum creatine kinase (SCK) is often somewhat raised to around 200–300 iu. This may be due to muscular anoxia (Blum and Brauman 1975). But within a few days of birth levels are reached which are not very different from older children (Zellweger *et al.* 1970). In young boys there is no significant correlation with age (Passos *et al.* 1985). However, in adolescence higher levels are not infrequent and may possibly be a reflection of increased muscle mass and physical activity at this period, otherwise values are the same as in adults. The distribution of SCK levels in normal young healthy adult males is positively skewed with a few individuals having high levels (Emery and Spikesman 1970a, b). But most values in young healthy adult males are less than 200 iu which is a little higher than in females (p. 198) presumably because the latter have less muscle mass.

Sibley and Lehninger in 1949 were the first to note that a serum enzyme (in this case aldolase) could be raised in patients with muscular dystrophy. Some 10 years later Ebashi and his colleagues in Tokyo (Ebashi *et al.* 1959) also showed that creatine kinase activity is raised in the serum of patients with muscular dystrophy, and this was confirmed the following year by Dreyfus in Paris (Dreyfus *et al.* 1960). Even at birth and before the disease becomes clinically evident, SCK levels are considerably higher in Duchenne muscular dystrophy than in normal boys – up to a hundred times higher. They may even be raised in the affected fetus by the second trimester of pregnancy (Edwards *et al.* 1984). However, as the disease progresses, levels fall but only approach normal values in the very late stages of the disease (Fig. 4.1).

The most likely explanation for the very high SCK levels in Duchenne muscular dystrophy is that the enzyme originates in muscle and escapes into the serum. The much lower levels in the later stages of the disease are no doubt due to the decrease in functioning muscle tissue and reduction in physical activity. Levels certainly decrease most around the time (age 8–10) when affected boys become confined to a wheelchair.

Grossly elevated SCK levels (50–100 times normal) occur not only in Duchenne muscular dystrophy but also in the early stages of Becker muscular dystrophy (Emery and Skinner 1976), acute ischaemic muscle necrosis, and occasionally in the acute phase of polymyositis (Thomson 1971). Moderately elevated levels (up to 10 times normal) can occur in some other forms of muscular dystrophy (notably limb girdle and facioscapulohumeral), spinal muscular atrophy (juvenile and adult forms), some individuals predisposed

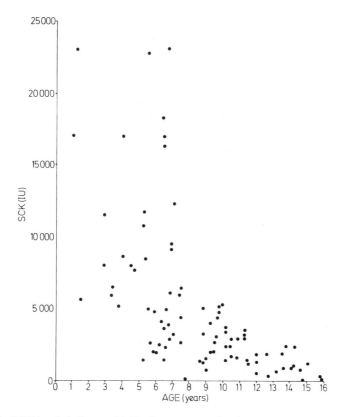

Fig. 4.1. SCK levels in boys with Duchenne muscular dystrophy.

to malignant hyperpyrexia, and in certain non-hereditary disorders such as motor neurone disease, severe hypocalcaemia, hypothyroidism, and after myocardial infarction. Thus, a boy with evidence of proximal muscle weakness, with a waddling gait and a positive Gowers' sign, who is otherwise well and does not have polymyositis, but has a *grossly elevated* SCK level, is almost certainly suffering from Duchenne or Becker muscular dystrophy.

Creatine kinase isoenzymes

Creatine kinase exists in three molecular forms or isoenzymes. Each isoenzyme results from the dimeric association of two sub-units referred to as M and B, and the three isoenzymes are designated as MM, MB, and BB (Dawson *et al.* 1965). The BB isoenzyme predominates in brain tissue, whereas the MM isoenzyme predominates in cardiac and skeletal muscle. The hybrid MB isoenzyme is a minor component in both cardiac and skeletal muscle (Dawson and Fine 1967). In normal serum the isoenzyme is very largely MM with only about 4 per cent being MB. This small MB fraction, however, is significantly increased in patients with Duchenne or Becker muscular dystrophy but does not distinguish between these two dystrophies (Vainzof *et al.* 1985). Though the MB form is found in cardiac muscle, its presence in serum in Duchenne muscular dystrophy is unrelated to cardiac involvement in the disease (Silverman *et al.* 1976) and presumably originates in dystrophic muscle in which there is more MB activity than in normal muscle.

Other muscle enzymes which exist as isoenzymes, and have been studied in detail in Duchenne muscular dystrophy, are lactate dehydrogenase, aldolase, and pyruvate kinase. Lactate dehydrogenase (LDH) exists as five isoenzymes (LDH 1–5). In the serum of patients with Duchenne muscular dystrophy there is a relative increase in the proportions of LDH 1–3 which reflects changes in the isoenzyme pattern in affected muscle tissue (Somer *et al.* 1973). There are muscle, brain, and liver forms of aldolase and the serum activity in Duchenne muscular dystrophy is predominantly that of the muscle type (Tzvetanova 1971). Pyruvate kinase (PK) exists as three isoenzymes (M_2, M_1, and L). In patients with Duchenne muscular dystrophy serum activity is mainly of the M_1 type which is the only PK isoenzyme found in skeletal muscle and brain and the major component in cardiac muscle (Zatz *et al.* 1978). Finally, carbonic anhydrase III and β-enolase are skeletal *muscle specific* enzymes, and these too are elevated in the serum of affected boys (Carter *et al.* 1979, 1980; Mokuno *et al.* 1984). Thus, in all these instances the enzyme pattern in the serum of patients is similar to that in muscle tissue.

Other serum enzymes

Following the early studies in Paris (Schapira and Dreyfus 1963), several other enzymes have been found to be raised in Duchenne muscular dystrophy, though none to the same extent as creatine kinase. The highest levels (10–20 times normal) occur with aldolase, pyruvate kinase, carbonic anhydrase III, and β-enolase. Less dramatic increases have been found in a number of other enzymes including:

Lactate dehydrogenase
Phosphoglycerate mutase
Alanine aminotransferase (glutamic-pyruvic transaminase, GPT)
Aspartate aminotransferase (glutamic-oxaloacetic transaminase, GOT)
Phosphohexose isomerase
Phosphoglucomutase
α-Hydroxybutyrate dehydrogenase
Malate dehydrogenase.

Most of these are major 'soluble' (sarcoplasmic) muscle enzymes. Their increase in serum in Duchenne muscular dystrophy probably reflects increased efflux through the muscle membrane, possibly augmented later in the disease process by release from fibres undergoing necrosis. Evidence supporting this idea has been critically assembled by Rowland (1980), who also provides an extensive bibliography. The evidence may be summarized as follows. (1) As already seen, the isoenzyme pattern of certain enzymes in serum closely resembles that of muscle tissue. (2) Under certain experimental conditions, it has been shown that enzymes are released from viable muscle tissue *in vitro*. (3) In patients aldolase levels have been shown to be slightly higher in the venous return than in the corresponding arterial supply of the lower limb. (4) Almost all of the enzymes that are increased in the serum of patients are cytoplasmic, whereas enzymes which are bound in some way to intracellular structures are not ordinarily found in the serum. (5) When the activity of an enzyme is increased in the serum of patients with Duchenne muscular dystrophy, it is almost always decreased in affected muscle, thus indicating that the enzyme originated from muscle. (6) The decline in serum enzyme levels as the disease progresses correlates well with the diminishing muscle mass. Finally, the idea is further supported by the fact that at least in some cases release is related to molecular size. The molecular weights of creatine kinase (81 000 daltons) and aldolase (150 000 daltons) are considerably less than in AMP deaminase (320 000 daltons) and phosphofructokinase (400 000 daltons), which are also major muscle enzymes but which are virtually absent in serum of patients with Duchenne muscular dystrophy. However, some proteins with small molecular weights either do not appear at all in the serum of patients (adenylate kinase, 21 000 daltons), or only in relatively small amounts (myoglobin, 17 000 daltons).

The situation is therefore not simple and cannot be explained purely in terms of leakage from affected muscle. The serum level of an enzyme will be affected by its clearance rate, and its efflux from muscle will depend on its relative concentration in this tissue, its binding to intracellular structures and possibly some form of selective force at the level of the muscle membrane but about which little is yet known (Pennington 1977a).

From a practical point of view attempts to distinguish Duchenne and Becker types of muscular dystrophy on the basis of serum levels of various enzymes have been uniformly unsuccessful. The changes are of greater interest in attempting to understand more of the pathogenesis of these diseases, a subject which will be discussed later (p. 132).

Electromyography (EMG)

When muscle fibres contract they generate electrical activity. The electrical activity created by a group of muscle fibres activated by a single neurone, the

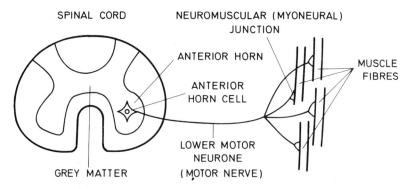

Fig. 4.2. The motor unit consists of an individual motor neurone (anterior horn cell) and the muscle fibres which it activates.

so-called motor unit (Fig. 4.2), produces a motor unit action potential or simply action potential. Electromyography (EMG), among other things, is a technique for studying the electrical activity of contracting muscle fibres and provides useful information about the structure and functioning of motor units. It can therefore be a valuable diagnostic aid in neuromuscular disorders. It has the advantage over a biopsy that many different muscles and different parts of the same muscle can be studied. However, although changes in motor unit activity can give an idea of the severity and distribution of muscle involvement, it has been recognized for many years that these changes are not specific for any particular disease entity (Denny-Brown, 1949). Furthermore, although some information can be gained from surface electrodes, usually the electrode is inserted into the muscle and cooperation by the patient is important. It can, therefore, be a difficult procedure to carry out on young children.

The technique of EMG involves inserting a fine concentric needle electrode through the skin into the muscle. The electrode is essentially a hollow needle surrounding an insulated core which is bared at the tip. The electrical activity generated when the electrode is inserted (insertion activity), when the muscle is at rest (spontaneous activity), and during voluntary muscle contraction is suitably amplified and displayed on a cathode ray oscilloscope and often reproduced through a loudspeaker. A permanent record can be made on tape, and the information can also be fed into a computer for automated analysis.

The interpretation of electromyographic records requires much experience and in all but the most straightforward cases is best left to the expert. Here only a brief review can be given of the essential EMG changes helpful in diagnosing a suspected case of Duchenne muscular dystrophy. Further details, along with more sophisticated approaches, can be found for example in Buchthal and Rosenfalck (1963), Lenman and Ritchie (1970), and Yu and Murray (1984).

The normal EMG

When a needle electrode is inserted into a muscle, this evokes a discharge of action potentials, but this only lasts a brief period and is probably due to mechanical excitation of adjacent muscle fibres. At rest there is virtually no activity and the record is flat. However, on weak voluntary contraction of the muscle, action potentials are generated. They represent the potentials derived from groups of muscle fibres which are contracting nearly synchronously and are situated fairly close together and frequently activated by a single neurone. With minimal contraction and with the electrode position carefully adjusted, it is possible to record single action potentials. The wave form of the potential is determined by the number of phases or deflections across the base line (Buchthal *et al.* 1954a). A potential with more than four phases is referred to as being polyphasic (Fig. 4.3).

The duration of the action potential, measured from the first deflection from the base line to its subsequent return to the base line, is averaged over a number of recordings, and in health ranges from about 4 to 15 ms. (Buchthal, 1957). The amplitude (peak-to-peak) ranges from 100 μV to 1 mV, and normally less than about 5 per cent of the action potentials are

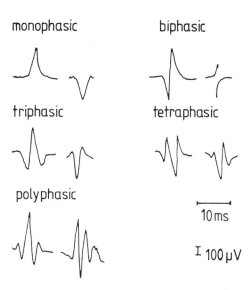

Fig. 4.3. Variations in the wave forms of action potentials recorded on minimal contraction of the gastrocnemius muscle in normal healthy adults.

polyphasic. However, these parameters are influenced by a number of factors including the type of electrode used, the depth of its insertion, the age and sex of the individual, the state of fatigue of the muscle, the ambient temperature, and the particular muscle being studied (Buchthal *et al.* 1954b). Ideally, control values should be established using the same equipment, under the same conditions, and on individuals matched as closely as possible with the patients being investigated. Some representative normal values for the quadriceps and deltoid muscles in healthy young adults are given in Table 4.1. Values obtained in healthy children are less (Buchthal and Pinelli 1951; Buchthal 1957).

As the strength of voluntary contraction is increased, so more motor units are recruited and activated, giving rise to what is referred to as an *interference pattern* on the oscilloscope screen. The interference pattern is reduced whenever the *number* of (activated) motor units is reduced as occurs in spinal muscular atrophy and in the late stages of muscular dystrophy.

The EMG in muscular dystrophy

Stemming from the early work of Buchthal and Kugelberg in the 1940s (Buchthal and Clemmesen 1941; Kugelberg 1947) the electromyographic features of muscular dystrophy came to be recognized: action potentials are smaller (reduced duration and amplitude) and polyphasic potentials more frequent than in normal. Many subsequent studies confirmed these earlier findings and have been reviewed by Buchthal and Rosenfalck (1963). Although muscular dystrophy may be suspected from inspection of the record as displayed on the oscilloscope, measurements of individual action potentials are less subjective and far more valuable (Gilliatt 1962). The changes observed are due to a general loss of active muscle fibres so that the *size* of each motor unit is reduced and as a result the action potentials are smaller. Later, as the disease progresses and muscle tissue is replaced by fat and connective tissue, so the *number* of motor units decreases and eventually there may be areas where very little if any activity can be recorded.

Table 4.1 *Some values (mean ± s.d.) for the amplitude and duration of motor unit action potentials in healthy young adults (Emery et al. 1973a)*

| | Quadriceps | | | Deltoid | | |
	No.	Amplitude (μV)	Duration (ms)	No.	Amplitude (μV)	Duration (ms)
Males	15	384 ± 99	8.3 ± 1.2	12	318 ± 58	8.4 ± 0.8
Females	17	332 ± 61	7.2 ± 1.1	11	274 ± 37	8.6 ± 0.9

More recently several other electromyographic techniques have been introduced which can be of diagnostic value. The *single fibre EMG* electrode records activity from only a few fibres of a motor unit. It gives an idea of the spatial distribution of muscle fibres and in Duchenne muscular dystrophy indicates an increase in fibre density early in the disease. However this and other sophisticated techniques such as *macro-EMG* and *scanning-EMG* are outside the scope of this discussion.

The EMG in other disorders

The EMG in other disorders which may have to be differentiated from a suspected case of Duchenne muscular dystrophy may be summarized as follows:

Other forms of muscular dystrophy

Other forms of dystrophy presenting in childhood and the various congenital myopathies all show a myopathic EMG which cannot usually be distinguished from Duchenne muscular dystrophy.

Spinal muscular atrophy

The electromyographic findings in this group of disorders are usually quite different from those found in myopathies. Characteristically there is prolonged insertion activity and fibrillation potentials are recorded at rest. These are small potentials with a duration of 0.5–2 ms and an amplitude of 30–150 μV, and occur at a rate of about 2–10 per second. They are probably, at least in part, due to the response of 'sensitized' denervated fibres to circulating acetylcholine. Occasionally these fibrillation potentials are reflected in a fine tremor of the base line of an ECG recording. In one case this drew my attention to the possible diagnosis (Fig. 4.4). This is rarely found in records from healthy individuals or patients with other neuromuscular disorders.

Other characteristics of the record in neurogenic atrophy include a reduced interference pattern, occasional 'giant' action potentials (high amplitude and long duration), and the mean action potential amplitude and duration is generally increased (Gardner-Medwin *et al.* 1967; Hausmanowa-Petrusewicz *et al.* 1968a). These various changes find an explanation, at least in part, in the changes which result when denervation is followed by reinnervation from surviving neurones. In some regions denervated muscle fibres become subsequently reinnervated by adjacent nerve fibres (collateral reinnervation) so increasing the size of the surviving motor unit.

The various features of the electromyographic record in neurogenic atrophy are compared with normal in Fig. 4.5. However, in such diseases the electromyographic record may sometimes appear almost normal or may even

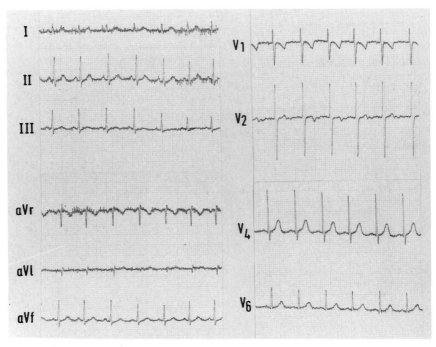

Fig. 4.4. ECG record of a boy aged 9 with Wohlfart–Kugelberg–Welander (type III) spinal muscular atrophy. Note the fine tremor particularly in the limb leads.

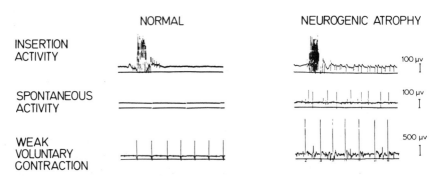

Fig. 4.5. Electromyographic features in neurogenic atrophy compared with normal: prolonged insertion activity, fibrillation potentials at rest, and occasional 'giant' potentials on voluntary contraction.

exhibit some myopathic features when the differentiation from dystrophy can be difficult.

Polymyositis

The other major disorder to be considered in the differential diagnosis is polymyositis (Kagen 1984). In the early stages of this disease there is prolonged insertion activity, and fibrillation potentials are present. The mean action potential duration and amplitude are reduced and polyphasic potentials are frequent.

Electromyographic features characterizing muscular dystrophy (and myopathies in general), spinal muscular atrophy and polymyositis are summarized in Table 4.2. It would seem that the differentiation of muscular dystrophy from spinal muscular atrophy is fairly clear-cut, and in most cases this is true. It would also seem that polymyositis can be differentiated from muscular dystrophy on the basis of spontaneous activity. In general this is also true but it is not an entirely reliable difference because it may occur in dystrophy or be absent in polymyositis (Buchthal and Rosenfalck 1963).

Table 4.2 *The usual electromyographic features differentiating muscular dystrophy, spinal muscular atrophy, and polymyositis*

	Muscular dystrophy	Spinal muscular atrophy	Polymyositis
Insertion activity	Very brief	Prolonged	Prolonged
Fibrillation potentials	−	+	+
Action potentials			
duration	↓	↑	↓
amplitude	↓	↑	↓
Polyphasic potentials	+	−	+
Giant potentials	−	+	−

Muscle pathology

A great deal has been written about the pathology of muscle in various neuro-muscular disorders. Some texts give a concise account of the essential changes observed in such disorders (Bethlem 1970; Hughes 1974) whereas others are extensive monographs which deal in detail with the various changes observed in the course of these diseases (Adams 1975); Mastaglia and Walton 1982; Schröder 1982; Carpenter and Karpati 1984; Dubowitz 1985; Kakulas and Adams 1985). Here only a brief description will be given of those changes in muscular dystrophy which are helpful in establishing the diagnosis. The subject, however, will be referred to again when pathogenesis is considered (p. 139).

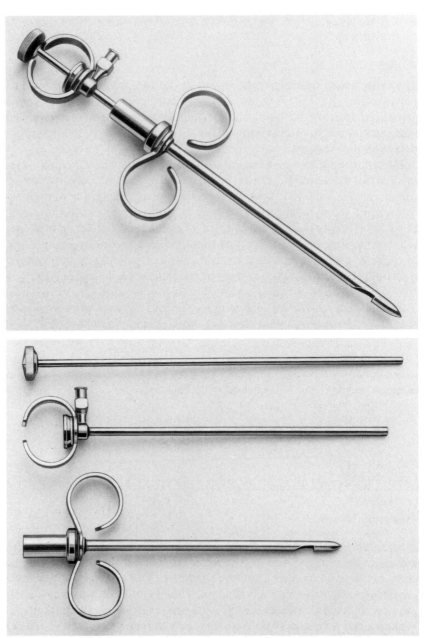

Fig. 4.6. The UCH skeletal muscle biopsy needle. (*Above*) the assembled instrument. (*Below*) the constituent parts which include the cutting cannula, with a side arm for applying suction, and the outer needle. (Instrument supplied by NI Medical, Redditch, Worcs., England.)

Biopsy technique

A muscle biopsy is best carried out on a muscle which is moderately affected clinically. If a minimally affected muscle is chosen then the changes may be too slight to establish the correct diagnosis. On the other hand, if a severely affected muscle is selected it may also be impossible to establish a diagnosis because little may remain apart from fat and connective tissue. In the past the method of open excision under general anaesthesia was the method of choice. This was despite the recognized anaesthetic risks in patients who often have compromised respiratory and cardiac function. Although Duchenne himself had advocated the use of a biopsy needle 100 years ago, for a long time this did not meet favour, largely because of the fear that being a 'blind' procedure, there might be the danger of damaging nerves or blood vessels. In fact, however, this has not proved the case and most now favour the use of a biopsy needle (Fig. 4.6) introduced with local anaesthesia under sterile condition (Edwards *et al.* 1980). Paraffin embedding of fixed material is still largely employed, but better results are obtained with liquid nitrogen and isopentane and studies made on cryostat sections. The latter procedure is associated with fewer artefacts and has the advantage that histochemical studies can also be carried out on the material. This is the method used here. Transverse sections are in general more informative than longitudinal sections, and useful stains are haematoxylin and eosin, or Gomori trichrome.

In a well established case of Duchenne muscular dystrophy, the changes observed in, say, the quadriceps or gastrocnemius muscles, include increased variation in fibre size, fibre necrosis with phagocytosis, and eventually replacement by fat and connective tissue (Fig. 4.7).

It is worthwhile considering some of these changes in a little more detail and tracing their development during the course of the disease.

Preclinical stage

Before there are any obvious clinical manifestations of the disease, there are already significant abnormalities in muscle pathology (Pearson 1962; Hudgson *et al.* 1967a; Bradley *et al.* 1972). Very early on the only significant abnormalities may be an increased variation in fibre size, and an increase in the number of prominent rounded fibres staining more densely with eosin – here referred to as *eosinophilic fibres*. In normal muscle these fibres are absent or very infrequent, and when present occur at the periphery of sections, indicating that they are artefactual. On the other hand, in Duchenne muscular dystrophy, they are seen throughout sections and in some cases can be particularly frequent (Fig. 4.8). These same fibres contain increased intracellular calcium as revealed by histochemical staining with alizarin red S, or a fluorescent method with pentahydroxyflavone (Morin) (Fig. 4.9).

Increased intracellular calcium in skeletal muscle in Duchenne muscular dystrophy has been demonstrated not only histochemically (Engel 1977;

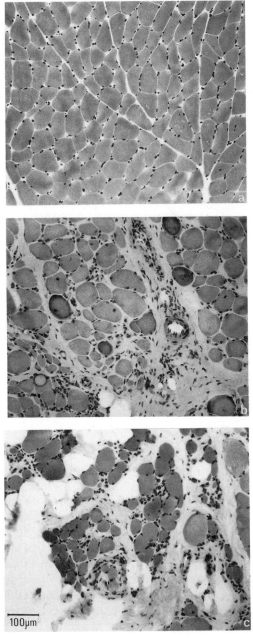

Fig. 4.7. Transverse cryostat sections of gastrocnemius muscle from (*a*) a healthy boy; (*b*) an early case of Duchenne muscular dystrophy; and (*c*) an advanced case of Duchenne muscular dystrophy (haematoxylin and eosin).

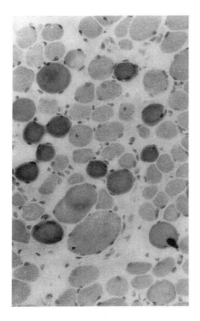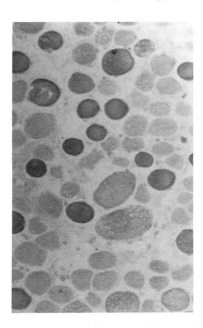

Fig. 4.8. Serial sections of gastrocnemius muscle in a preclinical (2-year-old) case of Duchenne muscular dystrophy, stained with (*left*) haematoxylin and eosin, and (*right*) alizarin red S. Note the numerous eosinophilic/calcium-positive fibres, but no evidence of muscle fibre necrosis.

Bodensteiner and Engel, 1978 Emery and Burt, 1980) but also by X-ray microanalysis (Maunder *et al.* 1977; Maunder-Sewry *et al.* 1980), and by chemical methods (Bertorini *et al.* 1982). The proportion of calcium-positive fibres in Duchenne muscular dystrophy is very variable and the highest proportion was found in a preclinical case (Table 4.3). A significant increase in calcium-positive fibres also occurs in Becker muscular dystrophy but to a much lesser degree in other muscular dystrophies (p. 139). The intracellular accumulation of calcium appears to be the prelude to the breakdown and death (necrosis) of the muscle fibre.

At this early stage in the disease process, *regenerating* fibres are also commonly found. They are recognized by their smaller size in cross-section, basophilic cytoplasm, high concentration of ribonucleic acid (RNA), large pale vesicular nuclei with prominent nucleoli (Mauro 1979). However, such fibres become less frequent as the disease progresses and as fibres undergoing necrosis become more obvious.

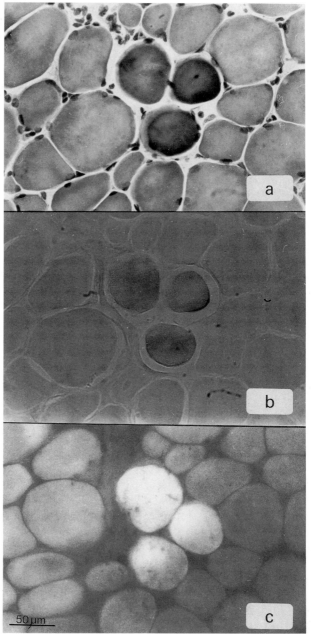

Fig. 4.9. Serial sections of muscle from an early case of Duchenne muscular dystrophy stained with (*a*) haematoxylin and eosin (note 3 centrally placed dark-staining eosinophilic fibres); (*b*) alizarin red S; and (*c*) fluorescent Morin. (From Emery and Burt, 1980, with permission.)

Table 4.3 *Proportion (%) of eosinophilic and calcium-positive fibres in cryostat sections of gastrocnemius muscle biopsy samples from boys with no neuromuscular disorder and boys with Duchenne muscular dystrophy (unpublished data)*

	Age (years)	Eosinophilic fibres	Calcium-positive fibres
Controls			
($N = 7$)	5–12	<0.2	<0.1
DMD			
B103	10	6.0	5.8
B110	9	1.4	1.8
B115	7	3.0	2.9
B111	6	2.7	4.4
B106	5	4.1	6.5
B117*	3	3.7	5.3
B159*	2	15.3	18.3

* Preclinical cases.

Later stages

The changes which take place as a muscle fibre undergoes necrosis are complex. As the intracellular structures are destroyed the fibre is invaded by phagocytic cells. In fact the '. . . most unequivocal evidence of necrosis is the presence of phagocytic cells within a disordered fibre' (Cullen and Mastaglia 1980). This is illustrated in Fig. 4.10.

As the necrotic fibres are phagocytosed they are replaced by fat and connective tissue so that eventually only small islands of muscle tissue remain.

Possible differences in muscle pathology between Duchenne and Becker types of muscular dystrophy have been described (Bradley *et al.* 1978). It seems unlikely, however, that any such differences point to any fundamental differences but are more likely to be reflections of the differing tempo in the two disorders.

The histological changes in muscular dystrophy are in general different from spinal muscular atrophy. In the latter group of disorders all those muscle fibres associated with the defective neurone gradually atrophy. This produces the classical picture of group atrophy and is pathognomonic of spinal muscular atrophy (Fig. 4.11).

The atrophy may be so profound as to present the appearance of 'nuclear clumps'. In spinal muscular atrophy, affected fibres undergo atrophy and tend to be grouped together. In contrast, in muscular dystrophy, affected fibres undergo structural changes and these occur in individual fibres at random. However, especially in the more chronic forms of neurogenic

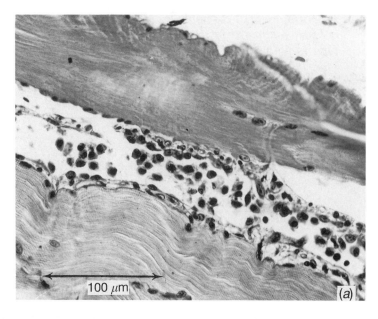

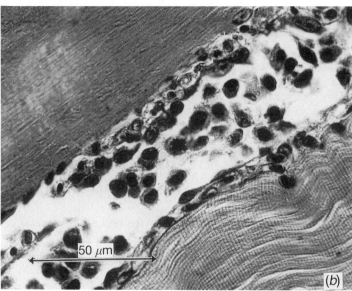

Fig. 4.10. Longitudinal sections of gastrocnemius muscle from a manifesting female carrier of Duchenne muscular dystrophy. (*a*) The upper fibre has lost most of the cross-striations which are still well defined in the lower fibre. Between the two fibres are the remains of a necrotic fibre which is undergoing phagocytosis. (*b*) Higher power magnification (haematoxylin and eosin).

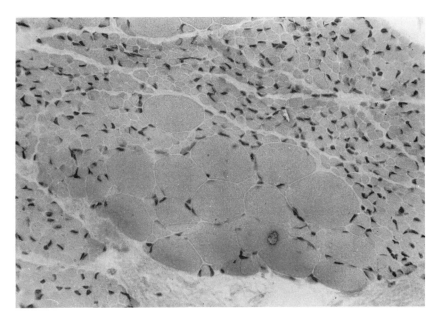

Fig. 4.11. Muscle fibre atrophy in spinal muscular atrophy (Werdnig–Hoffmann disease). Note large groups of atrophic fibres (haematoxylin and eosin).

atrophy, muscle fibres adjacent to groups of atrophic fibres, may undergo changes similar to those seen in muscular dystrophy; variation in fibre size, central nuclei, and even occasionally fibre necrosis and phagocytosis. It is possible that such changes result from faulty attempts at reinnervation: the metabolism of these abnormally innervated fibres is disturbed in some way which then results in the structural changes usually associated with muscular dystrophy (Drachman *et al.* 1967; Mumenthaler 1970). In their detailed and elegant studies Bradley and his colleagues (1978) noted in some biopsy specimens from cases of Becker muscular dystrophy, changes which can be associated with denervation. However, there are limits in attempting to define pathogenesis purely on the basis of morphological appearances. As these investigators pointed out there can be problems in interpretation:

. . . small, angular fibers can derive from fiber splitting, which can be the result of either a chronic myopathy, denervation, or tenotomy. Small groups of atrophic fibers can result from splitting or regeneration after necrosis. The changes described as characteristic of myopathy have been reported in biopsies from muscles affected by chronic denervation.   (Bradley *et al.* 1978)

In polymyositis there can also be muscle fibre necrosis and regeneration, but the distinctive pathological feature in this disorder is the infiltration of muscle tissue by inflammatory cells (mainly lymphocytes and plasma cells). This is usually focal and occurs in connective tissue, around blood vessels and within muscle fibres; a reaction which is not seen in Duchenne muscular dystrophy or cases of spinal muscular atrophy occurring in childhood. However, as Schmalbruch (1982) has emphasized, the distinction between groups of phagocytes engaged in phagocytosis, and perivascular infiltrates of lymphocytes and plasma cells is not always clear. Furthermore, in childhood polymyositis/dermatomyositis muscle histology may show only minimal changes or practically no significant changes at all. For this reason some advocate open biopsy in suspected polymyositis to ensure that as much tissue as possible can be examined. Dubowitz (1985) in fact suggests that in a suspected case of polymyositis in whom the muscle histology appears normal, a trial of therapy with steroids is advised because a positive response would be diagnostic, and also delay in treating this condition can seriously influence the prognosis.

Muscle histochemistry

On the basis of physiological experiments in animals, and biochemical and histochemical studies on muscle tissue, it is possible to classify human skeletal muscle fibres into three distinct types which are designated as 1, 2A, and 2B (Brooke and Kaiser 1970). Some of the differences between these fibre types are summarized in Table 4.4.

Animal experiments have shown that muscle fibres innervated by a single motor neurone possess similar physiological properties and identical histochemical characteristics. Thus there would appear to be at least three types of motor neurones. In Fig. 4.12 is illustrated diagrammatically the effects of

Table 4.4 *Some characteristics of different fibre types in human skeletal muscle*

	Type 1	Type 2A	Type 2B
Speed of contraction	Slow	Intermediate	Fast
Appearance			
(myoglobin content)	Dark	Dark	Pale
Size	Small	Intermediate	Large
Enzyme activities			
1. ATPase pH 9.4	+	+++	+ + +
2. ATPase pH 4.3	+ + +	+	+
3. Oxidative*	+ + +	+ +	+
4. Phosphorylase	+	+ +	+ + +

* NADH-tetrazolium reductase, succinic dehydrogenase.

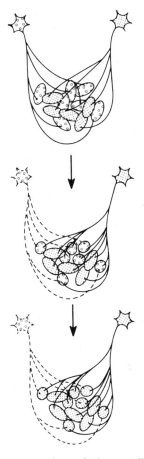

Fig. 4.12. Diagrammatic representation of the possible effects of denervation followed by reinnervation. For simplicity only two types of fibres are illustrated.

denervation as it occurs in spinal muscular atrophy. If this is rapidly progressive there may be little time for reinnervation. However, if reinnervation occurs, from nerve fibres from another neurone, this will lead eventually to groups of atrophic fibres being of the same histochemical type.

The appearance of fibre type atrophy in a case of Werdnig–Hoffmann disease is given in Fig. 4.13 in which type 2 fibres are predominantly affected. However, both fibre types can atrophy after denervation though most larger fibres tend to be of type 1. In muscular dystrophy and polymyositis no particular fibre type is predominantly affected and there is no grouping of fibre types. (Brumback and Leech 1984).

The reason why certain groups of muscles are especially affected early in the course of muscular dystrophy (p. 30) is not at all clear. This presumably reflects some difference in their biochemical/physiological properties compared with muscles affected to a lesser degree and only in the later stages of the disease. Johnson *et al.* (1973) approached this problem by considering the proportions of type 1 and type 2 fibres is normal skeletal muscles which in Duchenne muscular dystrophy are either severely affected or relatively unaffected. They found that there was a tendency for the proportion of type 2 fibres to be higher in muscles which are more *severely* affected, but there was no simple correlation between fibre type composition of individual muscles and their being affected or spared in the disease. Using their extensive data, there would also appear to be a slight excess of type 2 (or deficiency of type 1)

Table 4.5 *Mean proportion (%) of type 1 and type 2 fibres in various normal human muscles (Johnson* et al. *1973) divided into those muscles clinically affected early or late in the course of Duchenne muscular dystrophy*

		Type 1	Type 2
Affected early			
Sternomastoid		35.2	64.8
Pectoralis major			
(sterno-costal)		43.1	56.9
Triceps			
(surface)		32.5	67.5
(deep)		32.7	67.3
Brachioradialis		39.8	60.2
Extensor digitorum		47.3	52.7
Extensor digitorum brevis		45.3	54.7
Latissimus dorsi		50.5	49.5
Iliopsoas		49.2	50.8
Gluteus maximus		52.4	47.6
Vastus medialis			
(surface)		43.7	56.3
(deep)		61.5	38.5
Rectus femoris			
(lat. head surface)		29.5	70.5
(lat. head deep)		42.0	58.0
(medial head)		42.8	57.2
Tribialis anterior			
(surface)		73.4	26.6
(deep)		72.7	27.3
	Mean	46.68	53.32
	s.d.	–	12.74

Affected later			
Trapezius		53.7	46.3
Pectoralis major			
(clavicular)		42.3	57.7
Biceps brachii			
(surface)		42.3	57.7
(deep)		50.5	49.5
Biceps femoris		66.9	33.1
Flexor digitorum brevis		44.5	55.5
Flexor digitorum profundis		47.3	52.7
Gastrocnemius			
(lat. head surface)		43.5	56.5
(lat. head deep)		50.3	49.7
(medial head)		50.8	49.2
Soleus			
(surface)		86.4	13.6
(deep)		89.0	11.0
	Mean	55.63	44.37
	s.d.	–	16.42

fibres in those muscles affected *early* in the disease, but there is considerable variation, and the difference from those muscles affected later in the course of the disease is not statistically significant (Table 4.5). Whatever may be responsible for the differential involvement of muscles in Duchenne muscular dystrophy, this is not a simple matter of histochemical fibre type.

Muscle innervation

A most useful technique for diagnosing neurogenic atrophy is the intravital or supravital staining of motor nerve filaments and end-plates with methylene blue (Coërs and Woolf 1959). The motor end-plate is a complex structure at the site where excitation is transmitted from the motor nerve to the muscle fibre (Fig. 4.14).

In spinal muscular atrophy there is branching of subterminal intramuscular nerve fibres (Fig. 4.15) with collateral reinnervation, and degeneration of motor end-plates (Pearce and Harriman 1966; Hausmanowa-Petrusewicz *et al.*, 1968).

Branching of nerve fibres in this way is found in all forms of spinal muscular atrophy, but is very rarely seen in normal or dystrophic muscle. Studies of muscle innervation may therefore be useful in establishing a diagnosis in cases where routine histology in normal or if apparent 'myopathic' features predominate (Meadows *et al.* 1969).

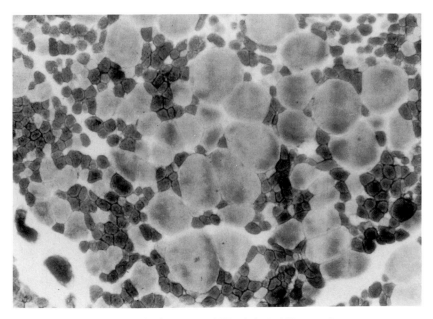

Fig. 4.13. Fibre type atrophy in a case of Werdnig–Hoffmann disease (ATPase pH 9.4).

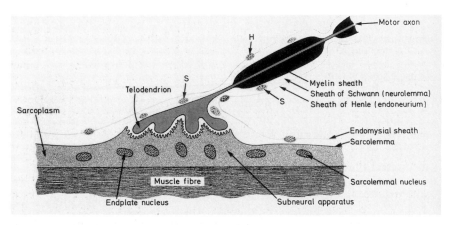

Fig. 4.14. The structure of the normal human motor end-plate. (H, nucleus of sheath of Henle; S, nucleus of sheath of Schwann.)

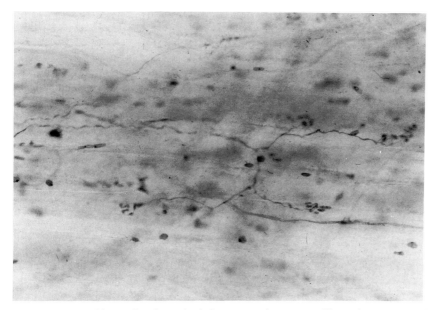

Fig. 4.15. Branching of subterminal intramuscular nerve fibres in a case of Wohlfart–Kugelberg–Welander spinal muscular atrophy (supravital staining with methylene blue).

Electronmicroscopy

Electronmicroscopy of muscle has provided details of the ultrastructural changes which take place in muscular dystrophy and spinal muscular atrophy (Mair and Tomé 1972; Hudgson *et al.* 1987). In Duchenne muscular dystrophy these changes include distention of the sarcoplasmic reticulum, Z band degeneration ('streaming') and disruption and loss of myofilaments, followed later by complete disarray of the band structure (Fig. 4.16). These changes however are not specific to Duchenne muscular dystrophy but occur in other forms of dystrophy. Various alterations in the sarcolemma have also been described early in the course of the disease (Cullen and Mastaglia 1980; Carpenter and Karpati 1984), and include defects in the plasma membrane and reduplication of the basement membrane. The molecular basis for these reported changes however is unknown but may be of relevance to the pathogenesis of the disease (p. 132). The motor end-plates and muscle microvasculature are essentially normal.

Other investigations

The diagnosis of Duchenne muscular dystrophy can be established in almost all cases on the basis of the clinical findings, SCK level, EMG examination,

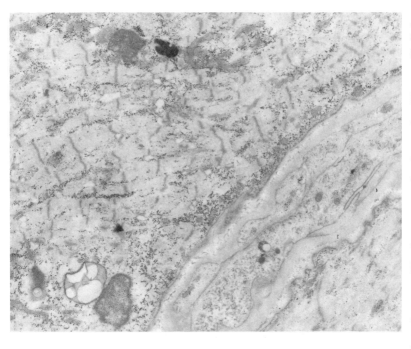

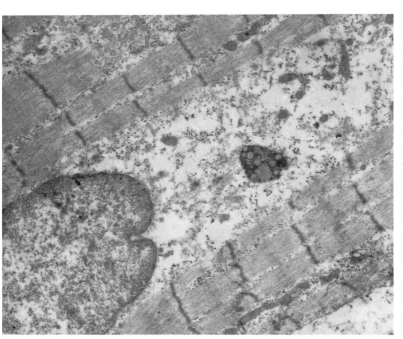

Fig. 4.16. Electronmicroscopy of skeletal muscle in: (*Left*) relatively early stage of Duchenne muscular dystrophy. The myofibrils have lost some myofilaments with widening of the intermyofibrillar space which contains a lysosome (phosphotungstic acid x14 000). (*Right*) later stage showing disorganization of the band structure (2% uranyl acetate and lead citrate x7000). (Reproduced by kind permission of Dr J. Trevor Hughes and Lloyd-Luke, publishers.)

and muscle biopsy. However, additional investigations may be useful in help-ing to differentiate the disorder from other conditions. Thus nerve conduc-tion studies will be important if a neuropathy is suspected since this will be associated with a reduced nerve conduction velocity. Electrocardiography (p. 95) may help to distinguish between autosomal recessive and X-linked recessive forms of childhood dystrophy (Skyring and McKusick 1961; Emery 1972).

Nuclear magnetic resonance (NMR) is a painless and non-invasive technique which is proving valuable in studying certain aspects of the bio-chemistry of muscle, such as ATP levels (Newman *et al.* 1982; Griffiths *et al.* 1985). However, the equipment is expensive and no defects detected in this way have so far proved to be diagnostic for Duchenne muscular dystrophy.

Ultrasound (Heckmatt *et al.* 1982) and more recently computed tomo-graphy (CT scanning) (Kawai *et al.* 1985), have been used to demonstrate and localize muscle loss by showing areas of changed density. They too have the advantage of being non-invasive, and CT scanning seems sufficiently sensitive to detect significant abnormalities in a proportion of carriers (Rott and Rödl 1985; Stern *et al.* 1985; de Visser and Verbeeten 1985a, b). It also offers a method of assessing inaccessible muscles such as the psoas and erector spinae (Smith *et al.* 1986a). These techniques, however, are unlikely to replace more conventional methods of establishing a diagnosis of muscular dystrophy, but with further refinements might well prove to be useful adjuncts in patient assessment.

Summary and conclusions

In the case of an otherwise healthy little boy who presents with evidence of proximal limb girdle muscle weakness and who has a grossly elevated SCK level (50–100 times normal), the diagnosis of Duchenne muscular dystrophy is almost certain. However, because of the importance of not missing poly-myositis which is treatable, and the need to exclude other disorders which can be inherited differently, electromyography but certainly a muscle biopsy is indicated in all cases. This is best carried out using a biopsy needle under local anaesthesia. The characteristic features of muscle histology are necrosis and phagocytosis of scattered individual muscle fibres in muscular dystrophy, muscle fibre group atrophy in spinal muscular atrophy, and infiltration with inflammatory cells (mainly lymphocytes and plasma cells) in polymyositis.

A significant feature of Duchenne muscular dystrophy is the presence of prominent, rounded fibres which stain densely with eosin, so-called eosinophilic fibres, which contain increased intracellular calcium.

Other investigations, such as muscle histochemistry, motor end-plate and muscle innervation studies, electronmicroscopy, electrocardiography, and computed tomography can all provide useful additional information helpful in differential diagnosis and also in understanding more about the nature of the disorder.

5 Differential diagnosis

Disorders which could possibly be confused with Duchenne muscular dystrophy include polymyositis, which must always be considered because it is treatable (p. 62), other forms of muscular dystrophy which may present in early childhood, various congenital myopathies, and spinal muscular atrophy.

The congenital muscular dystrophies

This is a relatively ill-defined group of disorders which is clearly very heterogeneous. In all cases the disorder is evident at birth or in the neonatal period, with hypotonia and muscle weakness (Fig. 3.1, p. 25). The muscle weakness is generalized and may affect the face but never the extraocular muscles. Tendon reflexes are usually reduced and joint contractures may be present at birth or develop later in childhood. Intelligence is unimpaired and the disorder is inherited as an autosomal recessive trait. In some instances progression is rapid and death occurs in infancy or early childhood (Short 1963; Wharton 1965; Claes *et al.* 1968). In other cases the disease is either non-progressive or only slowly progressive (Pearson and Fowler 1963; Claes *et al.* 1968; Vassella *et al.* 1967; Zellweger *et al.* 1967; Ketelsen *et al.* 1971; Donner *et al.* 1975; Lazaro *et al.* 1979). However, the distinction between severe and benign forms may not be entirely justified, and it is often difficult to predict at the time the diagnosis is first made what the ultimate prognosis may be (McMenamin *et al.* 1982).

Relatively slowly progressive forms of congenital muscular dystrophy have been described in association with mental handicap (Fukuyama *et al.* 1960), infantile cataracts and hypogonadism (Bassöe 1956), CNS malformations (Kamoshita *et al.* 1976), congenital heart disease (Lebenthal *et al.* 1970), and certain dysmorphic features associated with hyperhidrosis and recurrent upper respiratory tract infections (Furukawa and Toyokura 1977). Since some of these associations have been described in multiple affected sibs, they may well represent different rare autosomal recessive forms of congenital muscular dystrophy. Lewis and Besant (1962) have also described a rapidly progressive form of the disease in sibs in which the dystrophic process was almost entirely limited to the diaphragm.

The SCK level in congenital muscular dystrophy may occasionally be comparable to levels found in Duchenne muscular dystrophy (Donner *et al.* 1975). But why in many cases the SCK level is normal or only slightly elevated yet the muscle histology appears to be no different from other cases of congenital muscular dystrophy and Duchenne muscular dystrophy in which the SCK level is grossly elevated, is not at all clear.

Congenital myopathies

In recent years useful reviews of this heterogeneous group of disorders have been given by Heckmatt and Dubowitz (1983a), Bundey (1985), and Baraitser (1985), who consider their differential diagnosis in detail and provide extensive bibliographies. Some of the more important types are listed in Table 5.1.

None of these myopathies however is likely to be confused with a case of Duchenne muscular dystrophy because most, but not all, present at birth or in the neonatal period with hypotonia and generalized muscle weakness, often associated with respiratory problems and feeding difficulties. Facial features may be dysmorphic (nemaline myopathy, myotubular myopathy), and marked fatigability (mitochondrial myopathy), or muscle cramps (glycogenoses, carnitine palmityltransferase deficiency) may be important features. Serum enzyme levels are usually normal and a specific diagnosis is based on muscle histology with special stains or electronmicroscopy.

Table 5.1 *Some defined congenital myopathies and their suggested modes of inheritance*

	AR	AD	XR
Central core disease		+	
Nemaline myopathy	+	+	
Myotubular (centronuclear) myopathy	+	+	+
Minicore (multicore) disease	+		
Congenital fibre type disproportion	+	+	
Mitochondrial myopathies	+	+	
Kearn–Sayre syndrome	+		
Muscle carnitine deficiency	+		
Carnitine palmityltransferase deficiency	+		
Muscle glycogenoses (II, III, IV, V, VII)	+		

AR, autosomal recessive; AD, autosomal dominant; XR, X-linked recessive.

Other X-linked muscular dystrophies

Over the years several other X-linked muscular dystrophies have been recognized, all relatively more benign than Duchenne muscular dystrophy. The commonest of these is Becker muscular dystrophy which occasionally presents in childhood when it can then be confused with Duchenne muscular dystrophy.

Becker type muscular dystrophy

This disease was first clearly delineated by Becker some thirty years ago (Becker and Kiener 1955; Becker 1962) since when there have been many reports of affected families. The condition has been extensively reviewed by Rotthauwe and Kowalewski (1966), Zellweger and Hanson (1967a), Heyck and Laudahn (1969), Shaw and Dreifuss (1969), Markand *et al.* (1969), Conomy (1970), and more recently by Emery and Skinner (1976), Ringel *et al.* (1977), and Bradley *et al.* (1978).

The distribution of muscle wasting and weakness is very similar to Duchenne muscular dystrophy and like this latter disorder the hip flexors and quadriceps muscles tend to be affected early in the lower limbs, while in the upper limbs the serrati, pectoralis, biceps, brachioradialis, and triceps muscles are usually affected first (Fig. 5.1).

Although weakness almost always begins in the lower limbs, eventually the upper limb musculature becomes affected. Calf enlargement is invariably present and contractures are a late development. Cardiac involvement, if it occurs at all, is usually a late manifestation, although not always (Kuhn *et al.* 1979). A proportion, as yet not precisely determined, have some impairment

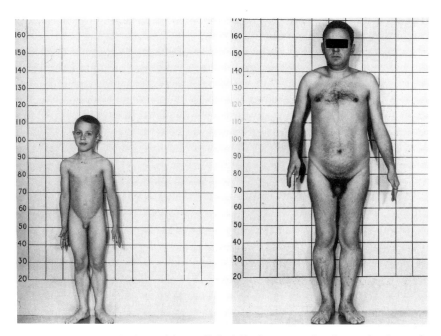

Fig. 5.1. A 6-year-old boy with preclinical Becker muscular dystrophy (note the enlarged calves) and his affected 26-year-old uncle. (From Emery (1983) with permission.)

of intellect. The SCK level is substantially raised, especially in the early stages and gradually falls as the disease progresses. In the preclinical stage of the disease, which may last 10 years or more, when the only abnormality is calf enlargement and there is no apparent muscle weakness, the SCK level is grossly elevated to levels comparable to those found in boys with Duchenne muscular dystrophy of the same age but who are clinically affected. Why in Becker muscular dystrophy there should be this lag period before the onset of muscle weakness remains unexplained.

Because of the very high SCK levels early in the course of Becker muscular dystrophy and overlap in age in onset with Duchenne muscular dystrophy, this can present a diagnostic dilemma in an isolated case. Points of possible distinction between the two disorders are revealed by comparing details of the course of the disease in the two disorders. A proximal myopathy occurring in an isolated male, or in families with only affected brothers, could possibly be adult onset limb girdle muscular dystrophy which is usually inherited as an autosomal recessive trait. For this reason we have restricted our definition of Becker muscular dystrophy to families in which a proximal muscular dystrophy affects males *in at least two generations of a family, the pattern of inheritance being consistent with that of an X-linked recessive trait.* Excluding index cases (probands) the course of the disease in 10 large families (Emery and Skinner 1976) has been compared with the findings in cases of established Duchenne muscular dystrophy.

Penrose (1951) has shown that if two approximately normal curves overlap the point of overlap (*x*), measured in standard deviation units from either mean, can be determined from the means (m_1 and m_2) and standard deviations (s_1 and s_2) of the two curves (Fig. 5.2):

$$x = \frac{m_1 - m_2}{s_1 + s_2}$$

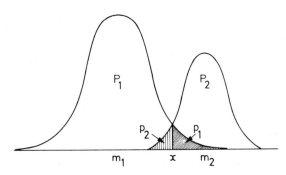

Fig. 5.2. Method for calculating the point of overlap in two normally distributed curves. The point of overlap (*x*) is such that $p_1/P_1 = p_2/P_2$. (From Emery (1986) with permission.)

Thus, if the point where two curves overlapped corresponded to 1.96 standard deviations from the means of either then, since 95 per cent of observations lie within 1.96 standard deviations on either side of the mean of a normal curve, 2.5 per cent (one-tail) will lie outside and therefore be misclassified.

By calculating the point of overlap (x) in terms of the number of standard deviations from the mean, it is possible to determine the percentage misclassification from appropriate tables of the normal probability integral (Fisher and Yates 1967). When this is applied to data for Duchenne and Becker types of muscular dystrophy, the value of x and the percentage misclassification (in parentheses) for age at onset is 1.182 (11.9 per cent), for age at becoming chairbound is 1.753 (4.0 per cent), and for age at death is 1.533 (6.3 per cent). Thus in (100–11.9) or 88.1 per cent of boys with Duchenne muscular dystrophy onset is before the age of 3.3 + (1.182) (1.7) or 5.3 years, whereas in 88.1 per cent of males with Becker muscular dystrophy, symptoms develop *after* the age of 5.3 years. Similarly, (100–4.0) or 96.0 per cent of boys with Duchenne muscular dystrophy become chairbound before the age of 9.4 + (1.753) (1.7) or 12.4 years, whereas 96.0 per cent of males with Becker muscular dystrophy become chairbound *after* the age of 12.4 years. Finally, (100–6.3) or 93.7 per cent of boys with Duchenne muscular dystrophy die before the age of 16.3 + (1.533) (3.1) or 21.1 years, whereas 93.7 per cent of males with Becker muscular dystrophy die *after* the age of 21.1 years (Table 5.2).

The two disorders are therefore best distinguished on the age at becoming confined to a wheelchair, and further help may be afforded by electrocardiography. Whereas there is electrocardiographic evidence of right ventricular preponderance in most boys with Duchenne muscular dystrophy (*see* p. 95) we have found no significant difference in the algebraic sum of $|R-S|$ in V_1 between 102 healthy males and 19 males with Becker muscular dystrophy (Emery and Skinner 1976). Thus, if an affected boy with no family history is still walking at the age of 12 and there is also no electrocardiographic evidence of right ventricular preponderance, he is more likely to have Becker muscular dystrophy than Duchenne muscular dystrophy, and the prognosis is therefore much better.

If other relatives are affected, then usually the diagnosis will be easier to make. But manifesting female carriers in a family of X-linked Becker muscular dystrophy may give the appearance of dominant inheritance which could then cause some confusion in establishing a diagnosis (Aguilar *et al.* 1978) but this appears to be an uncommon occurrence. Although usually inherited as an autosomal recessive trait, limb girdle muscular dystrophy of adult onset may occasionally be inherited as an autosomal dominant trait, and in some such families can sometimes be limited to males. However, this latter form of muscular dystrophy is unlikely to prove a serious diagnostic

Table 5.2 *Clinical course in Duchenne and Becker types of muscular dystrophy*

	Onset				Chairbound				Death		
	No.	Mean age (yrs)	s.d.	No.	Mean age (yrs)	s.d.	No.	Mean age (yrs)	s.d.		
Duchenne	144	3.3	1.7	120	9.4	1.7	129	16.3	3.1		
Becker	27	11.1	4.9	9	27.1	8.4	10	42.2	13.8		
P		*P*<0.001			*P*<0.001			*P*<0.001				
'*x*'		1.182			1.753			1.533				
Misclassification (%)		11.9			4.0			6.3				

problem because it appears to be very rare, having so far been described in only three families (De Coster *et al.* 1974; Hastings *et al.* 1980).

Apparent Duchenne and Becker muscular dystrophies in the same family

For many years a distinction between Duchenne and more benign X-linked forms of muscular dystrophy was questioned. It was really only when several large families were described in which all affected males had a consistently benign disease did the concept become accepted. Nevertheless, there have been occasional reports in recent years in which cases of presumed Duchenne and Becker muscular dystrophy occurred in the same family (Robert and Vignon 1972; Jackson *et al.* 1974; Furukawa and Peter 1977; Hausmanowa-Petrusewicz and Borkowska 1978; Gardner-Medwin 1982b). It is possible that these families could represent different mutations from the usual Duchenne and Becker forms of dystrophy. However, since there is considerable clinical variation in both these disorders it is perhaps to be expected that occasional families may be found in which affected males at opposite ends of the spectrum of severity may occur.

Mabry type muscular dystrophy

In 1965 Mabry and his colleagues described a large family from Kentucky with an X-linked muscular dystrophy with prolonged survival and associated with relatively severe disability and myocardial involvement. However, there appears to have been no further reports of any families with exactly this clinical picture.

X-linked muscular dystrophy with early contractures and cardiomyopathy (Emery–Dreifuss type)

In 1961, Dreifuss and Hogan described a large family in Virginia in the United States with an X-linked form of muscular dystrophy which they considered at the time to be a benign type of Duchenne muscular dystrophy. However, on reinvestigating the family a few years later, I was convinced that this was a very different disease from either Duchenne or Becker muscular dystrophy and a report setting out the differences was published in 1966 (Emery and Dreifuss 1966). This same disorder may well have been first described by Cestan and Lejonne in 1902 in two affected brothers, and has been reviewed more recently in a number of studies (Mawatari and Katayama 1973; Cammann *et al.* 1974; Rowland *et al.* 1979; Hopkins *et al.* 1981; Serratrice *et al.* 1982; Fowler and Nayak 1983; Dickey *et al.* 1984; Dominici *et al.* 1984; Oswald *et al.* 1986). The onset is in early childhood and is marked by progressive muscle wasting and weakness which, in the beginning, affects the lower limbs more than the upper limbs. The progression is relatively slow and most affected individuals survive into middle age with varying degrees of incapacity. There does not appear to be any intellectual impairment. The

SCK level is usually slightly raised but even in the early stages never approaches the grossly elevated levels found in Duchenne muscular dystrophy. The distinctive features of this disorder are: Firstly, *early* contractures of the elbows and Achilles tendons and later the posterior cervical muscles. Secondly, muscle weakness is more proximal (scapulo-humeral) in the upper limbs and distal (anterior tibial and peroneal muscles) in the lower limbs, at least in the beginning. Thirdly, there is no calf pseudohypertrophy. Fourthly, myocardial involvement with cardiac conduction defects is a frequent and important feature (Fig. 5.3). Provided the diagnosis is made

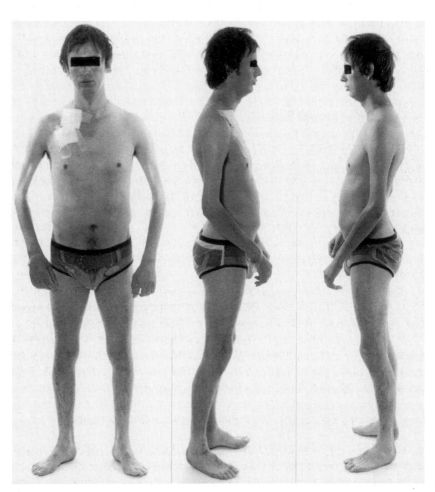

Fig 5.3. A 17-year-old boy with X-linked muscular dystrophy with early contractures and cardiomyopathy. Note the flexion contractures of the elbows, and wasting of the lower legs. A cardiac pacemaker has been inserted.

sufficiently early, the insertion of a cardiac pacemaker can be life-saving.

The interpretation of the electromyographic findings and muscle histology in the disorder have been somewhat controversial, but the accumulated evidence most favours a muscular dystrophy (Rowland *et al.* 1979; Hopkins *et al.* 1981). Also in a family described by Thomas *et al.* (1972), the spinal cord was normal in one affected individual who came to autopsy. Finally, although most cases described so far have been X-linked (Table 5.3), rare, somewhat similar variants of the syndrome may be inherited as an autosomal dominant trait (Chakrabarti and Pearce, 1981; Fenichel *et al.* 1982; Miller *et al.* 1985). The occurrence in an isolated female reported by Takamoto *et al.* (1984) could represent either an autosomal form or the heterozygous expression of the X-linked form. Some distinguishing features between the X-linked and autosomal forms are summarized in Table 5.4, but the differences in predominant muscle involvement may be more apparent than real.

X-linked scapulo-peroneal muscular dystrophy

This has previously been considered a possible separate disease entity. However, reports of the condition by Rotthauwe *et al.* (1972) and Thomas *et al.* (1972) have been considered by others (Rowland *et al.* 1979; Hopkins *et al.* 1981) to be cases of X-linked muscular dystrophy with early contractures and cardiomyopathy. Two further families (Waters *et al.* 1975) previously considered to have X-linked scapulo-peroneal muscular dystrophy were subsequently restudied by one of the authors who then decided that these too represented the form with early contractures and cardiomyopathy (Hopkins *et al.* 1981). Some confusion may have arisen because in the original report of Emery and Dreifuss (1966) weakness of the anterior tibial muscles was not emphasized. However, a scapulo-peroneal syndrome clearly exists which is inherited as an autosomal dominant trait and can be either neurogenic (Kaeser 1965) or myopathic (Thomas *et al.* 1975) in origin. However, in these cases onset is in adult life (a rare recessive neurogenic form may begin in childhood) and *early* contractures and cardiac conduction defects are *not* associated features. The myopathic form can be confused with facioscapulohumeral muscular dystrophy (Kazakov *et al.* 1976).

Autosomal recessive limb girdle muscular dystrophy of childhood

Two of Duchenne's original 13 cases of muscular dystrophy were in fact girls; and there have been many similar reports since. However, in the past many cases of girls with purported muscular dystrophy may well have had some other cause for their muscle weakness, such as a congenital myopathy or spinal muscular atrophy (Penn *et al.* 1970). Nevertheless, with improvements in diagnostic techniques it is now clear that muscular dystrophy can occur in

Table 5.3 *More recent reports of X-linked muscular dystrophy associated with early contractures and cardiomyopathy (Emery–Dreifuss type) (+, present, in at least some; −, absent in all; NR, not recorded.)*

Reference	Number		Onset	Contractures (early)			Calf pseudo-hypertrophy	Muscle weakness		Cardiac involvement	Comments
	Families	Total cases		Elbows	Tendo achilles	Post-cervical muscles		Proximal (UL)	Distal (LL)		
Emery & Dreifuss (1966)	1	8	4–5	+	+	NR	−	+	?	+	See text
Rothauwe et al. (1972)	1	17	<10	+	+	+	−	+	+	+	See text
Thomas et al. (1972)	1	5 (6)	<5	+	+	(1)	−	+	+	+	See text
Mawatari and Katayama (1973)	1	5	7–10	NR	+	+	NR	+	+	+	Considered to be SMA (but see Rowland et al. 1979)
Cammann et al. (1974)	1	8	7–11	+	+	NR	−	+	+	?+	
Waters et al. (1975)/ Hopkins et al. (1981)	2	37/35	2–15	+	+	NR	−	+	+	+	
Wadia et al. (1976)	1	5	10–?32	+ (late)	+ (late)	NR	+3/4	+	−	+	Possibly a different disorder
Rowland et al. (1979)	1	7	7	+	+	+	NR	+	+	+	
Tomelleri et al. (1980)	1	2 (brothers)	Early childhood	+	NR	+	−	+	+	+	Considered to be possibly neurogenic
Serratrice et al. (1982)	1	10	2–10	+	+	Limited extension	NR	+	+	+	
Fowler & Nayak (1983)	1	2	Early childhood	+	+	+	−	+	+	+	
Dickey et al. (1984)	2	6 (1 isolated)	1–5	+	+	+	NR	+	+	+	
Dominici et al. (1984)	1	5	Childhood	+	+	NR	NR	+	+	+	
Dubowitz (1985) (pp. 341–2)	1	3	11–12	+	+	?+	NR	NR	NR	?+	
Oswald et al. (1986)	1	8	Early childhood	+	+	+	NR	+	+	+	
Merlini et al. (1986)	1	5	Early childhood	+	+	+	−	+	+	+	See Dominici et al. 1984
Johnston & McKay (1986)	1	3	Early childhood	+	+	+	−	+	+	+	

Table 5.4 *Some distinguishing features between the X-linked and autosomal forms of muscular dystrophy with early contractures and cardiomyopathy (Emery–Dreifuss type)*

| Inheritance | Childhood onset | Course | Contractures | | | Calf pseudo-hypertrophy | Predominant muscle weakness | Cardio-myopathy | Reference |
			Elbows	Tendo achilles	Cervical				
XR	+	Slow	+	+	+	−	Scapulo-humero-peroneal	+	–
AD	+	Rapid (mostly)	+	+	+	−	Scapulo-peroneal	+	Chakrabarti & Pearce (1981)
AD	+	Slow	−	+	+/−	−	Humero-pelvic	+	Fenichel et al. (1982)
Isolated female	+	Slow	+	+	+	?	Humero-pelvic	+	Takamoto et al. (1984)
AD	+	Slow	+	+	+	+	Humero-peroneal	+	Miller et al. (1985)

XR, X-linked recessive; AD, autosomal dominant.

little girls, for which there are several possible explanations. This may be a manifestation of X-linked Duchenne muscular dystrophy. Firstly, she may be homozygous for the mutant gene, her mother being a carrier and a new mutation having occurred on her paternally derived X-chromosome. Such a perturbation, although theoretically possible, would be extremely rare depending on the mutation rate in sperm. Secondly, she may be a manifesting carrier of the disease as a result of random X-inactivation (p. 190). Thirdly, she may have a sex chromosomal abnormality or an X/autosome transloca-tion (p. 166). These possibilities will be discussed later. However, apart from in some way manifesting X-linked Duchenne muscular dystrophy, there is now clear evidence that an autosomal recessive form of a clinically similar disorder exists. This accounts for the disease in isolated affected girls, and families with affected sisters, or brothers and sisters; and presumably also a proportion of isolated cases of affected boys or families with only affected brothers. Very rarely a limb girdle type myopathy *limited to females* may be inherited as an autosomal dominant trait (Henson 1967; Yoshioka *et al.* 1986).

One of the earliest and most detailed accounts of the autosomal recessive condition was given by Dubowitz in 1960, since when there have been many reports of the disorder which have recently been reviewed (Gardner-Medwin and Johnston, 1984; Somer *et al.* 1985; Yoshioka *et al.* 1986). Gardner-Medwin and Johnston (1984) considered that although the X-linked and autosomal recessive forms were very similar, some points might be helpful in differentiation: in the autosomal recessive form toe walking is a prominent early feature before significant difficulties in walking occur, the course of the disease is relatively milder, affected children often not becoming confined to a wheelchair until their early teens or even later, the deltoids are relatively more affected than the biceps or triceps muscles, and intelligence is usually normal. Calf enlargement is often present and SCK levels are about the same in both disorders for individuals of the same age. In our own limited experience with two unrelated girls with muscular dystrophy, the one feature they seemed to share was a relatively more benign course compared with the X-linked form (Table 5.5). Both girls had normal karyotypes.

To these clinical differences it should be added that although most boys with X-linked Duchenne muscular dystrophy have significantly taller R waves in the right praecordial lead of the electrocardiogram (p. 95), at least after the age of 6, this is never found in the autosomal recessive form (Skyring and McKusick 1961; Emery 1972). Furthermore, the changes in muscle pathology have been reported to be perhaps more 'focal' than in X-linked Duchenne muscular dystrophy (Gardner-Medwin and Johnston 1984), and the two forms may also differ in muscle polyribosomal non-collagen protein synthesis (Ionasescu and Zellweger 1974).

The distinction between the two disorders, however, is often not at all clear

Table 5.5 *Clinical features in two girls with limb girdle muscular dystrophy of childhood. There was no consanguinity in either family*

Family	Age (years) Onset	Age (years) Chairbound	Calf enlargement	IQ	ECG	Comments
S	< 4	9	+ / −	N	N	Similarly affected older brother chairbound at 13
C	? 2	−	+ / −	N	N	Just ambulant at 18

in the individual case (Somer *et al.* 1985). If a brother and sister are affected and the parents are cousins, then the autosomal recessive form would seem most likely. However, in Britain and North America, the X-linked form would seem to be at least 20 times commoner than the autosomal recessive form (Emery 1964a). So in these countries it is probably better to assume that the X-linked form is more likely until proved otherwise. Certainly any affected girl should be fully karyotyped and all affected boys and girls should have an ECG examination for evidence of right ventricular preponderance. The situation in some other countries, however, may well be different. The autosomal recessive form seems common and may be more severe in certain Arabic communities in Tunisia (Ben Hamida *et al.* 1983), and the Sudan (Salih *et al.* 1983). Interestingly, those inbred communities in North America in which cases of the autosomal recessive form have been reported (Jackson and Strehler 1968; Shokeir and Kobrinsky 1976; Shokeir and Rozdilsky 1985) originated from Switzerland where this form of muscular dystrophy seems to be particularly common (Moser *et al.* 1966).

It is, of course, disturbing that these two disorders are so similar, because confusion between the two will lead to some normal sisters of isolated affected brothers being given inappropriate genetic advice. Also perhaps some of the clinical variability seen in what is assumed to be the X-linked form may in fact be partly the result of admixture with autosomal recessive cases. Finally, the existence of the autosomal recessive form could be a confounding factor in studying the aetiology and possible pathogenesis of Duchenne muscular dystrophy.

The manifesting carrier of Duchenne muscular dystrophy

Female relatives of boys with X-linked Duchenne muscular dystrophy may occasionally manifest certain features of the disease. This appears to have been first recognized by Kryschowa and Abowjan in 1934 who described a large family with the disease, one of the female carriers having noticably enlarged calves. Later Sidler (1944) described a 23-year-old woman (case 4) who had increasing difficulty climbing stairs from the age of 19, and on examination her right quadriceps was found to be atrophied. She had a brother and three maternal uncles with Duchenne muscular dystrophy. There have been many similar reports since, manifestations of the disease ranging from calf enlargement, through varying degrees of muscle weakness, to occasionally severe incapacity (Fig. 5.4).

Onset of weakness also varies considerably and may develop in childhood or may not become evident until adult life, and the weakness may be progressive or remain static. In many ways the distribution of weakness resembles that seen in adult limb girdle muscular dystrophy, but differs in that pseudohypertrophy is usually present, the weakness is often asymmetric, electrocardiographic abnormalities similar to those seen in affected boys can

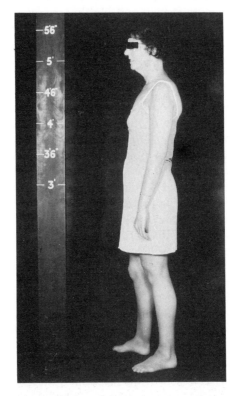

Fig. 5.4. A manifesting female carrier of Duchenne muscular dystrophy, aged 36, with lumbar lordosis, some enlargement of the calves, weakness of the anterior tibialis, quadriceps, and gluteal muscles, and to a lesser extent the shoulder girdle muscles. By age 47 weakness had progressed to such an extent that she became confined to a wheelchair.

occur, and the SCK level is invariably very high and occasionally may even approach levels found in affected boys. On the other hand, some female carriers may have very high SCK levels yet have no muscle weakness at all (Fig. 5.5).

It is important to distinguish a manifesting adult female carrier from a woman with autosomal recessive limb girdle muscular dystrophy, both of which occur with very roughly the same frequency (Moser and Emery 1974; Yates and Emery 1985), because genetic counselling in these two situations will be quite different (Zellweger *et al.* 1980). The risks to the sons of a manifesting carrier of X-linked Duchenne muscular dystrophy will be 50 per cent, but the risks to the offspring of a woman affected with autosomal recessive limb girdle muscular dystrophy will be negligible (Table 5.6).

Such manifestations in heterozygous females can be explained in terms of random inactivation of the X-chromosome: in those women with no clinical manifestations and a low SCK level, the active X-chromosome in most cells is presumably the one bearing the normal gene, whereas in those women with

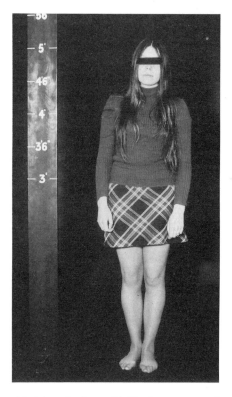

Fig. 5.5. A 19-year-old sister of a boy with Duchenne muscular dystrophy who has SCK levels in excess of 1500 iu, yet has no clinical manifestations of the disease.

Table 5.6   *Differentiation between a manifesting carrier of Duchenne muscular dystrophy (DMD) and a woman with limb girdle muscular dystrophy (LGMD)*

Symptom or sign	DMD carrier	LGMD
Pseudohypertrophy	>80%	Rare
Muscle weakness	Often asymmetric	Rarely asymmetric
ECG abnormalities		
(R–S in V_1 increased)	5–10%	–
SCK level elevated	>95%	<50%
	Often very high	Rarely high

manifestations of the disease and a high SCK level, the active X-chromosome in most cells is presumably the one bearing the muscular dystrophy gene (Emery 1963; 1965). This would explain why occasional heterozygous identical twin girls have been discordant for clinical manifestations (Fraser 1963; Gomez *et al.* 1977; Pena *et al.* 1982; Burn *et al.* 1986). There is often familial concordance for such manifestations, mothers and daughters or sisters often being affected (Moser and Emery 1974). This would suggest that X-inactivation, at least in these women, may not be entirely random but is perhaps under genetic control (p. 191).

A particularly confusing situation arises if the manifesting female happens to be a young girl and the weakness is progressive (Aymé *et al.* 1979; Held *et al.* 1980; Olson and Fenichel 1982). If she is the only affected individual in the family or is the sister of an isolated case of Duchenne muscular dystrophy, this could be confused with autosomal recessive limb girdle muscular dystrophy of childhood (p. 79). Features which might indicate a manifesting female carrier would be asymmetric muscle involvement and electrocardiographic evidence of right ventricular preponderance (Hazama *et al.* 1979). However, until the biochemical defects are known the only way of distinguishing the two conditions with certainty would be to demonstrate mosaicism in clones of cultured fibroblasts or use a gene specific DNA probe for Duchenne muscular dystrophy which would then indicate that the affected girl was a manifesting carrier.

The spinal muscular atrophies

The spinal muscular atrophies may be defined as a group of inherited diseases in which there is degeneration of the anterior horn cells (lower motor neurones) of the spinal cord and often the bulbar motor nuclei, but with no evidence of pyramidal tract of peripheral nerve involvement (Emery 1971). There is therefore no evidence of spasticity or hyper-reflexia, the plantar response is flexor and there are no sensory changes or any reduction in the peripheral nerve conduction velocity. This group of diseases excludes motor neurone disease (progressive bulbar palsy, progressive muscular atrophy, and amyotrophic lateral sclerosis), and its variants, as well as the peripheral neuropathies. In any event motor neurone disease in childhood is exceptionally rare and when it does occur is unlikely to be confused with muscular dystrophy because spasticity is usually the predominant clinical feature (Emery and Holloway 1982).

The spinal muscular atrophies are a very heterogeneous group of disorders and vary considerably in their clinical presentation and mode of inheritance. The clinical features and the relationships of these disorders have been much

Table 5.7 *A clinical and genetical classification of the spinal muscular atrophies (SMA)*

---

1. *Proximal SMA*
   (*a*) Infantile (type I)
       Autosomal recessive
         (*i*) Usual form (Werdnig–Hoffmann)
         (*ii*) With arthrogryposis multiplex congenita
   (*b*) Intermediate (type II)
       Autosomal recessive
   (*c*) Juvenile (type III)
       Autosomal recessive
         (*i*) Usual form (Wohlfart–Kugelberg–Welander)
         (*ii*) 'Ryukyuan' SMA
         (*iii*) With microcephaly and mental subnormality
       Autosomal dominant
       X-linked recessive (very rare)
   (*d*) Adult (type IV)
       Autosomal recessive
       Autosomal dominant
       X-linked recessive
2. *Distal SMA*
   Autosomal recessive
   Autosomal dominant
3. *Juvenile Progressive Bulbar Palsy*
   Autosomal recessive
         (*i*) Usual form (Fazio–Londe)
         (*ii*) With nerve deafness (Van Laere)
4. *Scapulo-peroneal SMA*
   Autosomal recessive
   Autosomal dominant
5. *Facioscapulohumeral SMA*
   Autosomal dominant

---

discussed in recent years (Pearn 1983; Russman *et al.* 1983; Hausmanowa-Petrusewicz *et al.* 1984; Serratrice *et al.* 1984). A classification favoured by the author is given in Table 5.7, details of which are given in Emery (1987). However until the primary biochemical defect(s) underlying these disorders is known, such a classification must remain tentative. Nevertheless, a classification based on both genetic and clinical differences. is the best that is possible with our present state of knowledge.

The only forms which might possibly be confused with Duchenne muscular dystrophy are those in which muscle weakness is predominantly *proximal* in distribution. This group is much commoner than the others. Whether it is possible to separate the so-called infantile and juvenile forms of proximal spinal muscular atrophy on clinical grounds has been hotly debated in the past. Much of the confusion arose because of overlap in the age at onset which is notoriously difficult to assess accurately. If other features are also taken into account, such as the course of the disease and age at death, then it would seem quite legitimate to separate these disorders. The frequency of spontaneous activity on electromyography (Buchthal and Olsen 1970), and the degree of collateral reinnervation (Hausmanowa-Petrusewicz *et al.* 1968), have also been found to differ in the infantile and juvenile forms. Features which can be used clinically to distinguish not only these two forms of proximal spinal muscular atrophy but also intermediate and adult forms are summarized in Table 5.8.

The severe infantile (type I, Werdnig–Hoffmann disease) and the intermediate (type II) forms are quite distinct from Duchenne muscular dystrophy because of the very marked hypotonia and weakness from an early age, the presence of fasciculations and an SCK level which is rarely raised and then only slightly. However differentiation from the juvenile form (type III, Wohlfart–Kugelberg–Welander disease) on clinical grounds may not be so easy. In fact this was first regarded as pseudomyopathic because of its similarity with muscular dystrophy (Wohlfart *et al.* 1955; Kugelberg and Welander 1956). Furthermore, although usually inherited as an autosomal recessive, or less commonly as an autosomal dominant trait, males are more often affected than females (Emery *et al.* 1976a, b; Hausmanowa-Petrusewicz *et al.* 1984). This form of spinal muscular atrophy is more benign than Werdnig–Hoffmann disease with onset in early childhood and with survival into adulthood (Namba 1970) (Fig. 5.6).

The clinical presentation may closely resemble Duchenne muscular dystrophy: weakness first affects the pelvic girdle musculature and patients often present with a tendency to fall and a waddling gait. Later, the pectoral girdle, neck, trunk, and distal limb muscles also become affected. Interestingly muscle weakness, at least in the early stages, is often asymmetric which is unlike muscular dystrophy, pseudohypertrophy of the calf muscles is uncommon, and muscle fasciculations are often present and are a useful

Table 5.8 *Some distinguishing features of the various forms of proximal spinal muscular atrophy*

Type	Age (usual)		Ability to sit without support*	Muscle fasciculations	SCK
	Onset	Survival			
I (Infantile)	<4 mths	<4 yrs	Never	+/−	Normal
II (Intermediate)	<2 yrs	>4 yrs	Usually	+/−	Usually normal
III (Juvenile)	>2 yrs	Adulthood	Always	+ +	Often raised
IV (Adult)	>30 yrs	50 yrs +	Always	+ +	Often raised

* At some time during the course of the illness.

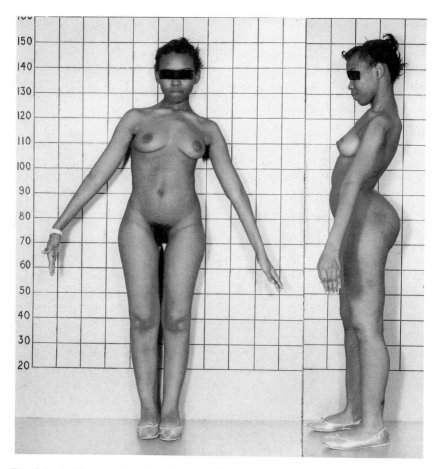

Fig. 5.6. A 17-year-old girl with type III spinal muscular atrophy (Wohlfart–Kugelberg–Welander disease). Note the marked lordosis and wasting of the left deltoid muscle. An older and two younger brothers were also affected.

diagnostic sign. A fine tremor of the outstretched hands is common and *minipolymyoclonus*, intermittent and irregular movement which is sufficient to produce visible movement of the joints and head, may also be present (Spiro 1970). The progression of the disease is very variable, even within families, although the majority require a wheelchair in their twenties or thirties. The SCK level is very rarely grossly elevated, but it can be moderately elevated. In most cases electromyography, muscle histology, and histochemistry confirm the neurogenic nature of the disorder.

Summary and conclusions

Several disorders can mimic Duchenne muscular dystrophy. They include certain other forms of muscular dystrophy which may present in early childhood, various congenital myopathies, and spinal muscular atrophy. Among the muscular dystrophies, the congenital forms are unlikely to lead to confusion because in general they are evident at birth or in the neonatal period with severe hypotonia and generalized muscle weakness. Similarly, the congenital myopathies are unlikely to pose a problem in differential diagnosis because most cases present in early life with generalized muscle weakness, often associated with respiratory problems and feeding difficulties, or may have distinctive clinical features, serum enzymes are normal and the diagnosis is established on muscle histology. Among the other X-linked muscular dystrophies, the benign form associated with early contractures and cardiomyopathy is so distinctive that this too is unlikely to cause confusion. But because of the very high SCK levels early in the course of the disease, overlap in age at onset and similar pattern of muscle involvement, Becker muscular dystrophy can present a diagnostic dilemma in the isolated case. However, possible points of distinction are that in the Becker form almost all affected males are still walking at 12, and there is no electrocardiographic evidence of right ventricular preponderance.

A particularly difficult problem is posed by autosomal recessive limb girdle muscular dystrophy of childhood when only a boy is affected in the family. The disease is relatively more benign than Duchenne muscular dystrophy and there are reported to be some minor clinical differences, and whereas most boys with Duchenne muscular dystrophy have electrocardiographic evidence of right ventricular preponderance, this is not found in the autosomal recessive limb girdle form. But the distinction is often not at all clear, although *a priori* in Britain and North America a case is much more likely to be Duchenne muscular dystrophy since this is much the commoner of the two disorders.

Finally, the only form of spinal muscular atrophy which might possibly be confused with Duchenne muscular dystrophy is the proximal juvenile form (type III, Wohlfart–Kugelberg–Welander disease). However, points which would suggest this disease rather than Duchenne muscular dystrophy would be some asymmetry of muscle involvement, absence of pseudohypertrophy, and evidence of muscle fasciculations. In most cases electromyography, muscle histology, and histochemistry will confirm the neurogenic nature of the disorder.

6 Involvement of tissues other than skeletal muscle

The muscular dystrophies have often been described as *primary* diseases of muscle. The term primary in this context could have two interpretations; either that muscle is the most obviously affected tissue which is certainly true, or that the fundamental molecular defect is expressed only in skeletal muscle, which is patently not true. In recent years it has been shown that significant abnormalities can be found in a variety of tissues quite apart from skeletal muscle. This is perhaps not unexpected since the abnormal gene is present in all cells of the body. However, why a particular gene is expressed in some tissues and not in others raises a fundamental question in molecular biology. There are indications that certain DNA sequences, so-called enhancer sequences, may well be involved in differential gene activity, but it seems likely to be some time yet before the full details are known.

The variety of manifestations of a genetic disease can also result from the pleiotropic effects of a single gene or, at the molecular level, either from the involvement of adjacent genes which control other phenotypic features or from different point mutations within the game gene.

Pleiotropy refers to the multiple effects that a gene mutation may have as a trail of consequences leading on from the basic defect. An excellent example of this is provided by sickle cell anaemia whereby the responsible gene mutation results in sickle cell haemoglobin which is less soluble than normal haemoglobin and therefore tends to crystallize out resulting in deformation of the red cell which becomes sickle shaped. These abnormal cells are then destroyed (haemolysed) resulting in anaemia. But at the same time they also tend to clump together, thereby obstructing small arteries, resulting in ischaemia of tissues with a variety of consequences including attacks of abdominal pain, splenic infarction, limb pains, osteomyelitis, cerebro-vascular accidents, haematuria, renal failure, 'pneumonic' episodes, and heart failure. The diversity of clinical manifestations in Duchenne muscular dystrophy can also be partly explained in terms of the pleiotropic effects of the responsible mutant gene.

An association of *different genetic disorders* in the same individual can occur purely by chance, such as the reported occurrence in Duchenne muscular dystrophy of haemophilia (Konagaya *et al*. 1982) and trisomy-21 (Moser, 1971). However, very occasionally such an association may result from the deletion of genetic material involving adjacent genes which are responsible for different diseases, Thus, Francke and her colleagues (Francke *et al.* 1985) have described a boy with Duchenne muscular dystrophy who also had chronic granulomatous disease and seemingly retinitis pigmentosa. Cytogenetic studies revealed that he had a small but visible interstitial deletion of the short arm of his X-chromosome which presumably involved the loss of genetic material from all three of the *adjacent* genes responsible for these different diseases (p. 169). In another case a smaller, but also visible deletion in the same region of the X-chromosome was found in a boy with Duchenne muscular dystrophy, glycerol kinase deficiency, and adrenal insufficiency (Bartley *et al.* 1986). It is possible that the reported associations of Duchenne muscular dystrophy with retinitis pigmentosa (Marandian *et al.* 1977) or with chronic granulomatous disease (Kousseff 1981) *could* also be due to a similar mechanism. However, this sort of molecular abnormality is rare and very much the exception. Much more likely is that the variations in clinical manifestations of the disease in different families are due to either submicroscopic deletions at various sites or of varying length within the Duchenne region itself, or to different point mutations within the coding region of the gene.

Whatever the mechanism, it is important in patient management to appreciate that Duchenne muscular dystrophy is a multi-system disease and that a variety of tissues other than skeletal muscle can be affected. It is also important in genetic counselling to acquaint would-be parents with the possible consequences of the disease in an affected child so that they can better appreciate the full extent of the problem.

Smooth muscle

Circumstantial evidence that smooth muscle may be affected in Duchenne muscular dystrophy comes from the occasional occurrence of bladder paralysis, paralytic ileus, and gastric dilatation in affected boys (Robin and Falewski 1963). More direct evidence is provided by detailed autopsy studies such as those carried out by Bevans (1945), Huvos and Pruzanski (1967), Jedrzejowska-Kulakowska *et al.* (1968), and Leon *et al.* (1986). These studies have shown that the smooth muscle of the gastrointestinal tract often shows variation in fibre size, atrophy and loss of muscle fibres, and areas of fibrosis. These changes are comparable in many ways to those seen in affected skeletal muscle and have occasionally been found in cases who did not have any relevant gastrointestinal symptoms in life. However, no lesions of the smooth muscle of the vascular system have so far been reported.

Cardiac muscle

There is overwhelming evidence from clinical, pathological and physiological studies (Hunter 1980; Hunsaker *et al.* 1982) that cardiac muscle is involved in Duchenne muscular dystrophy.

From an early age there is very often a persistent sinus tachycardia, arrhythmias and non-specific murmurs are common, and sudden death may occur from cardiac causes. Mitral valve prolapse has been recorded in up to a quarter of affected boys, auscultatory evidence of which can be confirmed by echocardiography (Biddison *et al.* 1979).

At autopsy microscopic studies of cardiac muscle reveal features which resemble those seen in skeletal muscle with variation in fibre size, fragmentation of muscle fibres, replacement by connective tissue and some fatty infiltration (Bevans 1945; Gilroy *et al.* 1963; Perloff *et al.* 1966). Such changes have even been found in patients who did not necessarily have any symptoms of heart disease during life. Fibrosis appears to be a particularly important feature (Fig. 6.1). It begins in the outer myocardium involving the more postero-basal part of the outer-free wall of the left ventricle. At first fibrosis appears in discreet small areas, but eventually becomes more diffuse and involves most of the outer half of the ventricular wall. The right ventricle and atria are rarely involved and this pattern of myocardial fibrosis does not seem to occur in any other disease (Frankel and Rosser 1976). The dystrophic changes may also involve the intracardiac conduction system (Sanyal and Johnson 1982).

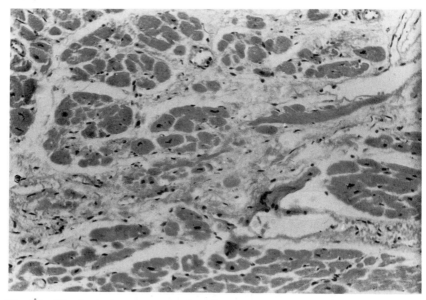

Fig. 6.1. Histological appearance of cardiac muscle from the left ventricle from a boy with Duchenne muscular dystrophy, age 21. Note the variation in fibre size and marked increase in connective tissue (haematoxylin and eosin).

Early in the course of the disease cardiac catheterization studies have shown few consistent abnormalities, but in severely affected boys approaching cardiac failure significantly elevated right atrial and right ventricular end-diastolic pressures have been recorded (Perloff *et al.* 1966, 1967; Demany and Zimmerman 1969). Non-invasive techniques such as ballistocardiography (Lowenstein *et al.* 1962), vectorcardiography (Ronan *et al.* 1972), echocardiography (Danilowicz *et al.* 1980), and particularly electrocardiography have all been used to study cardiac involvement in Duchenne muscular dystrophy, and to assess its extent and severity in the individual patient. Electrocardiography has proved particularly valuable and therefore merits some special consideration.

One of the earliest descriptions of electrocardiographic (ECG) abnormalities in muscular dystrophy was made by Schliephake in 1929. Since then a variety of ECG changes have been observed in Duchenne muscular dystrophy in particular, and these have been reviewed in detail (Lowenstein *et al.* 1962; Slucka 1968; Durnin *et al.* 1971; Jellett *et al.* 1974), and are listed in Table 6.1. Evidence of defective cardiac conduction has also been reported (Sanyal and Johnson 1982).

Numerous attempts have been made to determine if any particular ECG pattern is distinctive in Duchenne muscular dystrophy. Recently, Ishikawa and his colleagues in Japan have suggested that high frequency 'notches' on the QRS complexes can be used for estimating the extent and severity of cardiac involvement in Duchenne muscular dystrophy (Ishikawa *et al.* 1982), and Nigro *et al.* (1984) have found shortening of the PQ interval to be particularly valuable. These conclusions now await further evaluation. There is however general agreement that tall R waves in V_1 is a particularly frequent and consistent abnormality in the disease. A useful measure of this is the algebraic sum of the R and S waves in this lead (i.e. $|R\text{-}S|$ in V_1) which is abnormal in over 80 per cent of affected boys (Fig. 6.2). It is particularly interesting that the same abnormality has also been found in up to 10 per cent of female

Table 6.1 *ECG abnormalities arranged in decreasing order of frequency in Duchenne muscular dystrophy*

Tall R waves in V_1
    R/S ratio ↑
    $|R\text{-}S|$ ↑
Shortened P–R interval
Deep Q waves in $V_{5\text{-}6}$
Complex RSr^1, right bundle branch block
Altered T waves
Left axis deviation

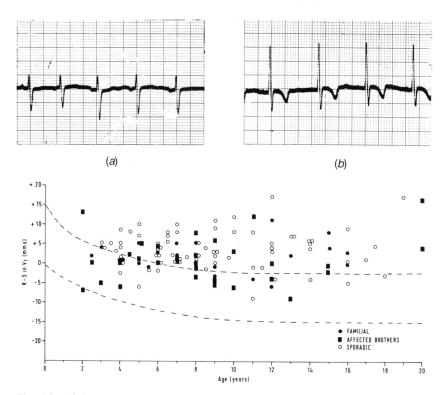

Fig. 6.2. Right praecordial lead (V₁) in: (*a*) a healthy boy, and (*b*) a boy with Duchenne muscular dystrophy, both age 10. Algebraic sum of R–S in V₁ for boys with Duchenne muscular dystrophy. Normal 90% confidence limits from Nadas (1963). (From Emery (1972) with permission.)

carriers of the disease (p. 192). It is uncommon in other forms of muscular dystrophy and spinal muscular atrophy which may occur in childhood (p. 88), and seems to be specific to Duchenne muscular dystrophy (Emery 1972). A variety of ECG abnormalities also occur in polymyositis but are different from those most commonly seen in muscular dystrophy (Stern *et al.* 1984).

The aetiology of the tall R waves in the right praecordial lead of the ECG is not clear. Various suggestions have been made including thoracic deformity, pulmonary hypertension, conduction defect due to myocardial dystrophy, and ventricular spetal hypertrophy. However none of these suggestions is entirely satisfactory. It seems (Perloff *et al.* 1967) that this anterior shift of the QRS complex is most likely due to the diffuse interstitial fibrosis in the postero-basal part of the left ventricle (Fig. 6.3). Involvement of the adjacent

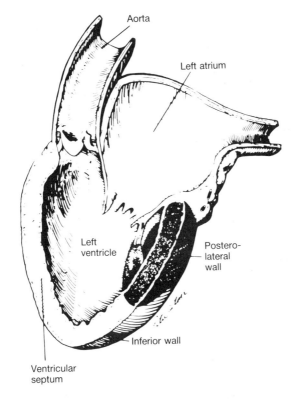

Fig. 6.3. Diagram of the left side of the heart illustrating the region of selective involvement in patients with Duchenne muscular dystrophy. (Reproduced by kind permission of Dr J. K. Perloff and the *American Journal of Medicine*.)

papillary muscle would account for mitral valve prolapse which can occur in the disease (Sanyal *et al.* 1980). Evidence supporting this idea comes from necropsy findings (Frankel and Rosser 1976) which have already been discussed, and also from two-dimensional echocardiography. The latter has revealed contraction abnormalities of the left ventricle in most patients which is first noted in the posterior free wall behind the mitral valve (Goldberg *et al.* 1982). But why this portion of the myocardium should be so selectively involved in this particular disorder is quite unknown.

Vascular system

Trophic changes in the skin of the extremities of patients with Duchenne muscular dystrophy are common, especially in the lower limbs and in the later stages of the disease. These changes include coldness and cyanotic mottling, and on occasions even scleroderma-like changes. Such changes most likely stem from inactivity, although Duchenne himself even raised the possibility that muscular dystrophy might have a vascular aetiology. This idea was diligently pursued some twenty years ago by Démos and colleagues in Paris, and later by King Engel in the United States.

Studies which have been designed to determine if the vascular system in involved in Duchenne muscular dystrophy focused, perhaps understandably, on muscle vasculature. Démos and colleagues measured the circulation time in patients in two ways: arm-to-arm using fluorescein as a marker and arm-to-tongue using sodium dehydrocholate. By subtraction the 'peripheral circulation time' in the upper limb was determined. This they found in boys with Duchenne muscular dystrophy to be above or below the 95 per cent range for normal children of comparable age, and to be significantly reduced in some female carriers (Démos 1961; Démos and Maroteaux 1961; Démos *et al.* 1962). However, there is no defect in the capillary nail bed (Dudley and Gibson 1964) and using venous occlusion plethysmography we failed to detect any significant changes in limb blood flow in affected boys at different stages of the disease or in carrier females (Emery and Schelling 1965).

However, since these early observations, more sophisticated methods have been developed for measuring blood flow, notably tracer clearance (^{133}Xe, ^{85}Kr, ^{125}I-antipyrine) and hydrogen electrode techniques (Moxley 1984). Using the ^{133}Xe clearance method, Paulson *et al.* (1974) and Bradley *et al.* (1975) found no significant difference in limb blood flow in affected boys compared with normal boys. However, in younger (less than 10 years old) affected boys though the number of capillaries per unit of muscle fibre area remains unchanged, capillary size is significantly increased (Jerusalem *et al.* 1974), and this would account for the slight increase in capillary diffusion capacity observed by Paulson *et al.* (1974). However, no structural abnormalities of the small arterial vessels or capillaries of the muscle have been detected with either light or electron-microscopy (Musch *et al.* 1975). More recently Mechler and colleagues, (1980) used the ^{133}Xe method to study blood flow in the tibialis anterior muscle in Becker muscular dystrophy. They found that whereas adrenergic beta-receptor responses of vascular smooth muscle to stimulation by adrenalin and blocking by propranolol was normal, there appeared to be some abnormality of alpha-receptor response to blocking by phentolamine which was not found in spinal muscular atrophy or polymyositis. The significance of this finding, however, is not clear.

The general concensus of both pathological and physiological studies seems to be that in the early stages of the disease there are no significant abnormalities in muscle vasculature apart from some slight increase in capillary size. Later any changes which do occur, such as diminution in capillary bed, are due to muscle replacement by fat and connective tissue which is relatively avascular.

Central nervous system

For some time there was, perhaps understandably, some reluctance to accept that boys with Duchenne muscular dystrophy could also be mentally handicapped. After all this was yet another misfortune for the affected child and his parents to bear. However, much research in the 1960s and 1970s confirmed the suspicion of many of the association, first noted in fact by Duchenne, that a proportion of affected boys can have some degree of mental handicap and that on occasions this can be severe. We have not systematically measured IQ in our patients although in one study we selected a group of boys who were *severely* mentally handicapped, some of them being ineducable (Emery *et al.* 1979), and at least two of our patients are highly intelligent having been accepted for university degree courses.

IQ of affected boys

There have been a great many studies of IQ in affected boys, the results of which are summarized in Table 6.2. There is considerable variation from

Table 6.2 *Studies of IQ in boys with Duchenne muscular dystrophy. Only the most recent or most detailed data included for any one centre*

			IQ		
Reference	No.	Mean	Range	≤70	≤50
Allen & Rodgin (1960)	30	82	14–117	9	5
Worden & Vignos (1962)	38	83	46–134	10	1
Schorer (1964)	28	79	–	–	–
Dubowitz (1965)	27	68	42–118	17	3
Zellweger & Niedermeyer (1965)	42	83	42–131	–	3
Cohen *et al.* (1968)	108	86	<50->120	21	3
Desai *et al.* (1969)	28	79	42–115	16	2
Prosser *et al.* (1969)	52	87	51–113	–	–
Kozicka *et al.* (1971)	52	76	35–114	21 (≤67)	3 (≤51)
Michal (1972)	74	85	39–122	–	–
Black (1973)	25	82	45–128	–	–
Marsh & Munsat (1974)	34	89	60–118	6	0
Florek & Karolak (1977)	129	79	30–127	27 (<68)	–
Leibowitz & Dubowitz (1981)	54	86	47–132	10	1
Total	*721*	*82*	–	*137* (19%)	*21* (3%)

those who are severely handicapped to a few with IQs above 130. The overall mean IQ is however about one standard deviation below the normal mean. Roughly 20 per cent have IQs below 70, and 3 per cent have IQs below 50.

This reduction in IQ is not due to any lack of educational opportunity as a result of their physical disability because it is not found in other diseases with comparable disability, such as juvenile spinal muscular atrophy. Furthermore, poor educational performance in Duchenne muscular dystrophy is often observed early in life when muscle weakness is relatively slight. Whatever causes the intellectual impairment must also operate at an early stage in development for it is not progressive and does not correlate with duration or severity of the disease though one recent study does suggest some possible relationship with age (Sollee *et al.* 1985). The fact that there is no difference in IQ of affected boys born to carrier mothers and those who are presumed to be new mutations, excludes a maternal factor from being responsible for depressing the IQ.

The most likely explanation is that the depression in IQ is yet another pleiotropic effect of the mutant gene. This is supported by the fact that unaffected sibs have normal intellect, and there is often a good correlation between affected brothers (Kozicka *et al.* 1971). Cohen *et al.* (1968) found a high concordance ($P < 0.001$) for intellectual function in 37 of 39 families and in the two apparent exceptions there were reasonable explanations for their being discordant, and Bortolini and Zatz (1986) found mental capacity to be concordant in 16 out of 22 (73 per cent) families they studied. Furthermore, we have found that whenever an index case is *severely* mentally handicapped (IQ < 50) and has an affected brother, the latter is very often also severely mentally handicapped (Emery *et al.* 1979; Emery 1984). The possibility that there might be bimodality in the distribution of IQ in affected boys was suggested by some earlier studies. But analysis of more recent and extensive data (from Cohen *et al.* 1968; Marsh and Munsat 1974; Vignos 1977a; Leibowitz and Dubotwitz 1981) makes this seem unlikely (Fig. 6.4).

Perhaps because the mean depression of IQ in affected boys is relatively moderate, the majority of female carriers have normal IQs (Prosser *et al.* 1969). However, Murphy *et al.* (1965) and Bortolini and Zatz (1986) indicate that mental impairment may very occasionally be present in those with clinical manifestations and/or a very high SCK level.

Partition of IQ

Following the work of Sherwin and McCully in 1961, attempts have been made to determine what aspect of intellect may be especially affected in Duchenne muscular dystrophy by comparing performance and verbal IQs (Table 6.3). With one exception (Black 1973), verbal IQ is more affected, the overall difference from performance IQ being about 7 or 8 points. There is no suggestion of bimodality in the distribution of the *differences* between performance and verbal IQs (Table 6.4).

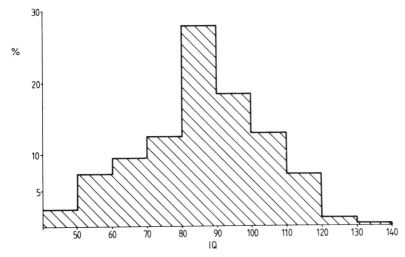

Fig. 6.4. Percentage distribution of IQ in Duchenne muscular dystrophy. (Data abstracted from Cohen *et al.* (1968); Marsh and Munsat (1974); Vignos (1977a); Leibowitz and Dubowitz (1981).)

Table 6.3 *Performance and verbal IQ in boys with Duchenne muscular dystrophy calculated from data given in various studies*

Reference	No.	Performance (P) Mean	s.d.	Verbal (V) Mean	s.d.	(P–V)
Zellweger & Niedermeyer (1965)	23	97.3	18.2	89.4	17.8	+7.9
Prosser *et al.* (1969)	39	88.0	14.2	87.1	16.5	+0.9
Black (1973)	25	80.2	22.4	84.8	19.1	−4.6
Marsh & Munsat (1974)	34	93.4	16.7	86.5	13.3	+6.9
Karagan & Zellweger (1978)	53	88.1	15.6	80.7	11.8	+7.4
Leibowitz & Dubowitz (1981)	54	91.5	16.0	83.7	19.3	+7.8

The impairment of verbal ability seems to be due to a defect in memory for patterns, numbers, and verbal labels, implying a particular deficit, in memory function (Karagan *et al.* 1980). Some depression of verbal IQ has also been found in Becker muscular dystrophy but not in limb girdle or facioscapulohumeral muscular dystrophy (Karagan and Sorensen 1981). Interestingly, it seems that those boys with Duchenne muscular dystrophy who survive longest may have the least depression of verbal IQ (Miller *et al.* 1985).

Table 6.4 *Distribution of the differences between performance and verbal IQs (P–V)*

Reference	39 to 30	29 to 20	19 to 10	9 to 0	−1 to −10	−11 to −20	−21 to −30
Marsh & Munsat (1974)	0	5	9	14	3	2	1
Karagan & Zellweger (1978)	2	5	17	13	12	4	0
Leibowitz & Dubowitz (1981)	2	11	12	16	4	7	2
Total	*4*	*21*	*38*	*43*	*19*	*13*	*3*
Percentage	*2.8*	*14.9*	*27.0*	*30.5*	*13.5*	*9.2*	*2.1*

Behaviour and emotional disturbances

Behaviour and emotional disturbances have been commented upon by a number of investigators (Schorer 1964; Cohen *et al.* 1968; Leibowitz and Dubowitz 1981; Pullen 1984). This seems likely to stem from a sense of failure, frustration, and distress generated by the progressive physical disability. However, in view of the nature of the disorder it is perhaps surprising that the majority of boys are not emotionally disturbed, and yet they are not. Nevertheless, allowing for age and IQ, boys with Duchenne muscular dystrophy do have a higher incidence of emotional disturbances than other physically handicapped children without cerebral involvement (Leibowitz and Dubowitz 1981), and it is just possible that this too could represent part of the disease. Epilepsy is not particularly frequent in Duchenne muscular dystrophy and visual and hearing acuity are normal (Allen 1973).

Neurological investigations

The failure to relate the impaired mental ability to any clear social or functional factors has lead to the search for an organic explanation. Electro-encephalography (EEG) has been reported as normal in a carefully controlled and blind study by Barwick *et al.* (1965). In some other studies, however, up to a half of the records have been considered abnormal in some non-specific way (Zellweger and Niedermeyer 1965; Cohen *et al.* 1968; Kozicka *et al.* 1971; Black 1973; Florek and Karolak 1977). But many patients with apparently abnormal EEGs have had normal IQs. Whatever, no specific EEG abnormality has been detected in the disease.

Ventricular enlargement on pneumoencephalography has been reported in two cases (Hovstad *et al.* 1976). More recently the non-invasive technique of computerized tomography (CT) has been used to study central nervous system (CNS) involvement. Yoshioka and colleagues (1980) found evidence of slight cerebral atrophy in two-thirds of the 30 cases they examined, and the older the patient the more severe was the atrophy. There were many with a low IQ in those with cerebral atrophy, but in those with apparently normal CT findings only three had a low IQ. Abnormal CT findings therefore seem to be associated with low IQ.

Finally, Rosman and Kakulas (1966) examined the brains of seven cases of Duchenne muscular dystrophy (two at least of these could have been Becker muscular dystrophy). In all cases with mental defect they found microscopic heterotopias in the cerebral cortex. However, in a more extensive study of 21 cases of classical Duchenne muscular dystrophy, Dubowitz and Crome (1969) could detect no consistent pathological abnormality and this view is now most generally accepted.

Skeletal system

A number of skeletal changes have been observed in Duchenne muscular dystrophy. They include progressive narrowing of the shafts of the long bones due to a reduction in the size of the medullary cavity and later thinning of the cortices. Since at the same time the head remains more or less the same size, the long bones assume a characteristic 'dumb bell' appearance (Fig. 6.5). There is often impaired development of the pelvic bones and scapulae, and various skeletal deformities occur including lumbar lordosis, scoliosis, and coxa valga. The bones themselves undergo progressive rarefaction and decalcification beginning at the ends of the long bones.

For a long time these changes were thought to be a direct consequence of a genetic defect, and such terms as 'bone dystrophy' and 'osteomyopathy'

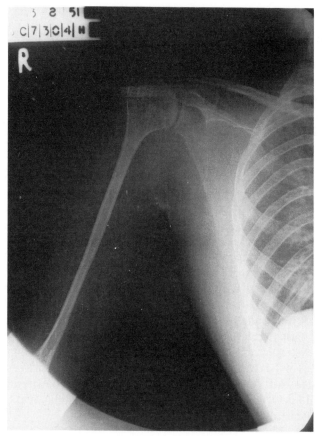

Fig. 6.5. Atrophy of the humerus in an advanced case of Duchenne muscular dystrophy. (Reproduced by kind permission of Sir John Walton.)

were used. However, Walton and Warrick (1954) showed quite clearly that these same changes can occur in any disorder associated with prolonged immobility. They are not due to an associated genetic factor but to disuse: to the absence of the normal stresses and strains imposed by muscular attachments, and to the adoption of abnormal postures of the body and positions of the limbs as a consequence of muscle weakness and contractures.

Gastrointestinal system

Apart from manifestations of smooth muscle involvement affecting motility of the gastrointestinal tract which has been mentioned already (p. 93), Bevans (1945) and Huvos and Pruzanski (1967) in reviewing the early literature referred to reports of recurrent diarrhoea and malabsorption in muscular dystrophy. Patterson *et al.* (1964) also furnished some evidence of intestinal malabsorption but this work does not seem to have been repeated or pursued further (Nowak *et al.* 1982). Constipation and halitosis are frequent symptoms, but these are likely to result from lack of physical activity and oral hygiene.

Other manifestations

Thymus hyperplasia has been noted in some cases (Bevans, 1945; Huvos and Pruzanski 1967), the relevance of which is not at all clear. Puberty can be delayed, hyperoestrogenaemia occurs (Usuki *et al.* 1985) and obesity is frequent. There is no evidence of pancreatic dysfunction and an early report of abnormal hepatic tests in some patients with muscular dystrophy (Morrell 1959) is difficult to interpret because no clear distinction was made between Duchenne muscular dystrophy and other forms of dystrophy occurring later in life.

However, apart from the study of skeletal muscle, cardiac muscle and the central nervous system, it has to be admitted that there have been few recent (Weiller 1985) systematic investigations of other systems, organs or tissues. There always remains, therefore, the possibility that in the rush to study the most obviously affected tissues, some significant defect may have been overlooked. As Houston Merritt commented to Lewis Rowland (1980) '. . . You could grind up spinal cord from now until Doomsday before you found that the abnormality of combined system disease (subacute combined degeneration) was in the stomach'.

With what is known so far, it is possible to construct a simple diagram of the pleiotropic effects of the Duchenne gene (Fig. 6.6). Some of the abnormalities found in the disease relate directly to skeletal, cardiac, and smooth muscle involvement. Others, however, are much more difficult to account for with our present knowledge.

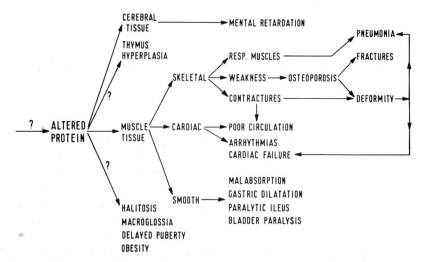

Fig. 6.6. Pleiotropic effects of the Duchenne gene. (From Emery (1983) with permission.)

Summary and conclusions

Most of the clinical features of Duchenne muscular dystrophy stem from involvement of skeletal muscle. However, there is incresing evidence that other tissues may also be directly affected by the disease.

Smooth muscle of the gastrointestinal tract and perhaps the bladder may be affected, and there is overwhelming evidence of cardiac muscle involvement, myocardial fibrosis being an important feature. This particularly affects the postero-basal portion of the left ventricle and accounts for the ECG changes of tall R waves in the right praecordial lead, changes which appear to be specific for Duchenne muscular dystrophy. They are evident from around the age of 6, and can be useful in the differentiation of Duchenne muscular dystrophy from other forms of motor disability in childhood. The vascular system does not appear to be affected and no consistent abnormalities in limb blood flow have been found.

There is clear evidence of a defect in cerebral function which is a direct consequence of the genetic defect most obviously expressed in a lowered IQ which on average is roughly one standard deviation below the normal mean, verbal IQ being more affected than performance IQ. Occasional behavioural and emotional disturbances may be associated with the disease. There are no obvious abnormalities of the brain to account for these manifestations which are likely to be biochemically induced.

The skeletal system is only secondarily affected by disuse atrophy, and so far there is no convincing evidence that any other tissues or organs are directly affected by the genetic defect.

7 Biochemistry of Duchenne muscular dystrophy

The literature on the biochemistry and possible pathogenesis of muscular dystrophy is overwhelming. Many biochemical abnormalities have been reported but none so far has been shown to be the basic defect. There are a number of reasons for this. Many abnormalities have proved not to be consistent, or to be present only in the later stages of the disease, or in other neuromuscular disorders as well. Also, unfortunately, many reported abnormalities have not been reproducable in other laboratories. These inconsistencies may be a reflection of the complex nature of muscle tissue and perhaps the molecular defect itself. It is also just possible that there is genetic heterogeneity (p. 163).

Selection of material, patients, and controls

One important problem is the selection of appropriate material for study. Muscle is clearly the obvious choice but there is then the problem of assessing the significance of any changes which could be secondary to the disease process. There is also the very serious practical problem of obtaining material for study. In the past this was a major restraint. Investigators were forced to store material against the day when it might be used for a particular study, but there was then the possibility of changes taking place during the period of storage. The use of needle biopsy technique (p. 55) avoids these difficulties to some extent because it can be repeated, though even this is not a procedure to be undertaken lightly in a small boy. The stage of the disease is also important for clearly abnormalities found early in the course of the disease are more likely to be closer to the basic biochemical defect. It is for this latter reason that studies have sometimes been extended to healthy female carriers in the belief that any abnormalities found in such individuals are more likely to be meaningful. But in carriers there is also the problem of X-inactivation, and some may be expected to exhibit no abnormalities at all if the majority of their active X-chromosomes are those bearing the normal gene.

It is a *sine qua non* that diagnosis in the affected individual has first to be clearly established, and of course material removed at biopsy can be used for both diagnostic histology as well as biochemical research. Unfortunately, all too often in the past Duchenne muscular dystrophy has not been differentiated from other forms of dystrophy or even from spinal muscular atrophy.

The choice of appropriate controls is also a problem for the diagnosis is usually established in an affected boy around the age of 3 to 5 years of age. Appropriate muscle tissue, usually the gastrocnemius, from a normal boy of this age is not too easily acquired. It is easier to obtain specimens of rectus abdominis muscle at laparotomy for example, but some would question whether it is valid to compare findings in this muscle with gastrocnemius muscle. Nor does it seem justified to use for comparisons only muscle tissue from other neuromuscular disorders such as spinal muscular atrophy or polymyositis, although such studies may later be necessary in order to establish whether or not an abnormality is specific to Duchenne muscular dystrophy.

For all these various reasons it has been with some relief that investigators have found in recent years encouragement to study other tissues, such as erythrocytes, peripheral blood leucocytes, cultured myoblasts, and fibroblasts.

Molecular basis

When the gene responsible for a particular disorder can be isolated and cloned, using an appropriate *in vitro* system such as a cell-free extract of rabbit reticulocytes (Pelham and Jackson 1976) it is possible to see what the gene synthesizes. The product can then be compared with normal and in this way the biochemical basis of the disease can be identified. This has sometimes been referred to as 'reverse genetics' for, in the past, it was necessary to start by identifying the product of the defective gene, but now it is possible to identify the mutant gene first and then determine its product. This will be discussed in more detail later (p. 176).

It could be argued that this is now the way to understand pathogenesis and that it is irrelevant to approach the problem through conventional biochemistry. I do not share this view. It would seem that the two approaches might well complement each other. What has been learned so far concerning biochemical changes in dystrophic muscle could well help to fill in details of the pathogenesis and the way in which the mutant gene leads to the development of muscle weakness. Why certain muscles are affected more than others, and why there is sometimes intellectual deficit will also have to be explained. Finally, the basic defect may reside in some complex genetic system, as in the β-thalassaemias, when it may not be so much the synthesis of an abnormal product which is involved but rather the abnormal synthesis of a normal product.

Conventional biochemical studies have concentrated on seeking the defect either in the accumulation of a particular metabolite, or in the deficiency of an enzyme or non-enzymic polypeptide. There have been many reviews of the subject, some of the most valuable and penetrating being provided by Ellis (1978), Rowland (1980), Lucy (1980), Pennington (1980, 1987), and Armstrong and Appel (1981). It would be impossible to review all the abnormal findings which have been reported in Duchenne muscular dystrophy, nor would this be valuable. Instead, the discussion will concentrate on those which have been found in *early* cases of the disease and preferably have been confirmed in several different laboratories.

Muscle tissue

It should be pointed out from the beginning that no specific or consistent abnormality has yet been found in any of the obvious candidate muscle proteins such as myoglobin, actin, myosin, tropomyosin, and troponin (Pennington 1987), although, admittedly, not all have yet been submitted to detailed investgation.

The various biochemical changes which have been observed in affected muscle can be conveniently considered as being the result of wasting, invasion by other tissue elements, and 'dedifferentiation'.

Muscle wasting

As the disease progresses so functioning muscle tissue degenerates, and is gradually replaced by fat and connective tissue. If the results are expressed in terms of *total* muscle weight then particular constituents may appear to be reduced when in fact the levels in *functioning* muscle tissue may be normal. A solution to this problem is to express results in terms of some specific reference base. In the past this has been total protein or better still non-collagen protein which corresponds to that fraction of the total muscle protein which is soluble in dilute alkali (Lilienthal *et al.* 1950; Pennington and Robinson 1968; Kar and Pearson 1972). In health the amount of non-collagen protein (expressed as non-collagen nitrogen) is roughly the same in different skeletal muscles (Table 7.1) and at least in later childhood and young adulthood it is not significantly affected by age or sex. Non-collagen protein represents over 90 per cent of the total protein of normal muscle but it may be less than 50 per cent in severely affected dystrophic muscle (Horvath and Proctor 1960).

More recently myosin or some similar contractile protein has been recommended as a reference base (Samaha *et al.* 1981). Whereas fibroblasts, macrophages, lipocytes, and other cells present in dystrophic tissue might contribute to non-collagen protein, they would not affect the myosin content. As would be expected, and known for a long time (Vignos and Lefkowitz 1959), as dystrophic muscle degenerates so its myosin content decreases. When levels of ATP and creatine phosphate are expressed in terms of myosin they are no different from normal (Samaha *et al.* 1981). This result

Table 7.1   *Non-collagen nitrogen (NCN) expressed as mg. (g wet weight)⁻¹, in various normal human skeletal muscles (unpublished data)*

Muscle	No.	NCN	
		Mean	s.d.
Rectus abdominis	20	23.3	6.2
Gastrocnemius	8	26.7	5.5
Deltoid	6	20.7	2.7
Pectoralis major	10	23.9	5.6
Miscellaneous*	9	24.0	3.6
Total	*53*	*23.7*	*5.3*

* Quadriceps (3); sternomastoid (2); sartorius (1); transversalis (1); diaphragm (1); latissimus dorsi (1).

is in stark contrast to several earlier studies which reported reduced levels using non-collagen protein as the reference base. Normal levels of ATP have also been confirmed by the technique of nuclear magnetic resonance (NMR) by Griffiths *et al.* (1985). That ATP levels are normal has important implications. It means that energy stores for muscle contraction are adequate, at least early in the course of the disease, and that this is therefore not the primary cause of muscle weakness (Edwards 1977). The latter seems more likely to be a reflection of the loss of muscle fibres due to their degeneration. However, recent studies using nuclear magnetic resonance (now sometimes referred to as magnetic resonance spectroscopy) seem to indicate that creatine phosphate may be reduced (Frostick 1986), but this finding awaits confirmation (Fig. 7.1).

As the amount of functioning muscle tissue decreases, this has several other consequences. Occasionally the glucose tolerance curve may be mildly abnormal, due to an inadequate disposal of glucose associated with the reduced muscle mass (Haymond *et al.* 1978), and plasma-free fatty acids may be raised (Takagi *et al.* 1970). More importantly, changes occur in creatine and creatinine metabolism, changes which have also been recognized for many years (Levene and Kristeller 1909). Creatine is largely synthesized in the liver and is delivered to the skeletal muscle where it is converted to creatinine which readily diffuses into the circulation and is excreted in the urine. In fact the amount of creatinine excreted each day by any individual is remarkably constant and is roughly proportional to the total body muscle mass.

Although the detailed picture may not yet be entirely clear (Fitch 1977), in general terms as muscle wastes from whatever cause, so the level of creatine in the plasma and especially the urine will increase, and the amount of

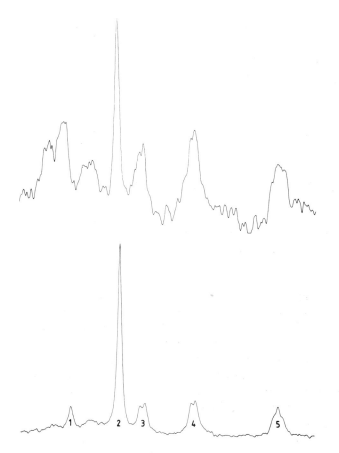

Fig. 7.1. Magnetic resonance spectrum of gastrocnemius muscle in a control (*below*), and a 15-year-old boy with Duchenne muscular dystrophy (*above*). In the affected boy there is a significant increase in intracellular pH (normal 7.01, affected 7.28) and an apparent reduction in the ratio of creatine phosphate to inorganic phosphate (1, inorganic phosphate; 2, creatine phosphate; 3–5, ATP peaks). (Reproduced by kind permission of Dr S. P. Frostick.)

creatinine in the urine will decrease. These changes however appear to be far removed from the basic defect in dystrophy, not only because they are not specific, but also because no abnormalities in creatine and creatinine excretion occur in female carriers of the disease unless they have significant muscle weakness (Emery 1963). Of 10 female carriers investigated, in only one who was a manifesting carrier with marked muscle weakness, was the creatine/creatinine ratio abnormally high (Fig. 7.2).

As skeletal muscle degenerates various breakdown products will be

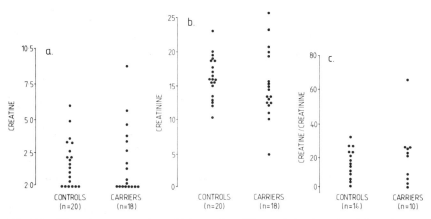

Fig. 7.2. The urinary excretion of (*a*) creatine, (*b*) creatinine (mg. kg^{-1} 24 h^{-1}), and (*c*) ratio of creatine/creatinine (x100) in healthy women and carriers of Duchenne muscular dystrophy. (Unpublished data.)

released and appear in the urine. For example, 3-methylhistidine is a known constituent of both actin and myosin, and as muscle breaks down the concentration in muscle decreases, and when expressed in terms of creatinine the urinary excretion increases (McKeran *et al.* 1977; Ballard *et al.* 1979). In fact the urinary excretion of 3-methylhistidine is an excellent measurement of myofibrillar protein catabolism (Mussini *et al.* 1984). Thus, while creatinine excretion may be taken as an index of total muscle mass, 3-methylhistidine excretion is an index of muscle breakdown.

Carnitine is largely synthesized in the liver and kidneys and is subsequently taken up by cardiac and skeletal muscle. As muscle breaks down so carnitine is released and concentrations in dystrophic muscle are significantly reduced (Berthillier *et al.* 1982). Since carnitine is an important co-factor in fatty acid oxidation, the reduction in muscle carnitine might also explain the accumulation of long-chain fatty acid derivatives in this tissue (Carroll *et al.* 1983).

Ionasescu and colleagues have reported increased muscle ribosomal protein synthesis and collagen synthesis *in vitro* not only in affected boys but also in some carriers (Ionasescu *et al.* 1977, 1980). The idea that this increased protein synthesis may reflect attempted regeneration is attractive. The investigators themselves believe that the increased amount of collagen present in Duchenne dystrophic muscle is related to the primary defect and is not due to secondary replacement fibrosis (Ionasescu and Ionasescu 1982). So far, however, similar results have not yet been reported by any other group.

The loss of contractile muscle protein in Duchenne muscular dystrophy could result from a reduced rate of synthesis, an abnormally high rate of degradation or a combination of both. *In vivo* protein synthesis has been measured by the intravenous infusion of labelled leucine, the incorporation of which into skeletal muscle is subsequently determined in needle biopsy specimens. These experiments have suggested that *total* muscle protein synthesis may actually be reduced in Duchenne muscular dystrophy (Rennie *et al.* 1982). However, these observations were made on boys aged 12 to 18 years when any attempts at regeneration are clearly failing. It would certainly be valuable to know what happens to *in vivo* protein synthesis in the very early stages of the disease.

Finally, although there is no doubt that many proteins are lost from dystrophic muscle, there is also evidence that some substances may actually *enter* affected muscle fibres. Experimentally, ingress of horseradish peroxidase (MW 40 000 daltons) (Mokri and Engel 1975), and Procion yellow (MW 674 daltons) (Bradley and Fulthorpe 1978) have been demonstrated, and evidence suggests that calcium (p. 139), IgG and complement (Engel and Biesecker 1982), and albumin (Cornelio and Dones 1984) enter affected muscle fibres. This has important implications for pathogenesis and will be discussed later (p. 144).

Enzyme changes in dystrophic muscle

There is general agreement that glycolysis as well as the activities of most individual glycolytic enzymes are reduced in muscle from patients with Duchenne muscular dystrophy as well as several other dystrophies (Ronzoni *et al.* 1960). Ellis' detailed studies indicate that in dystrophic muscle fructose in incorporated into the glycogen pathway at the expense of glucose and this results in increased lipogenesis (Ellis 1980). These changes, however, seem very likely to be secondary to the basic defect.

Fatty acid oxidation is also reduced but again this is not specific to Duchenne muscular dystrophy (Shumate *et al.* 1982). Mitochondrial oxidation on the other hand is unaffected until relatively late in the course of the disease.

A great many individual enzymes have been studied in muscle tissue from patients with Duchenne muscular dystrophy. (For example, Dreyfus *et al.* 1956; Vignos and Lefkowitz 1959; Heyck *et al.* 1963; DiMauro *et al.* 1967; Pennington 1962, 1977a, 1987; Kar and Pearson 1980.) In those instances where enzyme levels have been expressed in terms of non-collagen protein and studies made specifically on Duchenne muscular dystrophy, some general conclusions can be made. The level of activity of some enzymes appears to be normal, at least in the early stages of the disease (Table 7.2). These enzymes at least would seem to be excluded from playing any primary role in pathogenesis.

Other enzymes however have reduced activity (Table 7.3), in some cases even from very early on in the disease process as in the case of AMP deaminase (Kar and Pearson 1973). Interestingly, a deficiency of the erythrocyte form of phosphofructokinase is not associated with muscle disease but

Table 7.2   *Enzymes with* normal *activity in skeletal muscle tissue in Duchenne muscular dystrophy*

Aminotransferases (GPT, GOT)
Succinic dehydrogenase
Hexokinase
Phosphohexose isomerase
Aconitase
Cytochrome oxidase
Alkaline phosphatase
Acyl phosphatase
Fructose 1,6-diphosphatase
Lysolecithin phospholipase
Superoxide dismutase
Methylthioadenosine nucleosidase
Adenylosuccinase
Monamine oxidase
Glyoxalase II

Table 7.3   *Enzymes with* reduced *activity in skeletal muscle tissue in Duchenne muscular dystrophy*

Phosphoglucomutase
Phosphofructokinase
Aldolase
Triosephosphate isomerase
Phosphoglyceraldehyde dehydrogenase
Phosphoglycerate kinase
Enolase
Pyruvate kinase
Lactate dehydrogenase
Fumarase
Glycogen phosphorylase
Glycogen synthetase
Creatine kinase
AMP deaminase
Adenylate kinase

results in a non-spherocytic haemolytic anaemia (Etiemble *et al.* 1976).

The reduced activity of these various enzymes is probably largely the result of efflux from diseased muscle fibres though this cannot be the entire story. Thus, adenylate kinase, which has a relatively low molecular weight (21 000 daltons), is reduced in affected muscle but is not increased in serum (p. 47) and this is also of AMP deaminase. On the other hand, the aminotransferases are not significantly reduced in affected muscle but are increased in serum. Finally, acyl phosphatase is one of the smallest enzyme molecules known (MW 9400 daltons) and is abundant in skeletal muscle, largely in the soluble sarcoplasm, yet there is apparently normal activity in affected muscle (Kar and Pearson 1972a, but see Nassi *et al.* 1985). The explanation for these apparent contradictions may lie in the relative rates of synthesis (perhaps influenced to some extent by physical activity) versus destruction of different enzymes in affected muscle fibres, as well as their clearance rates from plasma. So far, however, very little is known of the relative importance of these different factors for individual enzymes (Pennington 1987).

Finally, and perhaps more interestingly, the activity of some enzymes is actually *increased* in Duchenne muscular dystrophy (Table 7.4). These changes are attributable to the invasion of affected muscle by macrophages and fibroblasts, as well as to the necrosis of affected muscle fibres. Macrophages and fibroblasts are known to contain several NADP-linked dehydrogenases (glucose-6-phosphate dehydrogenase, 6-phosphogluconate dehydrogenase, isocitrate dehydrogenase, and malate dehydrogenase), and other enzymes such as 5'-nucleotidase and ribonuclease. These cells also contain a number of proteases, including cathepsins, lysosomal acid hydrolases, and calcium activated proteases, which are all increased in dystrophic muscle (Pennington 1977b; Kar and Pearson 1972b, 1977). These enzymes attack and break down muscle protein and their increase in probably also an adaptive response of the muscle fibre to its degeneration and necrosis (Pennington 1987). However, such changes clearly are not primary but very much secondary to the disease process.

It should be noted, however, that this division into enzymes which are

Table 7.4 *Enzymes with* increased *activity in skeletal muscle tissue in Duchenne muscular dystrophy*

Glucose-6-phosphate dehydrogenase
6-Phosphogluconate dehydrogenase
Isocitrate dehydrogenase
Malate dehydrogenase
5'-Nucleotidase
Ribonuclease
Glutathione reductase
Prote(in)ases
Carnitine palmityltransferase
Lipid peroxidation
Phosphodiesterases

normal, reduced or increased in dystrophic muscle though convenient is somewhat arbitrary because it often depends at what stage in the disease process the assays are carried out. In almost all cases activity is normal at the beginning and abnormally low or high levels are found only later in the course of the disease. But some, such as acyl phosphatase, seem to remain at more or less normal levels right until the very late stages of the disease.

Membrane enzymes

Many muscle enzymes are free in the sarcoplasm but some are attached to membranes, such as the sarcoplasmic reticulum. The latter include adenylate cyclase, guanylate cyclase and Ca^{2+}, ($Na^+ + K^+$), and Mg^{2+}-ATPases. Until fairly recently enzyme studies have been limited to whole muscle homogenates which, at least later, are contaminated by extraneous adipose and connective tissue. It has therefore not been possible to study the activity in isolation of those enzymes which are attached specifically to muscle membranes. This is particularly important in investigating the possibility of a genetic defect in the sarcoplasmic membrane. To circumvent this problem minimally affected muscle should be studied, and recently the technique of using 'skinned fibres' has been developed, largely by Takagi and colleagues in Japan (Takagi and Nonaka 1981; Takagi 1984). In these preparations the surface membrane of the muscle fibre is removed mechanically or disrupted chemically. Using these techniques it seems that in the *early* stages of the disease the sarcoplasmic reticulum and contractile protein functions are normal (Wood 1984). However, whether or not there is any specific enzyme abnormality in dystrophic muscle membranes is as yet unresolved (Niebrój-Dobosz 1984) though it seems unlikely that calcium uptake by the sarcoplasmic reticulum membranes is abnormal (Takagi 1984). Furthermore, although based largely on the study of muscle homogenates, the weight of evidence suggests that any abnormality (such as the increase in Ca^{2+}-ATPase activity) is likely to be secondary. However, some subtle change in the composition of the muscle membranes cannot yet be excluded (p. 132).

'Dedifferentiation'

A number of observations indicate that in many ways dystrophic muscle resembles fetal muscle for which the term 'dedifferentiation' has sometimes been used. Firstly, it is less easy to distinguish different histochemical fibre types in dystrophic muscle (Engel 1970) which is also a feature of fetal muscle (Fig. 7.3), even at term (Toop 1975). Secondly, certain phospholipid changes in dystrophic muscle (more sphingomyelin, less lecithin plus choline plasmalogen, and more total cholesterol) are very similar to those found in fetal muscle (Hughes 1972). Thirdly, fetal myosins are found in muscle from patients with Duchenne muscular dystrophy and spinal muscular atrophy

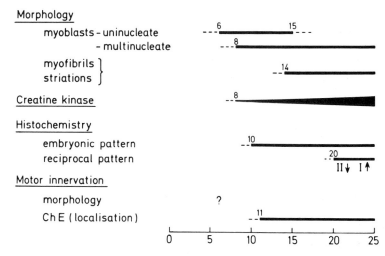

Fig. 7.3. Times (weeks of gestation) at which various aspects of muscle development become apparent. Ch E, choline esterase. (Data from various sources.)

(Fitzsimons and Hoh 1981). Finally, and most intriguingly, the isoenzyme patterns of dystrophic muscle resemble fetal muscle rather than adult muscle. This was first shown in the case of lactate dehydrogenase (LDH) (Dreyfus *et al.* 1962; Wieme and Herpol 1962). This enzyme is composed of five isoenzymes, each being formed by the tetrameric association of two sub-units, synthesized by two separate genes, referred to as M and H (Fig. 7.4). The M sub-unit predominates in adult skeletal muscle and the H sub-unit in cardiac muscle. On electrophoresis the most rapidly migrating isoenzyme (LDH-1) has the composition H_4, LDH-2 = H_3M, LDH-3 = H_2M_2, LDH-4 = HM_3, and LDH-5 = M_4. The amounts and proportions of the M

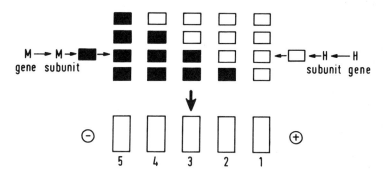

Fig. 7.4. The formation of the five isoenzymes of lactate dehydrogenase.

and H sub-units (LDH–M, LDH–H) can be determined in a number of ways including preferential inhibition by urea (Emery 1967a). The proportions of LDH–M and LDH–H in some normal skeletal muscles are given in Table 7.5.

Although there are some variations in different skeletal muscles, LDH–M clearly predominates. However, in fetal skeletal muscle LDH–H predominates, and the isoenzyme pattern resembles that seen in Duchenne muscular dystrophy even in the preclinical phase (Fig. 7.5). It may be that the normal adult pattern is never attained, in which case the term 'dedifferentiation' is hardly appropriate. Incidentally, there does not appear to be a complete absence of LDH–5 in all cases of Duchenne muscular dystrophy. A reduction in LDH–M is also found in some female carriers (Emery 1964b) but the change is not specific to Duchenne muscular dystrophy but is also found in a number of other neuromuscular disorders (Emery 1968).

Analogous changes in isoenzyme patterns have since been reported for creatine kinase, aldolase, isocitrate dehydrogenase, malate dehydrogenase, adenylate kinase, and enolase (reviewed by Ellis 1978).

The implication of these various findings is that dystrophic muscle synthesizes polypeptides not normally produced postnatally and that these changes are presumably a result of regenerative activity: newly synthesized peptides reflecting the activity of genes normally active only during fetal development. The enzyme hypoxanthine-guanine phosphoribosyltransferase is significantly increased in muscle in patients with Duchenne muscular dystrophy even from the age of 2, and this has been interpreted as being a means of enhancing increased protein synthesis and regenerative activity (Neerunjun *et al.* 1979). Finally, using immuno-histochemical techniques, the re-expression of fetal-specific myosins has now in fact been localized to regenerating fibres in Duchenne muscular dystrophy (Schiaffino *et al.* 1986).

Table 7.5 *Proportions (%) of LDH–M and LDH–H in various normal skeletal muscles (unpublished data)*

Muscle	No.	LDH–M	LDH–H
Rectus abdominis	5	87.0	13.0
Diaphragm	1	89.2	10.8
Gastrocnemius	3	86.7	13.3
Quadriceps	1	89.6	10.4
Latissimus dorsi	1	87.4	12.6
Pectoralis major	6	87.9	12.1
Deltoid	2	95.6	4.4
Soleus	2	67.1	32.9

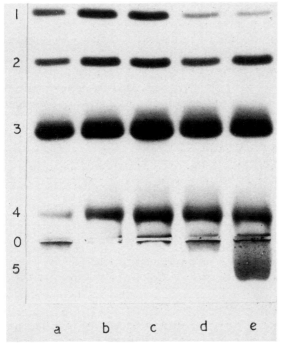

Fig. 7.5. LDH isoenzyme patterns in muscle extracts from: (*a*) 3-year-old boy with preclinical Duchenne muscular dystrophy, (*b*) 400 g fetus, (*c*) 7-month stillbirth, (*d*) neonate, (*e*) 3-month-old normal infant. O is the origin and the anode is at the top.

Cultured myoblasts

The study of myoblasts in tissue culture, free of all the possible confounding effects of extraneous factors, would seem to offer the ideal system for investigating the possible aetiology of Duchenne muscular dystrophy. Unfortunately, it soon became clear that there were serious technical difficulties to be overcome in this approach, not least of which was the presence of other cell types (mostly fibroblasts) which 'contaminate' such cultures. This was particularly a problem with primary explants where the biopsy material is first freed of any obvious fat and connective tissue, and then small fragments, about 1 mm in size, are grown in culture vessels with appropriate nutrient medium, usually enriched with chick embryo extract or fetal calf serum. To avoid problems of possible contamination with fibroblasts, cellular outgrowths from explants can be dissociated and the dissociated cells then transferred to secondary monolayer cultures, a procedure which can be repeated. In this way we chose to study fetal muscle in which fibroblast contamination is minimal in any event (Fig. 7.6).

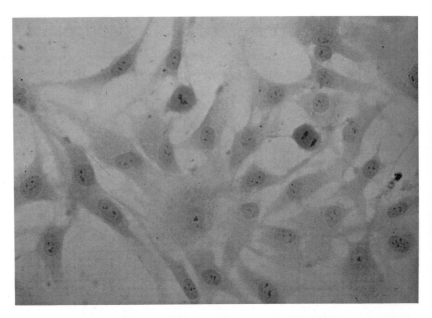

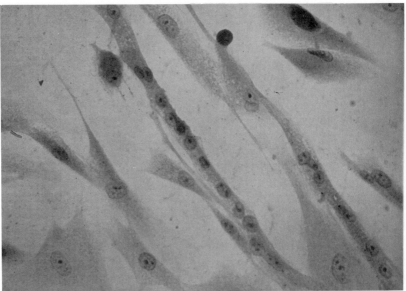

Fig. 7.6. Fetal muscle in tissue culture. (*Above*) dividing uninucleate myoblasts. (*Below*) fusion of myoblasts to form multinucleate myotubes.

As a further refinement *clonal* cultures can be set up whereby the progeny of single myoblasts can be studied. Finally, muscle-nerve co-cultures (e.g. Duchenne muscular dystrophy muscle and rodent spinal cord) can be used to study the possible effects of innervation *in vitro* (Askanas *et al.* 1985; Peterson *et al.* 1986).

The results of these various sorts of studies have been reviewed in detail (Hauschka 1982; Yasin *et al.* 1983; Miranda and Mongini 1984; Witkowski 1986a, b). Unfortunately, reports of abnormal growth, differentiation or morphology have often not been substantiated, and no clear picture has so far emerged. However, several reported biochemical abnormalities have been interpreted by Miranda and Mongini (1984) as indicating that dystrophic muscle in culture reaches a lesser degree of maturity than normal muscle. For example, in dystrophic muscle culture creatine kinase BB isoenzyme is significantly increased, although this is not specific to Duchenne muscular dystrophy (Franklin *et al.* 1981).

Also, a careful and detailed recent study, using a double-isotope labelling technique, indicates that the protein degradation rate in cultured muscle cells is normal in Duchenne muscular dystrophy which further supports the idea (p. 113) that the loss of contractile muscle proteins is perhaps largely the result of reduced synthesis rather than increased degradation (Neville and Harrold 1985).

Finally, analysis, of muscle satellite cells (mononucleated precursors of mature muscle cells) in clonal cultures indicates that their proliferative capacity may be reduced in Duchenne muscular dystrophy (Blau *et al.* 1983). This difficult but elegant approach to the study of muscle development *in vitro* may, one hopes provide more meaningful information in future.

Cultured fibroblasts

As we have seen the interpretation of the results of studies on muscle is often difficult because of contamination by other tissue cells and in whole muscle any changes observed could be secondary to the basic defect. For these reasons some have turned their attention to cultured skin fibroblasts and peripheral blood leucocytes in the conviction that the basic defect might be expressed in such tissues. Certainly the basic biochemical defects in many other metabolic disorders have been demonstrated in the past in skin fibroblasts (Davidson 1970), or peripheral blood leucocytes (Hsia 1970).

The growth, behaviour, morphology, and biochemistry of skin fibroblasts in tissue culture from patients with Duchenne muscular dystrophy have been studied intensely in recent years. Unfortunately, some earlier observations have either not been corroborated subsequently, or have not been repeated and it is often difficult to assess the relevance of an isolated finding.

Recent reports seem to substantiate some earlier indications that though the cells grow in size and divide normally (Hirsch-Kauffmann *et al.* 1985), intercellular adhesiveness may be reduced, although there is much overlap with controls (Jones and Witkowski 1983), and muscle cell motility *in vitro* is not significantly different from normal (Witkowski and Dubowitz 1985). Ribosomal protein synthesis has been reported to be reduced (Pöche and Schulze 1985).

The relevance of these findings to the pathogenesis of the disease is still a moot point, but that abnormalities occur at all indicates that the mutant gene may be expressed in skin fibroblasts, a tissue in which, unlike muscle, interference by other cellular constituents does not occur. But in all studies with skin fibroblasts a salutory warning of the need to use appropriate control material is provided by Thompson and colleagues (1983). They had previously reported finding a particular polypeptide present in cultured skin fibroblasts from normal males but apparently absent in Duchenne muscular dystrophy. However, they subsequently found that the polypeptide was also absent in normal skin fibroblasts obtained from sources other than the Repository of Mutant Human Cell Strains, Montreal, used as controls in their earlier studies. It transpired that the latter had been established entirely from preputial skin whereas the material in their patients had been derived from non-genital biopsies and therein lay the explanation for the apparent difference (Thompson *et al.* 1983)!

Peripheral blood leucocytes

There have so far been few studies directed toward studying the metabolism of peripheral blood leucocytes in Duchenne muscular dystrophy. Yet in many ways this provides an ideal tissue for such studies. The single most important disadvantage is that there is no *a priori* reason to believe that the mutant gene will necessarily be expressed in these cells.

Several individual enzymes, including phosphorylases, appear to have normal activity in leucocytes from patients with Duchenne muscular dystrophy (Scholte and Busch 1980). Our own studies of leucocytes in short-term culture have revealed no defect in glycolysis or the tricarboxylic acid cycle and electron transport chain (Emery *et al.* 1971). Furthermore there appears to be no *major* defect in fatty acid oxidation (β-oxidation) either (King and Emery 1973). Thus it would seem that none of the enzymes involved in these various metabolic pathways is primarily defective in the disease. This is further evidence that defective glycolysis in dystrophic muscle is a secondary phenomenon.

Serum

Most studies have concentrated on the levels of various muscle enzymes in the serum of patients with Duchenne muscular dystrophy. Elevated levels of most enzymes can be accounted for by their relative abundance in muscle tissue as compared with serum, and their release from dystrophic muscle into the circulation (p. 47). It has been suggested that enzymes may also be released from other organs, including the liver (Kleine 1970), but the evidence is not very convincing. Certainly the characteristic liver enzymes, γ-glutamyltransferase and sorbitol dehydrogenase, are normal.

Whatever the mechanism of muscle enzyme release, this is not a significant factor in producing muscle weakness because serum levels are highest when muscle weakness is least, and drugs like prednisone, thyroid hormones, diethylstilboestrol, and lithium carbonate when given orally for some time are associated with a decrease is serum enzyme activity in boys with Duchenne muscular dystrophy but there is no effect on muscle strength. How these diverse compounds affect enzyme release is not known (Rowland 1980).

Other serum proteins which are raised to varying degrees in the serum of patients with Duchenne muscular dystrophy include: α_2-globulin, myoglobin, and haemopexin which binds myoglobin and other haem compounds. However, all these various proteins also occur in normal serum, albeit often at very low levels. No abnormal metabolite has yet been detected in serum in Duchenne muscular dystrophy.

'Toxic plasma factor'

Although it seems most likely that the release of muscle proteins into the circulation is the result of muscle necrosis and/or a molecular defect in the muscle membrane, there is also the possibility that some circulating toxin might affect the membrane and increase its permeability. Evidence on this point is scanty. Sugita and Tyler (1963) incubated rat intact peroneus longus muscles in Krebs–Ringer-bicarbonate-glucose buffer to which they added fresh serum from controls and boys with Duchenne muscular dystrophy in the proportion of 1 ml to 30 ml of buffer. In the controls there was little creatine kinase activity in the buffer solution, but with serum from affected boys, creatine kinase activity progressively increased over a two hour incubation period. These interesting observations however do not seem to have been repeated. Also, it would be expected that if there were some substance in plasma which affects muscle membrane permeability then carrier mothers might be expected to transmit it to all their offspring.

The effects of dystrophic serum on normal erythrocyte ATPase activity have been studied by Peter *et al.* (1969) and Lloyd and Emery (1981). These investigators found that $(Na^+ + K^+)$ATPase activity in erythrocyte ghosts is inhibited by ouabain in normal controls but stimulated in Duchenne muscular dystrophy. However, if normal ghosts were incubated in Duchenne serum then their activity also became stimulated by ouabain. The serum 'factor' responsible for this effect was rendered inactive by deproteination.

Peter *et al.* (1969) have suggested that one possible explanation for these findings is that an auto-immune process may be involved whereby damaged muscle membranes induce an antibody response to membranes in general, but at present there is no experimental evidence for this interesting idea (but see p. 144).

Finally, a number of investigators have noted some increase in SCK activity when serum is diluted before assay, and it has therefore been postulated that there may be an inhibitor of the enzyme in plasma. However since the effect is observed in serum samples from normal women as well as carriers of Duchenne muscular dystrophy (Simpson *et al.* 1979) it is unlikely to be related to dystrophy *per se*.

Urine

As in the case of serum, no abnormal metabolites have yet been detected in urine specifically in Duchenne muscular dystrophy. The changes in urinary composition which have been observed can all be explained on the basis of the release of various breakdown products from degenerating muscle into the circulation and then excreted in the urine. As described previously (p. 110), the urinary excretion of creatine is increased, whereas the excretion of creatinine is decreased so that the ratio of creatine of creatinine in the urine is significantly increased.

Breakdown products excreted in increased amounts in urine, when expressed in terms of creatinine, include carnitine (DiMauro and Rowland 1976), various amino acids (Bank *et al.* 1971; Emery *et al.* 1979), and 3-methylhistidine (p. 112). The aminoaciduria in Duchenne muscular dystrophy is generalized with no consistent pattern (plasma amino acid levels are normal). Our own results determined by ion-exchange chromatography using a single-column gradient elution technique are given in Table 7.6. Frank myoglobinuria is not associated with Duchenne muscular dystrophy (Rowland 1984).

None of these changes in urinary composition are specific to Duchenne muscular dystrophy but may be found in any neuromuscular disorder in which muscle breakdown occurs. The increased urinary excretion of dimethylarginines in muscular dystrophy however has a different origin (Inoue *et al.* 1979; Lou 1979; Hirano *et al.* 1983). N^G, N^G-Dimethylarginine is mainly located in cell nuclei as a component of non-histone nuclear protein and its increased excretion reflects myosin turnover in muscle regenerating from satellite cells. It is therefore an index of regenerative activity and could be a useful parameter for assessing the value of any proposed therapy.

Table 7.6 *Urinary excretion of amino acids (mg.100 mg.α-amino*
N$_2^{-1}$.24 h^{-1}) in boys with Duchenne muscular dystrophy and
severe mental handicap (+MH, N = 12) and normal
intelligence (−MH, N = 7), and healthy boys of the same age
(N = 6) (unpublished data)

Amino acid	+MH		−MH		Controls	
	Mean*	s.d.	Mean*	s.d.	Mean	s.d.
Taurine	59.1	55.6	23.3	10.8	19.8	10.0
Hydroxyproline	0.0	0.0	0.6	1.5	0.0	0.0
Aspartic acid	1.3	1.9	1.5	1.3	2.3	3.0
Threonine	9.4	5.8	7.4	4.0	6.7	1.5
Serine	23.6	17.0	9.9	6.8	11.9	3.0
Glutamine	47.9	52.0	24.5	7.9	26.7	6.8
Asparagine	0.3	0.9	0.3	0.5	0.7	0.9
Glutamic acid	5.2	9.0	3.9	5.1	0.9	0.4
Proline	0.0	0.0	0.5	0.8	0.1	0.2
Glycine	92.8	86.8	33.0	12.6	24.5	4.1
Alanine	23.9	22.7	9.9	4.6	11.1	2.7
Cystine	7.7	10.3	2.0	2.3	2.6	3.4
Valine	4.9	3.9	5.6	10.8	1.8	0.8
Methionine	0.3	0.5	0.8	0.3	1.1	0.4
Isoleucine	1.2	1.5	1.1	0.9	0.5	0.1
Leucine	0.8	1.0	3.6	2.9	4.4	1.8
Tyrosine	11.6	8.8	6.4	3.3	6.4	3.7
Phenylalanine	7.0	5.0	3.5	1.8	3.1	0.9
β-Amino isobutyric acid	10.7	18.7	3.2	2.9	4.7	4.0
Ethanolamine	12.2	9.3	3.0	1.2	6.2	4.1
Ornithine	4.5	2.7	1.0	0.5	1.7	0.9
Lysine	7.9	5.4	6.3	4.5	4.5	2.7
Histidine	93.3	61.4	46.4	18.1	43.7	11.9
Tryptophan	5.1	9.6	4.5	2.5	2.5	1.6
Carnosine	6.9	12.9	6.4	3.1	8.0	0.9
Arginine	1.6	1.5	1.4	0.5	1.1	0.3

* Mean values exceeding the normal range (mean + 2 s.d.) are italicized.

Animal models

Various neuromuscular disorders have been described in many animals
including mink, sheep, duck, cow, and even perhaps the dog (Averill 1980).
Mainly because of the availability of animals and problems associated with
animal husbandry, only the diseases occurring in mouse, hamster, and
chicken have been studied in any depth (Harris 1979; Cosmos *et al.* 1980;
Harris and Slater 1980; Bradley *et al.* 1987).

In 1955, Michelson, then a student working at the Jackson Memorial Research Laboratory, Bar Harbor, Maine, identified a spontaneous mouse mutant with a myopathy in the inbred strain 129 (Michelson *et al*. 1955). This discovery was heralded with great enthusiasm by all workers in the field because a good mouse analogue of the human disease could conceivably provide an excellent model for investigating pathogenesis and even possible treatment (Fig. 7.7). But there were many problems to be overcome. It proved to be an autosomal recessive trait, and it was very difficult to maintain stocks of affected animals by breeding from homozygous affected parents. Furthermore, it gradually became clear that in the disease in this mutant (*dy*) as well as in a different milder allelic mutant (*dy*²ᴶ) indentified subsequently (another allele *dy*ᴷ has also been described very recently), there were morphological, functional, and electrophysiological abnormalities in the nervous

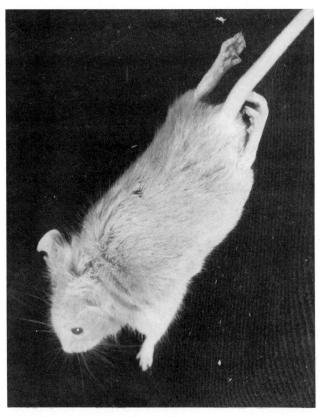

Fig. 7.7. Mouse mutant (Bar Harbor 129/ReJ *dy/dy*) with myopathy. Note the paralysed hind limbs and hunched forequarters.

system (Mendell *et al.* 1979; Bradley *et al.* 1987).

Similarly, mutant myopathies in the Syrian hamster (Homburger *et al.* 1962) and chicken (Julian and Asmundson 1963) have not proved to be strictly comparable to human muscular dystrophy. However, a recently isolated mouse mutant in the C57BL/10 inbred strain, referred to as *mdx*, seems more like the human disease. This is an X-linked mutant which has elevated serum creatine kinase and pyruvate kinase levels, and the muscle histology is similar in some respects to human muscular dystrophy (Bullfield *et al.* 1984).

In studies on animals we have bred from the original strain kindly provided by Dr Bullfield, central nuclei however seem to be *far* more evident than in Duchenne muscular dystrophy (Fig. 7.8). So far no abnormalities have been demonstrated in the peripheral and central nervous systems of this mutant. However, since the pathology is somewhat different and the disease is *not* progressive its use as a model for Duchenne muscular dystrophy has been cautioned (Dangain and Vrbova 1984) and in fact it may be more analogous to Emery–Dreifuss dystrophy (Caskey 1986; Hodgson *et al.* 1986b).

Although none of the animal models studied so far, with perhaps the exception of the mouse *mdx* mutant, is strictly analogous to human muscular

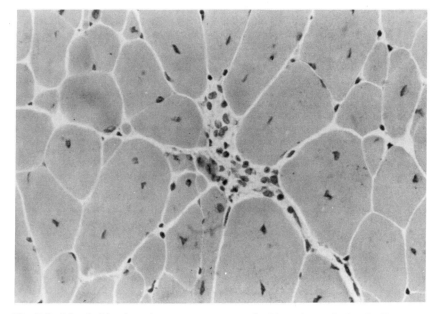

Fig. 7.8. Muscle histology in mouse mutant *mdx*. Note the variation in fibre size, central nuclei, and fibre necrosis and phagocytosis (haematoxylin and eosin).

dystrophy, there seems no doubt that certain aspects of pathogenesis might be profitably pursued in such animals (Mendell *et al.* 1979). For example, the tissue distribution of calcium in dystrophic mice (Nutting *et al.* 1980), and the relationship between increased intracellular calcium, defective mitochondrial oxidative phosphorylation, and the development of heart disease in the hereditary cardiomyopathy in the hamster (Proschek and Jasmin 1982). Finally, therapeutic trials in animal models might give clues to possible treatment of the human disease (Cosmos and Butler 1980). Sadly, however, despite the prodigious efforts of investigators working in this field, little light has been thrown so far on the cause of muscular dystrophy. One suspects that as in the case of many other hereditary disorders affecting both man and animals, more relevant information may come from studying patients themselves.

Summary and conclusions

Many biochemical abnormalities have been found in Duchenne muscular dystrophy but none so far has been shown to be the basic defect. Abnormal findings are likely to be relevant to pathogenesis only when they relate specifically to Duchenne muscular dystrophy and occur in the very early stages of the disease process before there is any significant muscle wasting and weakness.

Muscle tissue has been studied the most, and the observed biochemical changes are conveniently considered as being the consequence of three main processes. Firstly, there are those changes which result from wasting and degeneration, and these include the reduction in muscle myosin, carnitine, and most glycolytic enzymes. Secondly, there are changes attributable to the invasion of affected muscle by macrophages and fibroblasts as well as to the necrosis of affected muscle fibres. These include the increase in enzymes present in fibroblasts and macrophages (such as NADP-linked dehydrogenases) and proteases (cathepsins, lysosomal acid hydrolases, and calcium activated proteases). Thirdly, in many ways dystrophic muscle resembles fetal muscle (histochemically, and lipid, myosin, and isoenzyme patterns) for which the term 'dedifferentiation' has sometimes been used. The balance of evidence at present suggests that mitochondrial oxidation, sarcoplasmic reticulum and contractile protein functions are essentially normal, at least in the early stages of the disease. The results of studies on cultured myoblasts and fibroblasts have not yet revealed any very clear picture although there are indications that the mutant gene may b expressed in these tissues.

Studies on peripheral blood leucocytes suggest that there is no primary defect in glycolysis, the tricarboxylic acid cycle or electron transport chain, or fatty acid oxidation. No abnormal metabolites have yet been found in plasma or urine, and most of the changes which have been observed can be explained in terms of efflux from dystrophic muscle fibres.

Finally, so far there appears to be no animal analogue which is strictly comparable to Duchenne muscular dystrophy, though the *mdx* mouse mutant seems to be similar.

8   Pathogenesis

Ever since the disease was first described various ideas have been proposed to explain its possible cause. Duchenne himself considered the possibility of its having either a vascular or neurogenic basis. However, at the time many investigative procedures and experimental techniques were in their infancy and it was not really possible to pursue these ideas in any depth. In any event many early ideas, such as the disorder being due to a defect of the sympathetic nervous system, were fanciful with little, if any, supportive evidence. However, more recently several interesting suggestions have been proposed for which their advocates have adduced some evidence. Although most of these have now been shown to have little basis, they have nevertheless been valuable in stimulating much useful research. One also suspects that each may yet harbour at least a *soupçon* of truth for our complete understanding of the disease process. Thus, although a *primary* defect in muscle vasculature now seems extremely unlikely, nevertheless some minor changes in the microcirculation consequent on the replacement of muscle tissue by fat and connective tissue later in the course of the disease (Carry *et al.* 1986) could conceivably compromise the blood supply to any surviving muscle fibres and thereby aggravate the disease process. Or, even more likely, the ingress of calcium through the surface membrane of a fibre undergoing degeneration could well aggravate muscle fibre necrosis.

One other problem has been the frequent emphasis on anatomical or structural defects as the basis of the disease. This is perhaps because, as neurologists, many investigators have been trained to think of the anatomical location of a lesion. To biochemists and molecular geneticists, however, they view genetic disease in an entirely different manner; the identification of the biochemical expression of the defective gene in whatever tissue should be the primary concern of research in this field. In more recent years this philosophy has gained increasing converts.

Vascular hypothesis

Though the idea that Duchenne muscular dystrophy might have a vascular basis had been entertained in the past by a number of investigators, experimental evidence was not forthcoming until Démos in the early 1960s (Démos 1961; Démos and Maroteaux 1961; Démos *et al.* 1962) claimed to have demonstrated abnormalities in the circulation time in affected boys and some carriers (p. 98). Later King Engel and his colleagues approached the problem from a pathological point of view (Engel 1975). These investigators were impressed by the occasional clustering of necrotic muscle fibres which they interpreted as being the result of local ischaemia. They also considered that myocardial fibrosis in the disease was similar to that seen in ischaemic heart disease. Their most interesting evidence, however, came from the effects of aortic ligation in rats followed by the injection of vasoactive agents (such as serotonin or noradrenaline), or micro-embolization of muscle produced by injecting small dextran particles into the femoral artery of rabbits. In both cases a clustering of necrotic fibres was found accompanied by an elevation in serum enzymes. However, subsequent studies have shown that in Duchenne muscular dystrophy necrotic fibres are not significantly clustered but are randomly distributed. Also experimental ischaemic myopathy has been questioned as a model of Duchenne muscular dystrophy, mainly because muscle tissue is now recognized as having a very limited repertoire of responses to any injury. Finally, and most importantly, careful studies have revealed no significant abnormality either in the morphology of skeletal muscle blood vessels (Koehler 1977), or in muscle blood flow (p. 98).

Neurogenic hypothesis

In 1970 McComas and colleagues published a paper in *Nature* which generated considerable interest (McComas *et al.* 1970). The aim of their studies was to estimate the numbers of functioning motor units in the disease, and for various reasons they chose the extensor digitorum brevis of the foot, although later they extended their studies to other muscles. In essence what they did was to find the average amplitude of a single motor unit potential evoked by stimulation of the anterior tibial nerve at the ankle, then determined the amplitude of the muscle potential after a *maximal* stimulus of the nerve. By dividing the maximal amplitude by the average amplitude they estimated the number of motor units within the muscle. A significant reduction in the number of motor units was found in Duchenne muscular dystrophy, as well as several other muscular dystrophies, suggesting that there was loss of functioning motor neurones. This lead to the concept of the 'sick motor neurone' with the implication that perhaps a deficiency of some trophic neural factor might be the basic cause of the disease. McComas also drew attention to other observations which might support this idea, such as the occasional finding of abnormal motor end-plates and fibrillation potentials. A deficiency of some trophic neural factor might also provide a possible explanation for the associated intellectual impairment in the disease. However, the concept soon faced serious problems. No specific changes in motor end-plate morphology were found, and no abnormalities of motor innervation. Secondly, fibrillation potentials are not an absolute sign of denervation. Thirdly, there is no loss of anterior horn cells in Duchenne muscular dystrophy or in any other dystrophy. Finally, and most inportantly, the details of the electromyographic methodology adopted by McComas and his colleagues and the interpretation of the results have been seriously questioned (Bradley *et al.* 1975; Panayiotopoulos 1975). It now seems unlikely therefore that a 'neurogenic factor' plays any significant role in the pathogenesis of Duchenne muscular dystrophy. However, this is not to say that muscle innervation is of no consequence. The early experiments of Buller (Buller *et al.* 1960) demonstrated quite clearly that the physiological characteristics of fast and slow muscles depend on appropriate innervation and this has been confirmed by many studies since.

Membrane hypothesis

It is difficult to be sure when the idea was first considered that the basic defect in Duchenne muscular dystrophy might reside in the muscle cell membrane. Even in the 1950s this possibility was mooted when certain muscle enzymes were found to be increased in the serum of affected boys (p. 44). There is little doubt however that considerable impetus was given to the idea by the work of Roses and colleagues in the mid-1970s when they reported an apparent abnormality of the membrane-associated protein spectrin in *erythrocyte membranes* in Duchenne muscular dystrophy (Roses *et al.* 1975; Roses and Appel 1976; Roses *et al.* 1976a). This finding had instant appeal for many investigators working in the field. It not only satisfied the biochemists who needed a biochemical basis for any proposed membrane defect, but also those who expected that the basic genetic defect might possibly be expressed in tissues other than muscle.

Cell membranes in general consist of a lipid bilayer. On the extracellular surface are located various hormone receptor and ouabain binding sites as well as externally orientated enzymes, such as acetylcholinesterase. Within the membrane are located certain other enzymes, such as proteases, while on the intracellular surface are located other enzymes, such as glyceraldehyde-3-phosphate dehydrogenase, and cytoskeletal proteins, such as ankyrin, spectrin, and erythrocyte actin (Fig. 8.1).

If erythrocyte ghost protein is subjected to polyacrylamide gel electrophoresis (PAGE) then with appropriate staining a number of bands are revealed (Fig. 8.2). Band 2 is a component of spectrin and Roses and colleagues reported an apparent increase in phosphorylation of this peptide in Duchenne muscular dystrophy.

Since this original work a variety of other membrane abnormalities have been reported, not only in erythrocytes but also in lymphocytes, fibroblasts and muscle (Table 8.1).

The most obvious morphological abnormalities which have been reported include changes in erythrocyte shape, numbers of intramembranous parti-

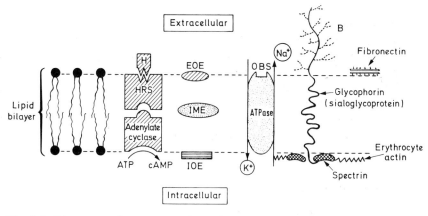

Fig. 8.1. Diagrammatic representation of a generalized cell membrane. HRS, hormone receptor site; EOE, externally oriented enzymes; IME, intramembrane enzymes; IOE, internally oriented enzymes; OBS, ouabain binding site; B, blood group specificities, virus receptor site. (From Emery (1983) with permission.)

Table 8.1 *Some reported membrane-associated abnormalities in Duchenne muscular dystrophy*

A. *Erythrocytes*
 1. Morphology
   echinocyte formation
   intramembranous particles ↓
 2. Biochemical
   K 'flux ↑
   Na, K-ATPase ouabain inhibition ↓
   Ca-ATPase ↑
   adenylate cyclase, epinephrine stimulation ↓
   phospholipids abnormal
   protein kinase (phosphorylation) ↑
   acetyl cholinesterase ↓
 3. Physical
   deformability ↓
   shear modulus ↑
   electron spin resonance abnormal
   osmotic fragility ↑
   electrophoretic mobility ↑
B. *Lymphocytes*
   capping ↓
C. *Fibroblasts*
   intercellular adhesiveness ↓

Table 8.1 *Cont'd*

D. *Muscle*
  1. Morphology
     membrane discontinuities
     intramembranous particles ↓
  2. Biochemical
     adenylate cyclase, epinephrine stimulation ↓
     phospholipids abnormal
     Na, K-ATPase ouabain inhibition ↓
  3. Physical
     penetration by dyes, etc. ↑

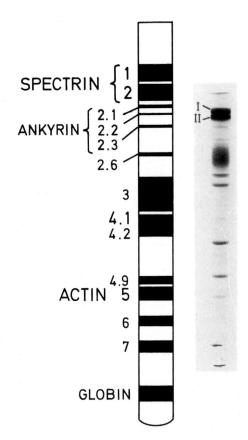

Fig. 8.2. SDS (sodium dodecyl sulphate) polyacrylamide gel electrophoresis pattern of the proteins in the erythrocyte membrane as visualized by staining with Coomassie blue.

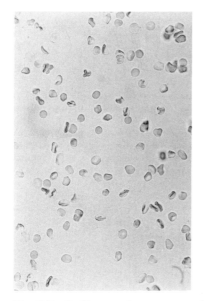 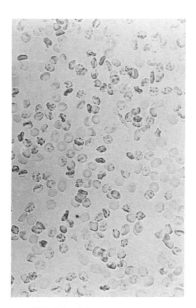

Fig. 8.3. (*Left*) normal appearance of erythrocytes. (*Right*) echinocytes.

cles, and lympocyte capping. Under certain *in vitro* conditions, erythrocytes may adopt a 'spiney' sea-urchin-like appearance which are therefore referred to as echinocytes, and such distortion has been reported to occur more frequently in Duchenne muscular dystrophy (Figs. 8.3 and 8.4). The membrane lipid bilayer may be freeze-fractured and on subsequent electronmicroscopy particles on both membrane fracture faces can be visualized and counted. In Duchenne muscular dystrophy it has been reported that the number of intramembranous particles, which represent membrane transport proteins, is reduced (Fig. 8.5).

Finally, protein receptors on the surface of peripheral blood lymphocytes can be visualized by using fluorescent-labelled polyvalent anti-human immunoglobulin producing so-called 'caps'. In Duchenne muscular dystrophy lymphocyte capping has been reported to be reduced compared with normal (Fig. 8.6).

Many of the reported physico-chemical abnormalities could be explained on the basis of reduced membrane fluidity – that in some way the membrane is more rigid than normal.

These various findings have been critically reviewed by Rowland (1976, 1980) who provides an extensive bibliography. It appears that in almost all cases, even including the original report of abnormal band 2 phosphorylation, the findings are controversial. Either the abnormality in question has

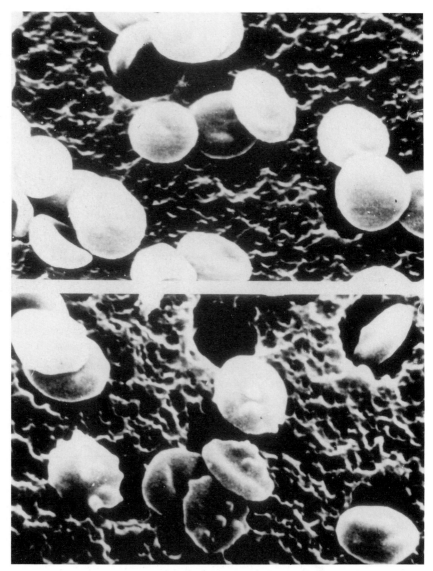

Fig. 8.4. Erythrocytes as seen with scanning electronmicroscopy. (*Above*), normal appearance, (*below*) echinocytes.

CONTROL   DUCHENNE

E

P

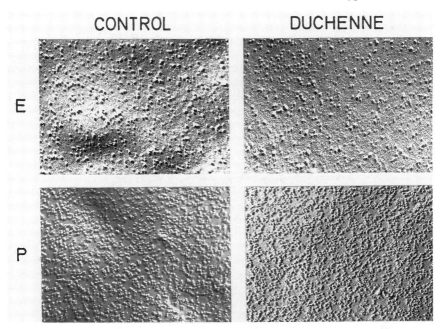

Fig. 8.5. Freeze-fracture electron micrograph of erythrocyte membranes showing the intramembranous particles on the P (protoplasmic) and E (external) faces. We have found no significant difference in the numbers of particles in controls and Duchenne muscular dystrophy (Lloyd *et al*, 1981).

not been reproducible in different laboratories, or it has been found to occur in normal as well as affected boys. Of 27 erythrocyte abnormalities reported from 102 different laboratories, 9 are single reports, and of the remaining 18 there is controversy in all but one, namely increased Ca^{2+}-ATPase activity (Rowland 1980). However, even this latter finding is something of an enigma. Although it appears the activity of this enzyme, responsible for pumping calcium out of the cell, may be increased in erythrocytes (Hodson and Pleasure 1977; Luthra *et al*. 1979; Ruitenbeek 1979), there is apparently no abnormality of calcium efflux (Shoji 1981; Szibor *et al*. 1981), and calcium levels are normal (p. 144). There is also no apparent abnormality in calcium exchange in cultured skin fibroblasts (Statham and Dubowitz 1979).

It is not at all clear why there should be much difficulties in reproducing observations in different laboratories, but it may be in part a reflection of the complexities of the various technologies involved as well as the need for their standardization A resolution of these problems is urgently needed. A membrane abnormality in affected muscle tissue could well be an epiphenomenon and therefore of little consequence to pathogenesis. However, a well documented and confirmed membrane abnormality in another apparently

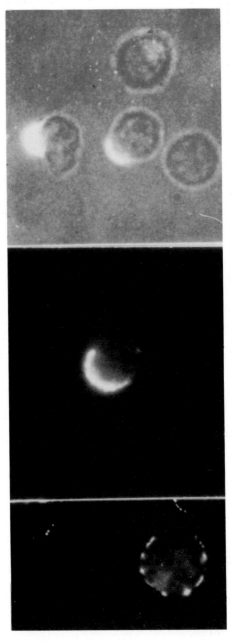

Fig. 8.6. Formation of 'caps' (from below to above) of fluorescent-labelled polyvalent anti-human immunoglobulin on peripheral blood lymphocytes.

unaffected tissue, such as erythrocytes, would be more difficult to explain away. It would be a very strong indication that the primary defect, or something very close to it, resides within the cell membrane itself.

Nonetheless, it is worth reflecting on the fact that enzyme efflux, which is perhaps the single most compelling argument in favour of a membrane defect, may well be limited to muscle. Enzyme (at least LDH) efflux from erythrocytes and lymphocytes is *not* significantly increased (Somer 1980).

Calcium hypothesis

Around the time that the idea was being seriously considered that a membrane defect might be the underlying cause of Duchenne muscular dystrophy, another idea was also gaining ground. This concerned the possibility that increased intracellular calcium might be a significant factor (Wrogemann and Pena 1976; Duncan 1978). There were a number of lines of evidence which favoured this idea.

There is histochemical and biochemical evidence of increased intracellular calcium in muscle in Duchenne muscular dystrophy, even from a very early age (p. 55), as well as in Becker muscular dystrophy, but apparently to a much lesser degree in other neuromuscular disorders (Table 8.2).

A significant increase in calcium-positive fibres has also been found in male fetuses at-risk for Duchenne muscular dystrophy (Emery and Burt 1980; Bertorini *et al.* 1984) when there is no evidence of muscle fibre necrosis

Table 8.2 *Proportion (%) of calcium-positive fibres in cryostat sections of gastrocnemius muscle biopsy samples in various neuromuscular disorders (unpublished data)*

Disorder	No.	Ca-positive fibres
Controls	7	<0.1
Muscular dystrophies		
Duchenne		
preclinical	2	5.3, 18.3
clinical	5	1.8–6.5
Becker	2	2.4, 5.5
limb girdle	2	–
facioscapulohumeral	2	–
Miscellaneous		
central core disease	2	–
nemaline myopathy	2	–
Werdnig–Hoffmann	2	0.0, 0.2

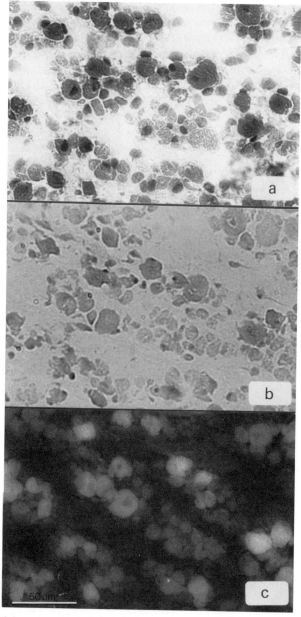

Fig. 8.7. Serial sections of muscle from an at-risk male fetus (B118) stained with (*a*) haematoxylin and eosin (note the dark-staining 'opaque' eosinophilic fibres), (*b*) alizarin red S, (*c*) fluorescent Morin.

(Fig. 8.7). We have examined 54 male fetuses at-risk for the disease with data on calcium-positive fibres in 37. Of these 37, 6 were considered to be affected, there being a good correlation between the presence of calcium-positive fibres and other variables (eosinophilic fibres and increased variance in muscle fibre size) which we have shown probably represent the earliest pathological manifestations of the disease (Toop and Emery 1974; Emery 1977a; Emery *et al.* 1979a) (Table 8.3).

The fact that increased intracellular calcium occurs in at-risk fetuses as early as the second trimester of pregnancy, clearly indicates that this must be a very early and significant biochemical change which precedes muscle fibre necrosis. Increased intracellular calcium could also explain several of the membrane changes which have been reported (references in Emery and Burt 1980). Also the efflux of creatine kinase from skeletal muscle, one of the most consistent features of the disease, can be induced *in vitro* by increasing the concentration of calcium in the incubating medium. The efflux of lactate dehydrogenase and alanine and aspartate aminotransferases is also increased (Anand and Emery 1980).

Finally, increased intracellular calcium might also account for muscle necrosis through the enhancement of calcium-activated proteases (Sugita *et al.* 1984). It might also explain the development of muscle contractures since the binding of calcium to troponin C allows myosin to bind with actin which results in muscle contraction.

However, although increased intracellular calcium is an early and seemingly significant abnormality, it is not likely to be the basic defect since it can occur under a variety of conditions. Normally the concentration of calcium in extracellular fluid is considerably greater than in the cytosol (Fig. 8.8), and therefore any defect in the calcium pump or the cell membrane would automatically result in a massive influx of calcium. For example, increased intracellular calcium has been shown to occur if the Ca^{2+}-ATPase pump is inactivated by an inhibitor, such as phenylhydrazine (Shalev *et al.* 1981), or if ATP is depleted due to anoxia, as in myocardial ischaemia following coronary occlusion (Nayler 1980). In Duchenne muscular dystrophy the increase in intracellular calcium is most likely a consequence of loss of the permeability-barrier of the muscle cell membrane. There then follows enhancement of calcium-activated proteases as well as mitochondrial calcium overload, resulting in a reduction in oxidative phosphorylation and eventually cell death (Fig. 8.9). The dependence of cell death on calcium influx in nicely demonstrated in the study of Schanne *et al.* (1979). These investigators showed that the exposure of rat hepatocytes in short-term culture to a variety of agents known to disrupt cell membranes in one way or another only resulted in cell death if the medium contained calcium (Table 8.4).

Taking into account all these various observations, it seems quite clear that

Table 8.3 *Male fetuses at-risk for Duchenne muscular dystrophy and considered to be abnormal. Values outside the normal range are italicized (unpublished data)*

| | P* | Gestation (weeks) | Fibre Diameter | | Eosinophilic fibres (%) | Ca-positive fibres (%) | |
			Mean (μm)	Variance		(1)	(2)
Controls (16)	–	14–21	6.9–10.7	0.8–3.6	0–5.0	0–3.9	0–7.0
At-risk							
B118	0.90	19	9.6	2.5	*8.0*	*12.0*	*10.5*
B132	0.20	16	10.0	*4.3*	*6.9*	*8.4*	*7.0*
B145	0.50	21	9.4	*5.4*	*9.9*	*6.8*	*7.5*
B150	0.18	12	9.5	3.2	*7.5*	*6.5*	*7.0*
B166	1.00	19	7.9	*4.0*	*6.1*	*4.3*	*7.5*
B188	1.00	20	9.1	*6.1*	*5.3*	*5.4*	*7.3*

* Probability of the mother being a carrier.
(1), alizarin red S; (2), fluorescent Morin.

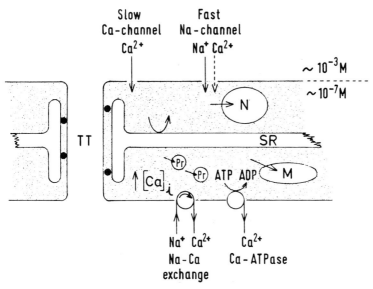

Fig. 8.8. Diagrammatic representation of a muscle cell and the factors which influence the intracellular concentration of calcium. (N, nucleus; M, mitochondria; SR, sarcoplasmic reticulum; TT, transverse tubule.)

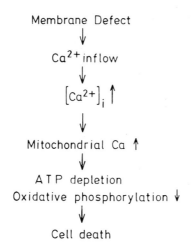

Fig. 8.9. Calcium influx and cell death.

Table 8.4   *Viability (trypan blue exclusion) of rat hepatocytes in short term culture in the presence or absence of calcium in the medium (from Schanne* et al. *1979, with permission)*

Treatment	Viability (%)	
	Medium plus Ca^{2+}	Medium minus Ca^{2+}
None	100 ± 3	101 ± 3
A23187 (ionophore)	6 ± 1	98 ± 5
Lysolecithin	19 ± 1	97 ± 9
Amphotericin B	30 ± 3	98 ± 3
Melittin	46 ± 1	103 ± 6
Phalloidin	38 ± 3	103 ± 5
Methylmethanesulphonate	48 ± 8	99 ± 2
Ethylmethanesulphonate	36 ± 6	106 ± 2
N-Acetoxyacetylaminofluorene	58 ± 3	101 ± 3
Silica	26 ± 9	100 ± 6
Asbestos	45 ± 6	104 ± 11

(Copyright, 1979, by the American Association for the Advancement of Science)

increased muscle intracellular calcium is a very early manifestation of the disease, which eventually triggers off muscle fibre necrosis. It has been suggested that intracellular calcium levels might possibly be increased in skin fibroblasts (Fingerman *et al.* 1984) but using electron probe X-ray micro-analysis we have been unable (Freeman and Emery, unpublished) to detect any consistent abnormality in calcium levels in *single* red cells in affected boys or carriers (Table 8.5), and levels in lymphocytes are normal (Klip *et al.* 1985). There is no evidence that cell death occurs in any tissue other than muscle in Duchenne muscular dystrophy.

'Autoimmune' hypothesis

Although most emphasis in the past has been on the efflux of protein from dystrophic muscle fibres, there is also experimental evidence which indicates that substances may actually *enter* affected muscle fibres (p. 113). Also, histochemical studies have demonstrated that *in vivo* there is ingress not only of calcium but also IgG, complement (Engel and Biesecker 1982), and albumin (Cornelio and Dones 1984). Based on the findings of Cornelio and Dones (1984) as well as our own unpublished data, it would seem that there is first an ingress of calcium and albumin into eosinophilic 'opaque' fibres (Table 8.6). The muscle fibre then begins to undergo necrosis and while still staining for calcium now also becomes positive for complement (Engel *et al.* 1984). This ingress of complement components with their subsequent activa-

Table 8.5 *Mean intracellular calcium concentrations (μmol.ml. cell water^{-1}) in single erythrocytes in healthy controls and affected boys and carriers of Duchenne muscular dystrophy (unpublished data)*

Controls	
females (5)	0.20, 0.46, 0.98, 1.01, 1.38.
males (2)	0.42, 1.56
Duchenne muscular dystrophy	
carriers (3)	0.55, 0.96, 1.52.
affected (5)	0.35, 0.49, 1.30, 1.64, 1.90

Table 8.6 *Histochemical reactions of muscle fibres in Duchenne muscular dystrophy*

	Muscle fibres			
	Normal	Eosinophilic 'opaque'	Necrotic	Regenerating
Calcium	−	+++	+/−	−
Albumin	−	++	++	−
Complement	−	−	+++	−
RNA (acridine orange)	−	−	−	++

tion would accentuate the process of muscle fibre lysis and destruction. Presumably when damage is incomplete, for whatever reason, the muscle fibre may attempt to regenerate which then does not stain for calcium, albumin or complement.

However, the question of fundamental importance is: 'what causes the ingress of calcium and triggers the train of events which eventually leads to necrosis?'. A primary membrane defect provided an attractive explanation but since much of the evidence for this is still controversial the possibility remains that some change in the biochemical composition of the muscle fibre itself may somehow initiate the process. Recent evidence suggests that this might be mediated through an autoimmune process.

It has been recognized for many years that necrotic fibres are invaded by macrophages. However, it has now been shown by immunocytochemical methods using labelled monoclonal antibodies to surface antigens on various mononuclear cells, that many of these are in fact T-cells (Arahata and Engel 1982), a view supported by ultrastructural studies (Fidziańska *et al.* 1984). This then raises the important possibility that cell necrosis may be initiated not from within but by T-cell-mediated injury as appears to occur in polymyositis (Rowe *et al.* 1983; Olsson *et al.* 1984). If membrane breakdown is caused by cytotoxic lymphocytes, then the primary defect could well reside in the muscle fibre itself and, as Engel has stated, '. . . abnormal muscle fibre components in Duchenne muscular dystrophy instigate a secondary autoimmune response' (Engel *et al.* 1984). That is, abnormal muscle fibre components could lead to a change in surface antigens which cytotoxic lymphocytes then recognize as foreign (non-self) and attack the muscle membrane which then results in the ingress of complement and calcium with subsequent fibre necrosis.

Support for this idea comes from the findings of Appleyard *et al.* (1985). These investigators have shown that HLA class I (HLA A, B, and C) antigens are *not* expressed in normal skeletal muscle or in congenital muscular dystrophy or spinal muscular atrophy. However they are expressed in polymyositis and various X-linked muscular dystrophies (Duchenne, Becker, Emery–Dreifuss). They are expressed to a lesser extent in limb girdle and facioscapulohumeral muscular dystrophies (Appleyard *et al.* 1985) and in other forms of dystrophy (Rowe *et al.* 1983). The expression of these surface antigens renders the muscle in these disorders susceptible to T-cell-mediated attack. Since T-cell attack is specific for a particular HLA antigen (see Gomard *et al.* 1986) the identification of the specific antigens being expressed by affected muscle fibres might well give a clue to the nature of the underlying intracellular defect. In any event, the use of immunocytochemical methods for demonstrating the presence or absence of expressed HLA class I antigens might well provide a useful additional diagnostic tool for these disorders.

The idea that a change in a muscle fibre component results in the expression of a surface antigen which then renders the cell susceptible to T-cell attack has a number of important implications. (1) Cell necrosis would be restricted to those tissues which not only express the antigen but are also exposed to possible T-cell attack, such as skeletal and cardiac muscle. It could be that though mononuclear cells may be associated with affected muscle fibres in a fetus (Fidziańska *et al.* 1984), cell destruction does not occur because of 'immaturity' of the immunological system. Also minimal muscle membrane damage at this stage in development is presumably adequate for the ingress of calcium but not for other factors (? complement) which are necessary to produce visible evidence of necrosis. (2) The expression of the genetic defect in an organ which is in an immunologically 'privileged' (protected) position, such as the brain, might interfere with its normal functioning but would not lead to T-cell attack with subsequent cellular necrosis. (3) The genetic defect may well not be expressed at all in some specialzed organs, such as the liver, which would therefore remain healthy. (4) Such a mechanism would explain why full expression of the genetic defect with muscle fibre necrosis does not occur in cultured myoblasts because of the absence in the system of immunologically competent cells, antibodies and complement coponents. The addition of these factors to culture media might possibly result in muscle cell necrosis. (5) It seems inescapable to conclude from these various studies that the basic defect must reside within the muscle fibre itself. That being so, the search should therefore continue for a significant biochemical abnormality in muscle tissue early in the course of the disease, and preferably in preclinical cases or even presumed affected fetuses. Any such abnormality might be expected to have a counterpart in cardiac muscle, brain tissue, and perhaps smooth muscle. Material from all these tissues should therefore be stored in cases which come to autopsy against the day when it can be used to assess the significance of any abnormal biochemical finding in skeletal muscle. It may well be that Duchenne muscular dystrophy is after all an inborn error of metabolism due to some subtle molecular abnormality of a muscle cell protein, or perhaps a glycoprotein as reported by Capaldi *et al.* (1985). Finally, if T-cell attack is a significant factor in muscle cell necrosis in certain forms of muscular dystrophy, possibly some therapeutic value might be obtained with monoclonal antibodies to T-lymphocytes, as has been discussed in general terms by Hohlfeld and Toyka (1985). Such monoclonal antibodies have been shown to induce tolerance to protein antigens in mice (Benjamin and Waldmann 1986).

However despite the obvious attractions of the 'autoimmune hypothesis', it has to be admitted that much of the evidence for it remains largely speculative at the present time.

Summary and conclusions

Over the years many ideas have been put forward as being the basic defect in Duchenne muscular dystrophy. Early theories were often fanciful with little if any supporting evidence. However, more recently several hypotheses have been proposed for which there has been at least some suggestive evidence, even if subsequently this has been shown to be faulty.

The first of these was the *vascular hypothesis* in which it was suggested that the basic abnormality was muscle ischaemia due to involvement of the small muscle vessels within the tissue. The *neurogenic hypothesis* on the other hand proposed that the disorder was due to a deficiency of some trophic neural factor as a result of so-called 'sick motor neurones'. Neither of these hypotheses has survived critical evaluation.

The idea that the disorder could be due to a widespread *membrane defect* caught the imagination when some early studies in the 1970s seemed to support this idea. Unfortunately almost all of the reported abnormalities in cell membranes in the disease have not been reproducible in different laboratories. It remains a possibility but is as yet 'non-proven'.

With regard to the so-called *calcium hypothesis*, there is no doubt that increased intracellular calcium in muscle tissue is an important and early biochemical feature of Duchenne muscular dystrophy. It is found not only in preclinical cases but also in presumed affected fetuses as early as the second trimester of pregnancy and precedes muscle fibre necrosis. However, for various reasons this is not likely to be the basic defect.

What does seem likely is that some change in muscle intracellular components leads to a change in surface antigens which cytotoxic T-lymphocytes then recognize as foreign (non-self) and attack the muscle membrane with all the consequent effects thereof. Recent evidence indicates that only dystrophic muscle fibres express HLA class I antigens on their surface, and that a proportion of the mononuclear cells associated with affected muscle fibres are in fact T-cells. There are several important implications of this *autoimmune hypothesis* including the possibility that Duchenne muscular dystrophy may after all be an inborn error of metabolism due to some subtle molecular abnormality of a muscle cell protein which results in changes in the antigenic properties of the cell surface.

9 Genetics

The familial nature of Duchenne muscular dystrophy was noted very early on by both Meryon (1852, 1864) and Gowers (1879b). In fact, as we have seen (p. 19), Gowers recognized that the disorder was limited to males and transmitted by healthy females, a mode of inheritance now recognized to be that of an X-linked recessive trait (Fig. 9.1).

Mode of inheritance

Evidence of X-linked recessive inheritance includes not only the typical pedigree pattern but also occasional female heterozygous carriers have had affected sons by different husbands. However, neither of these observations excludes the possibility that the disorder could be inherited as an autosomal dominant trait which is expressed only in males, so-called sex-limitation. But two lines of evidence refute this. First, the disorder has been recorded in females with XO Turner's syndrome (Walton 1957), XO mosaicism (Ferrier *et al.* 1965; Jalbert *et al.* 1966; Averyanov *et al.* 1977), or with a structurally abnormal X-chromosome (Berg and Conte 1974). Secondly, statistical evidence indicates that the proportion of cases due to new mutations more closely resembles that expected for an X-linked recessive trait than for an autosomal dominant trait with male limitation (Morton and Chung 1959). However, until relatively recently the disease locus did not appear to be

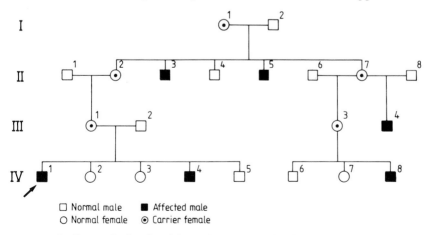

Fig. 9.1. Pedigree of a family with Duchenne muscular dystrophy.

within measurable distance of other known X-linked loci. No linkage was found with the Xg blood group locus, located at the end of the short arm (Clark *et al.* 1963; Blyth *et al.* 1965; Filippi and Macciotta; 1967), or with the loci for colour blindness (Emery 1966; Greig 1977), or G6PD (Zatz *et al.* 1974) which are closely linked to each other (Porter *et al.* 1962) and located toward the end of the long arm of the X-chromosome. But more recently, using DNA probes (Murray *et al.* 1982; Davies *et al.* 1983) as well as other information, the disease locus has now been shown to be located on the short arm of the X-chromosome around the position Xp21 (p. 167).

Penetrance

There have been occasional reports that the gene for Duchenne muscular dystrophy may not always be fully penetrant and that not all males hemizygous for the mutant gene may manifest the disease. For example, Thompson and her colleagues (1962) described two large families with Duchenne muscular dystrophy in which the gene appeared to the non-penetrant in certain males. In one family described in detail, a healthy brother of a known carrier had a daughter with an affected son. However, it is possible that the affected boy's mother was not a carrier and that her son was the result of a new mutation. Although two different mutations occurring in the same large family would be extremely uncommon, it is possible.

There have also been reports of minor abnormalities in muscle histology, electromyography, total body potassium, and urinary amino acids in some unaffected male relatives of affected boys. However, many of these findings were non-specific and based on few results, and they are therefore of doubtful significance. More importantly, several early studies indicated that a proportion of clinically unaffected male relatives of affected boys had slightly elevated SCK levels (reviewed in Emery and Spikesman 1970a, b), raising the possibility that these might represent subclinical cases of the disease. Unfortunately, in most of the these studies very few relatives were investigated and information on control values was rarely given. We investigated the problem in detail by studying 101 first degree male relatives of patients with Duchenne and Becker types of muscular dystrophy and in an equal number of age-matched healthy male controls. We found that around the same proportion of males in both groups had *slightly* elevated SCK levels. We concluded that an elevated SCK level in a male relative (excluding preclinical cases) is unrelated to muscular dystrophy. There is no evidence that this represents either a subclinical form of X-linked Duchenne muscular dystrophy or the heterozygous state of the autosomal recessive limb girdle form of muscular dystrophy occurring in childhood (Emery and Spikesman 1970a, b).

More recently, complex segregation analysis in a large number of families with the disease also indicates that the gene for Duchenne muscular dystrophy is always fully penetrant (Williams *et al.* 1983).

Heterozygous advantage and fetal loss

Of theoretical importance in Duchenne muscular dystrophy is whether heterozygous carriers exhibit increased reproductive fitness, and if there is increased prenatal or perinatal mortality which might be a reflection of an early manifestation of the disease. Evidence on both these points is still scanty and largely anecdotal.

With regard to the possibility that carriers might have larger families than normal, Danieli *et al.* (1980) found in their study that the mean family size of carriers was 5.38 ± 0.30 compared with 3.98 ± 0.24 in normal women (on the paternal side of the carriers' families), a difference which was statistically significant. However, in such studies there is always a problem of ascertainment: that at least some women may not have been designated as carriers until they had had at least one son who was affected. There are also theoretical reasons for doubting that significant heterozygous advantage occurs in any X-linked recessive disorder which is highly deleterious (Skolnick *et al.* 1977).

Danieli and colleagues (1980) in their extensive studies in Venetia (Italy) have suggested that the spontaneous abortion and male stillbirth rates in families with Duchenne muscular dystrophy may be increased. An apparent excess of male infant deaths was also observed by Lane *et al.* (1983). These interesting observations await further confirmation in other large population studies.

Incidence

In order to determine the frequency of the responsible gene and its rate of mutation it is necessary to determine the population frequency of the disorder. This information is also essential in order to determine if various preventive measures are being effective, and to help in the planning of adequate resources and welfare services for affected families.

Incidence refers to the number of *new* cases per unit of population. Prevalence on the other hand refers to *all* cases present in the population, either within a given period (so-called period prevalence rate) or at a particular point in time (so-called point prevalence rate) per unit of population at-risk at that time. In the case of Duchenne muscular dystrophy prevalence, particularly after early childhood, would be less than the true incidence at birth because of increasing mortality.

Since the disorder is not clinically recognizable at birth, birth incidence is usually derived from knowing the number of normal boys born in the same years that affected boys were born. However, a small proportion of normal boys may die by the age affected boys are diagnosed. It has therefore been argued that incidence should perhaps be related not to the number of normal live births but rather to the number of normal children who survive to the age affected boys are diagnosed. But some affected boys may also die before clinical manifestations become evident. The best compromise seems to be to calculate incidence from the assumed frequency at birth as a proportion of all births.

Incidence may also be derived from prevalence by taking into account the probability of ascertaining affected individuals in the population and the probability of an individual developing the disease by a given age (Morton and Chung 1959; Yasuda and Kondo 1980).

Some estimates of the incidence in 26 studies in various countries are given in Table 9.1. The estimates vary considerably from 130 to 390 per million male births. There are differences between different countries and even within a single country such as the United Kingdom or Italy. In Israel there appears to be a considerable difference in frequency between non-Ashkenazis and Ashkenazis (Kott *et al.* 1973).

Despite increasing awareness of the disease in recent years there has been no apparent increase in reported incidences (Fig. 9.2). It could be that in the past any inflation by the inclusion of other forms of dystrophy and perhaps even spinal muscular atrophy, has been balanced in more recent studies by improved ascertainment of true cases. The overall incidence based on nearly

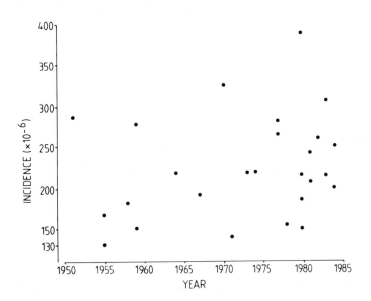

Fig. 9.2. Incidence of Duchenne muscular dystrophy and the years of reporting ($r = 0.23, P > 0.05$).

Table 9.1 *Estimates of incidence of Duchenne muscular dystrophy in various countries*

| Region | Period | Number | | Incidence ($\times 10^{-6}$) | Reference |
		Affected	Total		
Australia					
Victoria	1957–63	49	223 330	219	Lawrence et al. (1973)
NSW	1960–71	99	532 302	186	Cowan et al. (1980)
Canada					
Alberta	1950–74	110	420 374	262	Monckton et al. (1982)
Germany					
Südbaden	1918–32	21	125 000	168	Becker (1980); reported originally in 1955
Erfurt	1958–73	51	165 898	307	Spiegler & Herrmann (1983)
Italy*					
Venetia	1959–68	66	234 369	282	Danieli et al. (1977)
Piedmont	1955–74	73	301 283	242	Schiffer et al. (1981)
Emilia	1951–75	24	61 470	390	Lucci (1980)
Sud Tyrol	1960–75	8	39 980	200	Danieli (1984)
Campania	1960–71	156	721 163	216	Nigro et al. (1983)
Puglia	1956–75	121	805 335	150	Ferrari et al. (1980)
Japan					
Fukuoka	1949–58	9	46 465	194	Kuroiwa & Miyazaki (1967)
Chiba†	1979	–	–	217	Yasuda & Kondo (1980)
Netherlands					
Groningen	1963–74	357	1 420 962	251	van Essen & ten Kate (1984)
Poland					
Warsaw	1953–60	46	328 110	140	Prot (1971)
Rumania††	1961–68	214	1 387 694	154	Radu & Sarközi (1978)
Switzerland					
Bern	1939–54	26	119 395	218	Moser et al. (1964)

Table 9.1 *Cont'd*

Region	Period	Number		Incidence ($\times 10^{-6}$)	Reference
		Affected	Total		
UK					
England (NE)	1940–46	18	138 403	130	Walton (1955)
England (NE)††	1952–60	77	236 200	326	Gardner-Medwin (1970)
England (Midlands)	1939–49	7	46 210	151	Blyth & Pugh (1959)
England (Midlands)**	1976	27	110 434	244	Bundey (1981)
Scotland (SE)	1953–68	47	177 413	265	Brooks & Emery (1977)
Northern Ireland	1942–51	28	153 692	182	Stevenson (1958)
USA					
Utah	1931–41	18	63 000	286	Stephens & Tyler (1951)
Wisconsin†	1959	51	–	279	Morton & Chung (1959)
Colorado	1974	51	–	220	Lubs (1974)
	Total	*1652*	*7 858 482*	*210 ± 5*	*(mean ± SE)*

* Estimates for other regions given in Danieli (1984).
† Estimated from prevalence rate.
†† Boys attaining age 5.
** Prevalence in schoolboys.

8 million male births is $210 \pm 5 \times 10^{-6}$, or one case in 4762 male births. However, this figure includes several seemingly abnormally low estimates.

The birth incidence of the disease can also be determined by screening for raised SCK levels in the neonatal period and subsequently confirming the diagnosis by muscle biopsy (Guibaud *et al.* 1981). This subject will be discussed in more detail later (p. 181), but from the present point of view the overall incidence from these studies is $241 \pm 30 \times 10^{-6}$ (Table 9.2). However, in one of these studies the figure may be somewhat inflated by the inclusion of families who volunteered for screening, sometimes because a member of the family had been affected already. On the other hand, in a limited but very carefully controlled study of *every* male birth in a single maternity hospital (Skinner *et al.* 1982) the incidence was comparable.

At present it is really not possible to say if there are any significant differences within countries or even between different countries because of the confounding effects of variations in ascertainment. Certainly the incidences in two Japanese studies are roughly the same as values obtained in several European countries. Although certain types of consanguinity may result in an increase in female homozygosity for X-linked loci, such inbreeding has no effect on gene frequency *per se* and therefore would have no effect on the incidence of a disorder such as Duchenne muscular dystrophy. In certain communities reproductive compensation, whereby families reproduce until they have a healthy male offspring, could conceivably lead to an increase in incidence (Templeton and Yokoyama 1980). On the other hand, preventive measures, such as family limitation and prenatal diagnosis, might be expected to lead to a reduction in incidence. Otherwise incidence will depend

Table 9.2 *Incidence of Duchenne muscular dystrophy derived from various neonatal screening programmes*

Region	Period	Number Affected	Number Total	Incidence ($\times 10^{-6}$)	Reference
France	1975–78	12	71 091	169	Dellamonica *et al.* (1983)
Germany (voluntary)	1977–84	48	176 600	272	Scheuerbrandt *et al.* (1986)
New Zealand	1978	2	10 000	200	Drummond and Veale (1978); Drummond (1979)
Scotland	1976–81	1	3 356	298	Skinner *et al.* (1982 and unpublished)
Total		*63*	*261 047*	*241 ± 30*	*(mean ± SE)*

on the rate at which new mutations occur, and this is likely to be similar throughout the world.

Changes in incidence in recent years

In recent years and perhaps more so in future, some reduction in the incidence of Duchenne muscular dystrophy might be expected as a result of several factors.

Beginning in the 1950s there was an increase in interest in genetic counselling, and the mid-1960s saw the advent of carrier detection tests. Later, prenatal fetal sexing became possible so that a mother who was at high risk of having an affected son could request selective abortion of any male fetus in any subsequent pregnancy. Finally, in the very recent past prenatal diagnosis of affected male fetuses has become possible by the use of DNA probes (p. 208). Although this latter development is too recent to have had any significant effect on incidence, genetic counselling and carrier detection studies in affected families might be predicted to have resulted in some reduction in incidence. Evidence on this point however is still not entirely clear. Hurse and Kakulas (1974) claim there has been a decrease in Perth, Australia, over the period 1950–69. However, latterly there was a decrease in isolated cases with no family history which can only mean that ascertainment may not have been complete. Some boys may have developed the disease subsequent to the completion of the study. Monckton and colleagues (1982) also noted an apparent decrease in incidence in the latter part of their study period (1970–74) and concluded that this might be due to some potential cases having been born during this period but which had not yet been diagnosed.

In these sorts of studies it is therefore important that the period covered should be such that there is a reasonable chance that all potential cases are likely to have developed clinical manifestations and to have been diagnosed. As a test of the completeness of the study, and provided the population itself remains the same, the number of isolated cases should remain unchanged. In the South East of Scotland, a small and well defined region which is well endowed with medical and genetic services, no familial cases have been reported since 1969, presumably as a result of genetic counselling, whereas the number of isolated cases has remained more or less the same (Table 9.3). Somewhat similar findings have been reported in Wales (Harper 1982).

Mutation rate

The rate at which the gene causing Duchenne muscular dystrophy mutates may be estimated either indirectly or directly.

Table 9.3 *Incidence of Duchenne muscular dystrophy in the South East of Scotland*

Period	Number Affected	Total	Incidence ($\times 10^{-6} \pm$ SE)
1953–56	12	41 254	291 ± 84
1957–60	9	44 347	203 ± 68
1961–64	13	46 300	281 ± 78
1965–68	13	45 512	286 ± 79
1969–72	10	41 118	243 ± 77
1973–76	9	40 358	223 ± 74

Indirect estimation of mutation rate

For any X-linked recessive disorder (Haldane, 1935) if the reproductive fitness of affected individuals is f, and the incidence of the disease is I, then the mutation rate is:

$$= \frac{1}{3} I (1 - f)$$

However, in Duchenne muscular dystrophy biological fitness is zero because affected boys do not procreate. Therefore the mutation rate is given by $I/3$. If the incidence of the disorder assumed to be around 240 to 300 $\times$ 10^{-6}, then the mutation rate is around 80 to 100 $\times$ 10^{-6} genes per generation.

Direct estimation of mutation rate

In the direct method an attempt is made to estimate the actual number of new mutations among isolated cases. If a out of b known female carriers have an abnormal SCK level, then the detection rate of carriers is a/b. If n isolated cases are born in a given period among N males born in the same period, and if c is the number of mothers of these n males who have an *abnormal* SCK level, then among these isolated cases (subject to sampling error) the number of *new* mutations will be:

$$n - \frac{bc}{a}$$

and therefore the mutation rate is:

$$\frac{\left(n - \dfrac{bc}{a} \right)}{N}$$

In one study (Gardner-Medwin 1970), 22 out of 35 known carriers had raised

SCK levels. Of 56 mothers of isolated cases, 15 had raised levels. Thus the proportion of new mutations (mothers are non-carriers) among isolated cases is:

$$\frac{[56 - (35/22)\,15]}{56}$$
$$= 0.574$$

Over a 9-year period (1952–60), 43 isolated cases were born and therefore the number of new mutations is:

$$(43)\,(0.574)$$
$$= 24.682$$

The total number of males born in this period who survived to age 5 (by which time almost all cases of Duchenne muscular dystrophy are diagnosed) was 236 200. Thus the mutation rate is:

$$\frac{24.682}{236\ 200}$$
$$= 105 \times 10^{-6}$$

The estimates of the mutation rate by both these methods are considerably greater than values obtained for other X-linked disorders (Vogel 1983). For comparison some representative values for various genetic disorders are

Table 9.4 *Average estimates of mutation rates for various genetic disorders (data from various sources)*

Disorder	Mutation rate ($\times 10^{-6}$)
Autosomal dominants	
Achondroplasia	10
Retinoblastoma	8
Tuberous sclerosis	8
Polyposis coli	13
Neurofibromatosis	70
Huntington's chorea	5
Myotonic dystrophy	10
Autosomal recessives	
Albinism	28
Total colour blindness	28
Phenylketonuria	25
X-linked recessives	
Haemophilia A	32–57
Haemophilia B	2–3
Duchenne muscular dystrophy	80–100

given in Table 9.4. The only disorder with a comparable mutation rate appears to be neurofibromatosis.

Parental age and mutation rate

In X-linked recessive disorders possible effects of maternal or paternal age on mutation rates can be assessed separately by considering respectively *maternal* age in the case of mutant males, and *maternal grandfather's* age in the case of mutant heterozygous mothers. The latter are mothers with no affected relatives other than sons (or have only one affected son but a significantly elevated SCK level) where the new mutation can have occurred in the X-chromosome she inherited from her father (Penrose 1955).

None of the studies which have considered this problem have found any significant increase in the age of mothers of presumed new mutants (Hutton and Thompson 1970; Pellié *et al.* 1973; Emery 1977b; Becker 1980; Yasuda and Kondo 1982).

With regard to presumed mutant heterozygous mothers, the mean ages of both grandparents at the birth of these mothers can be compared with the mean ages of the mothers' spouses' parents at the birth of their spouse. In one study the mean maternal grandfather's age seemed ($P = 0.05$) greater than expected from appropriate demographic data (Emery 1977b). Furthermore, in this study and in two others (Becker 1980; Yasuda and Kondo 1982) the mean maternal grandfather's age was greater than the mean paternal grandfather's age (Table 9.5), but the differences were not statistically significant.

If there is any paternal age effect on the mutation rate in this disorder it would seem to be negligible. The results of these studies do not support the idea that the mutation rate in males is significantly different from females.

Sex difference in mutation rate

It can be shown that if a mother has an affected son but no one else in the family is affected, then the probability of her being a carrier is:

$$\frac{\mu + \nu}{2\mu + \nu}$$

where μ = mutation rate in female germ cells,
and ν = mutation rate in male germ cells.

The probability that she is *not* a carrier and that the son is therefore a new mutation is:

$$1 - \frac{\mu + \nu}{2\mu + \nu}$$

$$= \frac{\mu}{2\mu + \nu}$$

Table 9.5 *Ages of grandparents of cases of Duchenne muscular dystrophy where the mother is presumed to be a mutant heterozygote*

MGF			PGF				MGM			PGM				Reference
No.	Mean	s.d.	No.	Mean	s.d.	Difference	No.	Mean	s.d.	No.	Mean	s.d.	Difference	
26	34.3	6.14	22	30.9	6.42	+3.4	26	30.5	4.87	24	27.8	5.47	+2.7	Emery (1977b)
15	35.1	7.03	15	31.4	6.43	+3.7	14	30.4	6.63	16	27.4	5.48	+3.0	Becker (1980)
82	34.4	7.33	81	33.9	7.56	+0.5	82	30.3	7.06	82	29.0	6.07	+1.3	Yasuda & Kondo (1982)

MGF, maternal grandfather; PGF, paternal grandfather; MGM, maternal grandmother; PGM, paternal grandmother.

which represents the proportion of new mutants, often designated as 'x' (Haldane 1956). If the mutation rates are the same in both males and females then x is a third; if mutations occurred more frequently in the male then x approaches zero; and if mutations occurred more frequently in the female then x approaches a half.

This is not just of academic importance because if mutations were found to occur exclusively in the male then all mothers with an affected son would be carriers, and this would be important in genetic counselling.

Several different methods have been devised for estimating x and these have been detailed by Moser (1984). Essentially there are three approaches:
(1) analysis of sibships (method of Haldane (1956), a modification of this (C), and an independent method (B) by Cheeseman *et al.* (1958), methods of Morton (1959) involving complex segregation analysis (Morton 1969) as well as maximum likelihood methods);
(2) sex ratio of unaffected sibs (Davie and Emery, 1978); and
(3) methods based on the results of carrier detection tests.

The statistical methods used in sibship analysis are somewhat complex and details are given in the relevant publications.

With regard to the sex ratio method, this is independent of ascertainment, and is based on the assumption that among offspring of a *carrier* affected boys, unaffected boys and girls will, on average, occur in the ratio 1:1:2. Therefore the sex ratio (M:F) among unaffected sibs will be 1:2 (or 1:1.89 if corrected for the deviation of the sex ratio from 1). However among the sibs of *new mutants* the sex ratio will be 1:1 (or 1:0.94 if corrected). The proportion of new mutants among isolated cases can be estimated by determining the sex ratio among the sibs of isolated cases.

Finally, with regard to carrier detection methods, this has usually been based on comparing the proportion of abnormal test results (the most reliable being the SCK level) in known carriers with mothers of isolated cases. Thus if:

i = proportion of mothers of isolated cases with an elevated SCK level;
d = proportion of known carriers with an elevated SCK level; and
P_i = proportion of isolated cases among all cases assuming *complete ascertainment* in a given population; then
$x = (1 - i/d) P_i$ (Moser, 1984).

There are also more sophisticated methods for tackling this problem (Winter 1980). Some representative values are given in Table 9.6, from which it will be seen that the 95 per cent confidence limits ($x \pm 1.96$ SE) of almost all these estimates would accommodate a value of 0.33 which assumes that mutation rates are equal in males and females. However, occasionally significantly lower values have been obtained, particularly with carrier detection methods other than SCK levels. But in these cases the value of the methods

Table 9.6 *Estimation of the proportion (x) of new mutants in Duchenne muscular dystrophy. Values have been rounded off to two decimal places*

Method	x ± SE	Reference
Sibship analysis		
Haldane	0.51 ± 0.08*	Cheeseman *et al.* (1958)
	0.52 ± 0.10†	
Cheeseman (B)	0.39 ± 0.16*	
	0.37 ± 0.19†	
Cheeseman (C)	0.34 ± 0.14*	
	0.40 ± 0.18†	
Maximum likelihood	0.32 ± 0.14*	Smith & Kilpatrick (1958)
	0.39 ± 0.17†	
Morton	0.35 ± 0.05	Morton & Chung (1959)
Haldane	0.29 ± 0.07	Danieli *et al.* (1980)
Cheeseman (B)	0.22 ± 0.08	
Cheeseman (C)	0.19 ± 0.07	
Maximum likelihood	0.29 ± 0.05	Yasuda and Kondo (1980)
Morton (modified)	0.17 ± 0.08	Bucher *et al.* (1980)
Cheeseman (B)	0.13 ± 0.11	Lane *et al.* (1983)
Segregation analysis	0.27 ± 0.08	Williams *et al.* (1983)
Maximum likelihood	0.23 ± 0.05	Danieli & Barbujani (1984)
Sex ratio in sibs		
	0.44 ± 0.12††	Davie and Emery (1978)
	0.32 ± 0.12**	
	0.23 ± 0.20††	Bucher *et al.* (1980)
Carrier detection		
(based on SCK)	0.32 ± 0.05	Gardner–Medwin (1970)
	0.32 ± 0.06	Moser (1971, 1977)
	0.12 ± 0.04	Roses *et al.* (1977)
	0.28 ± 0.04	Davie & Emery (1978)
	0.30 ± 0.09§	
	0.34 ± 0.06 (est.)	Caskey *et al.* (1980)
	0.12 ± 0.03	Danieli *et al.* (1980)
	0.35 ± 0.03	Zatz (1986)

* Northern Ireland data (Stevenson 1958).
† Utah data (Stephens and Tyler 1951).
†† Uncorrected, or ** corrected.
§ pedigree *and* SCK data.

used for detecting carriers (serum LDH–5 (Roses *et al.* 1977), lymphocyte capping (Pickard *et al.* 1978), and polyribosomal protein synthesis (Bucher *et al.* 1980)) have been questioned, and it is possible that they could lead to an excess of false positive results and thereby overestimate the proportion of carriers among mothers of isolated cases.

The increasing election by mothers, after the birth of an affected son, of family limitation and selective abortion of male fetuses in future pregnancies, may well invalidate the assumptions underlying these various approaches. These practices will lead to an increasing proportion of isolated cases and a decreasing sex ratio (M:F) in subsequent sibs. The study of DNA markers within families of isolated cases will eventually provide a definitive answer to this problem (p. 178). However, even now the evidence would seem overwhelmingly in favour of the mutation rate in Duchenne muscular dystrophy being essentially the same in both males and females.

So far it has been assumed that all cases result from a mutation in the germ cells. But if the male twins discordant for Duchenne muscular dystrophy reported by de Grouchy *et al.* (1963) were in fact identical, as the authors stated, then this raises the possibility that mutations may also occur at an early cell division *after* conception when the affected individual would then be a mosaic. There is no evidence at present as to whether such somatic mutations occur and lead to clinical disease.

Genetic heterogeneity

The concensus view is that Duchenne muscular dystrophy is a well defined and homogeneous disorder. However, we have seen already that there is a wide spectrum of clinical severity (see Chapter 3). Furthermore, the very high incidence of the disorder cannot be accounted for by heterozygous advantage (Skolnick *et al.* 1977), and seems more likely to be due to genetic heterogeneity with mutations at different loci, or at different points in the same locus or region of DNA, contributing to the clinical disorder.

Correlations between relatives regarding age at onset and of becoming confined to a wheelchair have also been interpreted as indicating heterogeneity (Feingold *et al.* 1971). In addition, Samaha and Congedo (1977) have reported two different patterns of muscle sarcoplasmic reticulum membrane proteins in affected boys, and Cohen *et al.* (1982) have shown that decay rates in muscle strength in affected boys are not homogeneous but may be bimodally distributed. Finally, we found that in affected boys with *severe* mental handicap (IQ < 50), the age at onset and of becoming confined to a wheelchair was somewhat later; the fall in SCK levels with age less marked; and the urinary excretion of certain amino acids somewhat greater than in a group of carefully *matched* affected boys with normal intelligence (Emery *et al.* 1979b). It was suggested that perhaps affected boys with *severe* mental

Table 9.7 *Age at onset and of becoming confined to a wheelchair in patients with normal intelligence (N) or with severe mental handicap (MH)*

	Onset							Chairbound							Reference
	N			MH				N			MH				
No.	Mean	s.d.	No.	Mean	s.d.	P	No.	Mean	s.d.	No.	Mean	s.d.	P	
15	2.20	0.78	15	2.43	1.03	NS	12	8.77	1.12	13	9.65	1.60	NS	Emery et al. (1979b)
29	3.64	1.72	10	3.61	2.01	NS	24	9.49	1.70	11	10.83	1.65	<0.05	Bortolini & Zatz (1986)

handicap might possibly represent a small subgroup of patients genetically distinct from most other patients with the disease. It was not suggested that the presence or absence of lesser degrees of mental handicap could be a criterion for dividing patients into different genetic groups because this is obviously not valid. Bortolini and Zatz (1986) have also examined the possibility of genetic heterogeneity on the basis of various clinical criteria and SCK levels in affected boys with normal intelligence or severe mental handicap. They felt their data did not reveal any evidence of heterogeneity though boys with severe mental handicap did become confined to a wheel-chair somewhat later than boys with normal intelligence. Comparable data from these two studies are summarized in Table. 9.7.

It seems, however, that this problem is unlikely to be resolved by simply considering various clinical criteria. Perhaps as the molecular pathology of the disease becomes clear it will be possible to compare various clinical and biochemical parameters in those with one molecular defect (say a gene deletion) with those with a different defect (Griggs *et al.* 1986). In any event it seems clear already that heterogeneity exists at the molecular level (p. 178).

Summary and conclusions

Evidence from various sources, including pedigree studies, affected girls with X-chromosome abnormalities, and statistical methods show that Duchenne muscular dystrophy is inherited as an X-linked recessive trait. The mutant gene is always fully penetrant and a subclinical, as opposed to a preclinical, form of the disease does not exist. There is a suggestion that the rates of spontaneous abortion and male stillbirths may be increased in affected families, but this requires further evaluation. Estimates of the incidence of the disorder, based on population surveys and neonatal screening, vary but are probably around 240 to 300 $\times$ 10^{-6}, or just under 1 in 4000 live male births. This puts the mutation rate at around 80 to 100 $\times$ 10^{-6} genes per generation which is considerably greater than any other X-linked disorder. A possible difference in mutation rates in male and female germ cells has been studied by considering maternal and grandpaternal age effects, as well as the proportion of isolated cases which could be due to new mutations. The results of these investigations indicate that the mutation rates in male and female germ cells do not differ significantly and that one-third of isolated cases of the disease are due to new mutations.

Finally, the wide spectrum of clinical severity, the high mutation rate, and correlations between relatives, suggest that there may be genetic heterogeneity. At present this problem cannot be resolved satisfactorily on the basis of clinical criteria alone, although it seems clear already that heterogeneity exists at the molecular level (see Chapter 10).

10 Molecular pathology

In order to unravel the molecular pathology of a disease where the basic bio-chemical defect is unknown, various approaches are possible. These have been detailed elsewhere (Emery 1985). Logically, and certainly the way research has progressed in the case of Duchenne muscular dystrophy, the following steps are usually involved. First, the gene has to be localized to a specific chromosome and then to a particular site on the chromosome. Secondly, armed with such information DNA markers can be selected which are located in this particular region of the chromosome and if they prove to be closely linked to the disease locus they can be used *indirectly* for carrier detection and prenatal diagnosis (p. 199). Thirdly, it may be possible, using molecular techniques, to 'walk the genome' from the DNA markers toward the mutant gene so as to eventually include the gene itself. As will be seen, however, there are several other strategies being pursued to isolated the Duchenne locus. Fourthly, having isolated the gene, or at least part of it, this can then be used as a 'gene-specific' probe for *direct* prenatal diagnosis and carrier detection. Finally, having isolated the gene then it will be possible by DNA sequencing and *in vitro* protein synthesis to define the nature of the molecular defect and its product. Each of these steps will be described, although much of the detail is really outside the scope of this book and is furnished in the relevant bibliography.

Localization of the Duchenne gene

An early clue as to the specific location of the Duchenne locus came from the study of rare cases of a Duchenne-like disorder in girls. The first cases were described in 1977 (Greenstein *et al.* 1977; Verellen *et al.* 1977), but there were soon many others. The salient features of some published cases are summarized in Table 10.1, although several others have been discussed. In each case the findings have been consistent with the diagnosis of a muscular dystrophy with grossly elevated SCK levels and myopathic changes on electromyography (EMG) and muscle pathology. Most have been clinically similar to Duchenne muscular dystrophy although in some cases the disorder seemed less severe and perhaps more like Becker muscular dystrophy. Some have been mentally retarded. All, however, have had a reciprocal transloca-tion between an autosome and the X-chromosome, and since these are balanced translocations with no apparent loss of chromosomal material these girls might have been expected to be normal. In such X/autosome translocations however it is the normal X which tends to be preferentially inactivated, with the result that genes on the derived (der) X are expressed. It could therefore be that the mothers of these girls were heterozygous carriers and the maternal X-chromosome carrying the mutant gene was involved in the translocation. However, this is unlikely because in only two instances (Canki *et al.* 1979; Verellen-Dumoulin *et al.* 1984) has there been any suggestion that the mother *might* be a carrier, and at least in one of these this now seems very unlikely (Verellen-Dumoulin 1986). Also the parents of these girls have had normal chromosomes and we are therefore left to conclude that both the translocation as well as the disease must have arisen *de novo* in the affected girls.

Since different autosomes were involved in the translocations but the breakpoint on the X-chromosome was always *in the region of Xp21*, the most likely explanation is that the translocation in some way disrupted the normal gene at Xp21 which then resulted in the disease. The mutant gene is therefore presumed to be located at this point on the X-chromosome (Fig. 10.1). X/autosome translocations involving this region of the X-chromosome have occasionally been described in which muscular dystrophy was *apparently* not

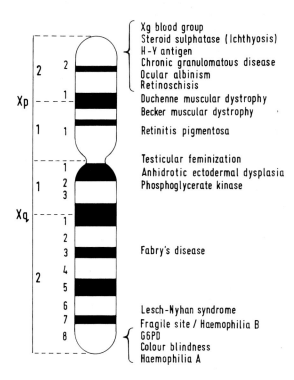

Fig. 10.1. Simplified gene map of the X-chromosome and its banding pattern.

Table 10.1 *Summary of some salient features in girls with a Duchenne-like disorder and various X/autosome translocations*

Autosome breakpoint	Parents' karyotype	Parental ages Maternal	Paternal	Probability mother is a carrier	Age Onset	Chairbound	At reporting
11q13	N	NR	NR	SCK normal	NR	NR	16 yrs
21p12	N	21	25	SCK normal	2 yrs	–	20 yrs
3q13	N	28	40	Possibly a carrier on SCK and EMG but no details	10 mths, generalized hypotonia	–	45 mths
1p34 (+ inversion)	N	NR	NR	$P = 0.01$	Walked at 15 mths, but unsteady	8 yrs	8 yrs
5q35	N	39	39	SCK normal	4 yrs	–	9 yrs
6q21	N (mother)	29	26	$P = 0.06$	5 yrs	10 yrs	$11\frac{1}{2}$ yrs
11q23	N	NR	NR	SCK normal	?	–	13 yrs
9p22	N	18	22	SCK normal	<2 yrs	–	9 yrs
2q36	N	NR	NR	NR	19 mths, generalized hypotonia and delayed milestones	Requires assistance in walking	14 yrs
6q16	N	NR	NR	SCK normal	<3 yrs	–	$4\frac{1}{2}$ yrs
9p21	N	NR	NR	SCK normal	<2 yrs	12 yrs	Died at 23
8q24	N	25	29	SCK normal	2–3 yrs	–	6 yrs
4q26	N	NR	NR	SCK normal	2 yrs	–	3 yrs
5q31	N	20	23	SCK normal	$2\frac{1}{2}$ yrs	–	$6\frac{1}{2}$ yrs
15q26	N	31	34	SCK normal	4–5 yrs	–	$9\frac{2}{3}$ yrs

N, normal; NR, not recorded; MH, mentally handicapped; ?, not clear.

a feature (for example, Laurent *et al.* 1975). However, the region identified by studies of banded chromosomes covers a relatively large segment of DNA and is likely to involve loci other than Duchenne muscular dystrophy.

There is considerable variation in clinical severity in girls with X/autosome translocations and a Duchenne-like disorder. It seems possible that the phenotype may well depend on the proportion of cells in which the der X is presumably active. The milder the phenotype the lower the proportion of cells in which the active X-chromosome is the der X, and therefore the greater the proportion of cells in which the active X-chromosome is the normal X. For example, the proportion of cells in which the active X is the der X is somewhat lower in two cases considered to be mild (Verellen-Doumoulin *et al.* 1984; Narazaki *et al.* 1985). Alternatively it could be that in these milder

Severity	IQ	Active der X (%)		Comment	Reference
		Fibroblasts	Lymphocytes		
?	NR	NR	NR	–	Greenstein *et al.* (1977, 1980)
Mild	N	95	93	–	Verellen *et al.* (1977, 1978)
					Verellen-Dumoulin *et al.* (1984)
					Verellen-Dumoulin (1986)
? Severe	MH	–	93	Certain dysmorphic features (hypertelorism, facial assymetry, etc.)	Canki *et al.* (1979)
Severe	N	–	100	–	Lindenbaum *et al.* (1979)
Severe	N	100	98	–	Jacobs *et al.* (1981)
Severe	N	–	98	–	Zatz *et al.* (1981a)
? Mild	N	–	?	–	Bjerglund Nielsen *et al.* (1983)
? Severe	MH	–	99	–	Emanuel *et al.* (1983)
? Severe	MH	NR	NR	Course has fluctuated with SCK ranging from normal to 27 000 iu	MacLeod *et al.* (1983)
? Severe	NR	NR	NR	–	Perez Vidal *et al.* (1983)
Severe	MH	–	100	Idiopathic ketonic hypoglycaemia; epilepsy and features of Turner's syndrome	Bjerglund Nielsen & Nielsen (1984)
Mild	N	98	75	–	Narazaki *et al.* (1985)
?	?	–	100	–	Saito *et al.* (1985)
Severe	MH	–	100	–	Nevin *et al.* (1986)
? Severe	N	95	93	–	Ribeiro *et al.* (1986)

cases the translocation has interrupted the chromosomal region concerned with Becker muscular dystrophy.

X/autosome translocations involving other breakpoints on the X-chromosome have also been described. In these cases as well the expression of various X-linked disorders could be attributed to the disruption of the normal alleles at the respective loci (Table 10.2).

While studies of X/autosome translocations in females with muscular dystrophy were in progress, a unique case was described which further confirmed the location of the Duchenne locus. This concerned a boy with Duchenne muscular dystrophy and some degree of mental retardation, but who also exhibited chronic granulomatous disease, McLeod syndrome (reduced antigenicity of the red cell Kell blood group), and a presumed

Table 10.2 *Expression of X-linked disorders in females with various X/autosome translocations*

Disorder	X breakpoint	Reference
Duchenne and ? Becker muscular dystrophy	Xp21	
Anhidrotic ectodermal dysplasia	Xq12	Gerald and Brown (1974)
Aicardi's syndrome	Xp22	Ropers *et al.* (1982)
Hunter's syndrome	Xq26 or Xq27	Mossman *et al.* (1983)
Aarskog syndrome	Xq13	Bawle *et al.* (1984)
Incontinentia pigmenti	Xp11	Gilgenkrantz *et al.* (1985)
Lowe's syndrome	Xq25	Hodgson *et al.* (1986a)

related retinitis pigmentosa (Francke *et al.* 1985). High resolution chromosome banding studies revealed that the band Xp21 appeared to be slightly reduced in size, and molecular studies confirmed that the affected boy had a small interstitial deletion in this region. This deletion presumably removed DNA sequences at the Duchenne muscular dystrophy locus as well as at other adjacent loci so producing the clinical phenotypes. This case further supported the idea that the Duchenne locus is at Xp21. It also indicated that the loci for these different disorders are clustered together. In fact various associations of these different disorders have been reported previously in males: chronic granulomatous disease with McLeod syndrome (Marsh 1978); McLeod syndrome with raised SCK levels (Marsh *et al.* 1981) and a subclinical myopathy (Swash *et al.*, 1983); chronic granulomatous disease with McLeod syndrome and raised SCK levels (Marsh *et al.* 1981); chronic granulomatous disease with Duchenne muscular dystrophy (but no mention of McLeod syndrome, Kousseff 1981); chronic granulomatous disease, McLeod syndrome, Duchenne muscular dystrophy, and possibly retinitis pigmentosa (Francke *et al.* 1985).

The gene for ornithine transcarbamylase (OTC) is also localized to Xp21 (Lindgren *et al.* 1984) and has been shown to be relatively closely linked to the Duchenne locus (Davies *et al.* 1985a, b). A small but visible deletion associated with OTC and glycerol kinase deficiencies and X-linked adrenal hypoplasia has been described (Hammond *et al.* 1985). Also, a small deletion in the same region of the X-chromosome has been found in boys with a myopathy, glycerol kinase deficiency, and adrenal insufficiency (Bartley *et al.* 1986; Saito *et al.* 1986). This triad has also been reported when there is no *visible* deletion (Renier *et al.* 1983), but a deletion may then be detected using an appropriate DNA probe (Dunger *et al.* 1986). The triad may also be associated with other abnormalities (Guggenheim *et al.* 1980). Glycerol kinase deficiency and adrenal hypoplasia have been recorded in different male members of a family but in the absence of a myopathy (Bartley *et al.* 1982).

It is tempting to order these overlapping phenotypes as shown in Fig. 10.2, although it is not yet certain if this is in fact the order of the gene loci themselves.

It should be noted that deletions in the region of Xp21 result in various abnormal phenotypes only in males. In females such deletions have minimal clinical effects, presumably because the deleted X is preferentially inactivated (Herva *et al.* 1979).

Cases of Duchenne muscular dystrophy with *no* other associated abnormalities but with a microscopically evident interstitial deletion at Xp21 are very much the exception. Such a case has been described by Wilcox *et al.* (1986) where the deletion was large enough to be visible but was presumably not sufficiently extensive as to include any adjacent gene loci. In the vast majority of cases however no deletion or any other alteration is microscopically evident in the region of Xp21 (Fig. 10.3) even with high resolution banding (Spowart *et al.* 1982). Such techniques reveal that the band Xp21 can be subdivided into three regions (Fig. 10.4) and when applied to lymphoblastoid cell lines from females with a Duchenne-like disorder and an X/autosome translocation, the breakpoint has been found to be in sub-band Xp212 or in Xp211 (Boyd and Buckle 1986). It can be calculated that the

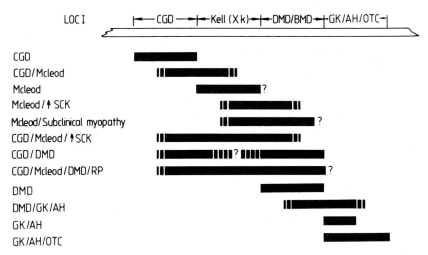

Fig. 10.2. Diagrammatic representation of *overlapping phenotypes* involving chronic granulomatous disease (CGD), McLeod syndrome, Duchenne and Becker muscular dystrophies (DMD, BMD), glycerol kinase deficiency (GK), adrenal hypoplasia (AH), ornithine transcarbamylase deficiency (OTC), and retinitis pigmentosa (RP).

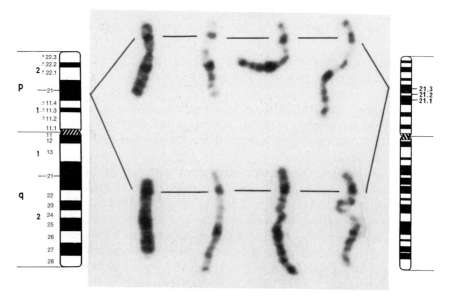

Fig. 10.3. High resolution banding patterns of X-chromosomes from boys with Duchenne muscular dystrophy (*top*), and healthy boys (*bottom*). The possible appearance with techniques which identify a total of 400 bands (*left*), and 850 bands (*right*) are also illustrated. (From Spowart *et al.* (1982) with permission.)

DNA represented in the sub-bands Xp211, Xp212, and Xp213 is around 5000 kb, 2000 kb, and 4000 kb respectively (1 kb = 1000 base pairs of DNA). The chromosomal region involved in some way with Duchenne/Becker muscular dystrophy would therefore appear to span several thousand kilobases of DNA. It may not of course be composed of a single unit but of several contiguous units. The very high mutation rate could find an explanation if the 'gene' were very large and therefore presents a large target for mutations. But there are also other possibilities. For example, one possibility is a contribution from gene deletions and duplications resulting from mispairing and unequal crossing-over. This could result if there was normally a pseudogene alongside the Duchenne locus. Mispairing between the two X-chromosomes during meiosis in the female might conceivably result in two different DNA strands: one with two Duchenne genes and a pseudogene, and one with only a pseudogene. The later DNA strand would represent a 'new mutation' due to a deletion of an active gene (Winter and Pembrey 1982). Certainly such unequal crossing-over leading to gene deletions and duplications is known to occur in α-globin, β-globin, and ABO gene loci, but as yet there is no evidence for this in Duchenne muscular dystrophy.

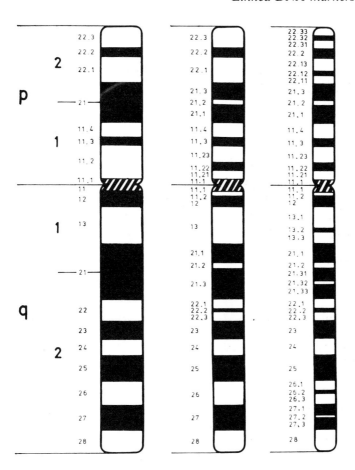

Fig. 10.4. Diagrammatic representation of the high resolution banding patterns which can be delineated on the X-chromosome by various techniques.

Linked DNA markers

Between functioning genes there are large stretches of DNA, the functions of which are still largely unknown. Within this DNA are variations in nucleotide sequences which have no apparent phenotypic effects on the host organism and are inherited in a Mendelian fashion. These changes in base sequence, which occur about once in every 100 base pairs, can be identified because they can alter the DNA site normally cleaved by a particular restriction enzyme since these enzymes cleave DNA at sequence specific sites. Thus, a change in base sequence in a segment of DNA will, with a particular restriction enzyme, result in different sized fragments in different individuals. These genotypic

changes can be recognized by the different mobilities of the restriction fragments on gel electrophoresis. The fragments are identified by using an
appropriate 'probe' which is a labelled DNA fragment that will hybridize
with, and thereby detect, complementary sequences among the DNA
fragments produced by a restriction enzyme (Southern blot). Details of the
technology are explained simply in Emery (1985).

These variations in nucleotide sequences are referred to as restriction fragment length polymorphisms (RFLPs). Their interest lies in the fact that the
demonstration of linkage between an RFLP and the locus for a particular
genetic disease can be useful for carrier detection and prenatal diagnosis.
Also, if the chromosomal site of an RFLP were already known then it could
furnish information on the site of a disease locus to which it proved to be
closely linked. A hypothetical example of the co-inheritance of an RFLP and

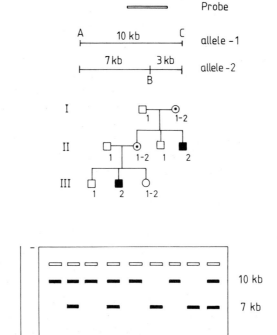

Fig. 10.5. Pedigree of an X-linked recessive disorder linked to an RFLP (the alleles of
which are represented below the pedigree symbols) and the appearance of the
corresponding Southern blot.

an X-linked recessive disorder is given in Fig. 10.5. Here it is assumed there is a polymorphism at restriction site *B*, the absence of the site is called allele-1 and the presence of the site is allele-2. When the restriction enzyme cuts the DNA in one chromosome at sites *A* and *C* it generates a single fragment of size 10 kilobases (10 kb) which corresponds to allele-1. If the enzyme cuts the DNA not only at sites *A* and *C* but also at *B*, two fragments will now be generated of sizes 7 kb and 3 kb which correspond to allele-2. Polymorphic genotypes can therefore be deduced from the pattern of bands on an electrophoretic gel. In this example, grandmother (I_2) and mother (II_2) are both heterozygous for the RFLP and both carry the X-linked recessive disorder. Since both affected males have allele-2 it would appear that allele-2 and the disorder are co-inherited. That is, they are both on the same X-chromosome. By studying individuals in a family in which an RFLP and an X-linked recessive disorder are inherited it is possible to estimate how frequently crossing-over occurs between them. Thus, in this example, if the unaffected son III_1 had also inherited allele-2 there would appear to have been at least one cross-over (or recombinant) out of four meioses. By studying a number of informative families in this way, the frequency of recombination can be determined. Recombination frequency, usually designated as θ, is related to the distance between the gene loci concerned – one per cent recombination being equivalent to a distance of one map unit, or one centiMorgan (cM), which is roughly equal to 1000 kb, or 10^6 base pairs. When loci are some distance apart then the error rate in diagnosis will be equal to θ at each meiosis. The details of the calculation of genetic distances from linkage data are explained in Emery (1986) and there are also computer programs, such as LIPED (Ott 1974) and LINKAGE (Lathrop and Lalouel 1984), for this purpose.

With regard to linkage with Duchenne muscular dystrophy, the first step was to isolate a relevant DNA sequence. In 1981, Davies and her colleagues isolated the first DNA sequences from cloned fragments derived from the human X-chromosome, so-called X genomic library. The location of these cloned sequences was then determined by various methods. These included studying somatic cell hybrids with a full complement of Chinese hamster or mouse chromosomes and different extents of the human X-chromosome. Another method of localizing a DNA sequence was by *in situ* hybridization whereby the sequence was labelled and hybridized directly to a metaphase chromosome preparation. One of the cloned sequences, designated RC8, turned out to be located on the short arm of X-chromosome. Using this as a probe, it detected a polymorphism with the restriction enzyme *Taq* I, and by studying several families the polymorphism detected by RC8 (now called DXS9) proved to be linked to Duchenne muscular dystrophy (Murray *et al.* 1982). Shortly afterwards a different probe (L1.28) detected another polymorphism (DXS7) on the opposite side of Xp21, and it was found that the

Duchenne locus lay between the two (Davies *et al.* 1983). Both markers eventually turned out to be about 15 cM on either side (referred to as 'flanking' or 'bridging') the Duchenne locus. This was in fact the first disorder shown to be linked to an RFLP.

At the same time Kingston and her colleagues (Kingston *et al.* 1983) showed that Becker muscular dystrophy was linked to DXS7 (L1.28). Subsequently it was also shown to be linked to DXS9 (RC8) and to other DNA markers at roughly similar genetic distances to Duchenne muscular dystrophy (Kingston *et al.* 1984; Fadda *et al.* 1985; Brown *et al.* 1985; Wilcox *et al.* 1985). These findings therefore indicated that Duchenne and Becker muscular dystrophies could either be allelic or the two loci be very close together in the same region of the X-chromosome. Interestingly, Emery–Dreifuss muscular dystrophy appears to be linked to colour blindness (Thomas *et al.* 1972), and to DNA markers located at Xq28 (Hodgson *et al.* 1986b; Thomas *et al.* 1986), which indicates that the responsible gene mutation may not be allelic with Duchenne and Becker muscular dystrophies.

A number of polymorphic loci have now been detected around the Duchenne locus. Their ordering and exact distances apart are not yet entirely certain but the current situation is summarized in Fig. 10.6. The subject of DNA markers in X-linked dystrophies has been reviewed in a series of articles in the *Journal of Medical Genetics* (1986, Vol. 23, No. 6, p. 481 *et seq.*).

Isolation of the Duchenne gene

The most obvious approach to eventually isolating the Duchenne gene itself would be to 'walk the genome' from a closely linked probe toward the gene, so as to eventually include it. This could be done by studying overlapping clones of DNA sequences. There are several reasons, however, why this approach is difficult. Even a very closely linked marker only 1 cM from the disease locus is a million base pairs away, and it would be extremely difficult to know if one was moving closer or further away by this strategy. Other methods seem more likely to succeed.

One approach pursued by Worton and his colleagues in Toronto, Canada, has been to isolate the junctional region in an X/autosome translocation associated with a Duchenne-like disorder in a female. They chose a translocation involving chromosome 21 (described by Verellen-Dumoulin *et al.* 1984), which they showed split the block of genes encoding ribosomal RNA on the short arm of chromosome 21 (Worton *et al.* 1984). They then used ribosomal DNA probes to identify the junctional fragment in clones derived from the region of the translocation site. The region spanning the translocation breakpoint, and which presumably contains at least part of the Duchenne (and ? Becker) locus, was then cloned. A sequence derived from the clone was found to detect an RFLP which is very closely linked to Duchenne muscular dystrophy. It also failed to hybridize with DNA from the occasional patient

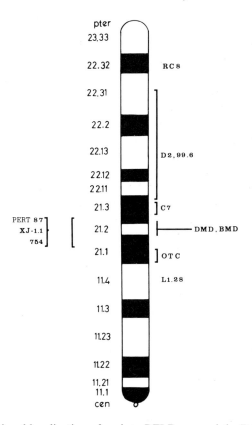

Fig. 10.6. Provisional localization of various RFLPs around the Duchenne/Becker locus. (Reproduced by kind permission of Dr Kay Davies.)

with Duchenne muscular dystrophy indicating that in these boys there is a deletion of the region complementary to the probe (Ray *et al.* 1985).

Kunkel and colleagues in Boston have approached the problem in a particularly ingenious way. They extracted DNA from a patient with the deletion described previously by Francke and her colleagues (p. 169). The DNA was then sheared by sonication which produces DNA fragments with irregular ends. DNA from a 49, XXXXY lymphoid cell line was cleaved with the restriction enzyme *Mbo* I. The two sets of fragments were then mixed and heated in order to disassociate the DNA strands. These were then allowed to reassociate in the presence of phenol (so-called phenol enhanced reassociation technique – PERT). Under appropriate conditions, and with the patient's DNA in excess, most of the reassociated molecules will have sheared ends and a few will be hybrid molecules with one sheared end and one *Mbo* I 'sticky end'. However, those sequences in the control *not* represented in the patient's DNA (where they are deleted) will not hybridize with the patient's

DNA. By perforce they will only hybridize between themselves and therefore consist of perfectly reassociated molecules with two *Mbo* I ends. Only the last can be ligated into an appropriately cleaved plasmid and be cloned (Kunkel *et al*. 1985). In this way a library of cloned sequences (referred to as PERT probes), corresponding to the portion of DNA deleted in the affected boy, have been produced. These have detected several RFLPs closely linked to the Duchenne locus and, like Worton's probes, they have also detected small deletions in a proportion of affected boys (Monaco *et al*. 1985) which are of different lengths in different families (Kunkel *et al*. 1986).

It should be noted that the probes isolated by Worton (XJ 1.1) and Kunkel (PERT) have shown recombination with Duchenne muscular dystrophy ($\theta \simeq$ 0.05) thus further indicating that the Duchenne 'gene' is very large, or consists of several genes or involves a region where chromosomal rearrangements are particularly frequent (Fischbeck *et al*. 1986).

Using these various probes it seems that around 5 to 10 per cent of affected boys may have a small submicroscopic gene deletion which in some cases can be familial. These findings have several important implications. First, since these probes are within (or extremely close to) the Duchenne locus it should be feasible to 'walk the genome' so as to eventually cover the entire locus (or 'gene cluster'). Secondly, boys with a deletion might be expected to mount an immune response if exposed to the missing gene product, and this could conceivably provide a means of identifying such a product. Thirdly, it is possible to identify new mutations with certainty in cases of the disease associated with a deletion. This is illustrated in Fig. 10.7 based on two families reported by Monaco *et al*. (1985). Using a particular probe (PERT 87-8) an RFLP was detected with the enzyme *Bst* XI reflected in two DNA fragments of sizes 4.4 kb and 2.2 kb (say allele-1 and allele-2).

In family A, grandmother (I_2) is either homozygous for allele-2 or hemizygous because one allele has been deleted. Her daughter (II_1) has no allele-2 which she should have inherited from her mother. She is therefore heterozygous for the deletion which is evident in her affected son (III_1) who is therefore *not* a new mutation.

In family B both grandmother and mother and heterozygous for the RFLP and neither allele is deleted. However, one of the alleles is deleted in the affected son who must therefore be a new mutation.

Another approach being pursued to isolate the Duchenne locus (Davies *et. al*.1986), is to screen an X-chromosome library with mRNA isolated from fetal and adult muscle. In this way it is hoped to isolate those X-chromosome sequences which are *expressed* in these tissues. Then, by using appropriate somatic cell hybrids or *in situ* hybridization, the selected sequences can be further screened for those which are located to Xp21. Kunkel and his colleagues have now, by chromosome walking on either side of PERT 87 for

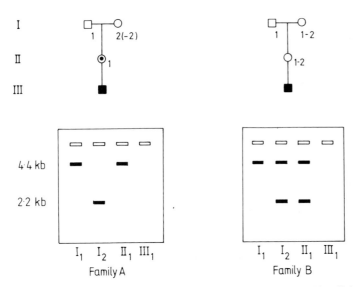

Fig. 10.7. Two families in which affected boys have a gene deletion. The alleles of an informative RFLP are represented below the pedigree symbols and the appearances of the corresponding Southern blots are diagrammed.

a distance of some 200 kb, identified two small regions which are conserved in several mammalian species. These were used to search for transcripts in RNA isolated from various fetal tissues, and one identified a 16 kb transcript in fetal skeletal muscle. From the study of the corresponding cDNA, the organization of the exons and introns predicts that the Duchenne 'region' may involve up to 2000 kb (Monaco *et al.* 1986).

Future prospects

In the not too distant future the Duchenne locus will be isolated, cloned, and sequenced. This will provide valuable information on molecular pathology, and generate gene-specific probes which can be used for carrier detection and prenatal diagnosis. Most importantly, having isolated the gene it will then be possible to determine its product which will then lead to rational approaches to treatment. However, such information may well prove to answer some more fundamental questions. In Duchenne muscular dystrophy the proximal muscles are most affected and therefore presumably their biochemistry and physiology is in some way different from other muscles, and in turn these differences are likely to reflect differences in gene activity in different muscle groups. The normal alleles of genes responsible for various different types of dystrophy (proximal, distal, ocular) are presumably important in the normal activity of different muscle groups. Such matters raise fundamental questions concerning differential gene activity in different muscles but at present virtually nothing is known about this. Undoubtedly knowledge of the nature and product of the gene(s) responsible for Duchenne muscular dystrophy will be a step forward in finding answers to such questions.

Summary and conclusions

Since the basic biochemical defect in Duchenne muscular dystrophy is unknown, this presents a problem in tackling the molecular pathology of the disease. Nevertheless, progress has been made. Several females with Duchenne muscular dystrophy and X/autosome translocations have now been described, the breakpoint on the X-chromosome always being at Xp21. This, and the fact that a unique case of Duchenne muscular dystrophy has been found with a deletion in this same region of the X-chromosome, points to the disease locus being located at this point. Several restriction fragment length polymorphisms (RFLPs), which are polymorphisms due to the presence or absence of a particular restriction site, have now been identified around Xp21 and linked to the Duchenne locus. In conjunction with SCK levels, information on linked RFLPs can be used in carrier detection. However, even the closest marker is too far for chromosome 'walking' and therefore other strategies are being devised to isolate the Duchenne gene.

One group has approached the problem by isolating and cloning DNA fragments from the junctional region in an X/autosome translocation associated with a Duchenne-like disorder in a female. In another approach the region corresponding to that deleted in an affected boy has been cloned. Both these techniques have generated a number of RFLPs very closely linked to Duchenne muscular dystrophy, and have also detected small, submicroscopic deletions in 5 to 10 per cent of affected boys. In these latter cases it is possible to identify new mutants among isolated cases of the disease.

Finally, in the not too distant future, the Duchenne locus (or possibly 'gene cluster') should be isolated, cloned, and sequenced. This will then provide valuable information on molecular pathology and yield gene specific probes for carrier detection and prenatal diagnosis. Most importantly, however, it should open up a rational approach to finding an effective treatment.

11 Prevention

Since Duchenne muscular dystrophy is a serious disorder for which at present there is no effective treatment, a great deal of emphasis has been given to prevention. This involves the ascertainment of women likely to have an affected son, and the provision of genetic counselling and prenatal diagnosis for such women.

Ascertainment of families at risk

The ascertainment of women at risk of having an affected child is the first prerequisite of prevention. Logically this would seem best achieved by screening all females to determine which ones are likely to be carriers. This is impractical, however, because there is as yet no single test which could be used to detect all carriers, and in any event the cost of such screening would be prohibitively expensive. Furthermore, as already observed, in one-third of cases the mother is not a carrier, the affected son being the result of a new mutation (p. 161).

Another approach might be to screen all pregnancies for affected males. However, quite apart from technical and economic considerations, this would raise a number of serious ethical problems. At present the only practical solution is to ensure that all affected boys in the community are ascertained, and that their mothers, and subsequently other female relatives, are then tested to determine their carrier status and the likelihood of the disorder recurring.

Population screening

Because SCK levels in affected boys are grossly elevated from birth, there is the potential for detection in the neonatal period. This can be achieved by determining the SCK level in dried blood spots obtained from a heel prick. The blood spots are placed on a filter paper card and the air-dried specimen can then be assayed immediately or stored. Enzyme activity remains stable for up to two weeks at room temperature provided direct heat and sunlight are avoided. Specimens can therefore be conveniently sent by post. It should be emphasized, however, that it is not possible to screen for female carriers in this way because the probability of any female at random *not* being a carrier far outweighs the possibility of her being a carrier based on a slightly elevated SCK level.

A sensitive assay for creatine kinase activity in minute quantities of dried blood was first introduced by Antonik and further developed by Scheuerbrandt (Zellweger and Antonik 1975; Beckmann and Scheuerbrandt 1976). This is a bioluminescence assay and depends on the generation of ATP by creatine kinase (p. 43). The ATP then reacts with luciferin in the presence of the enzyme luciferase to produce light – a reaction employed by fireflies. A sensitive but less expensive fluorimetric/electrophoretic method has also been developed for measuring creatine kinase activity in dried blood spots (Adriaenssens and Vermeiren 1980; Lloyd *et al.* 1982). Essentially, this method consists of separating creatine kinase isoenzymes from the haemoglobin of the blood spot and from each other by electrophoresis, the enzyme substrate being in a gelatin or agarose matrix. The activities of creatine kinase isoenzymes (particularly the MM isoenzyme) are determined by comparing the UV fluorescence of the samples with standards of known activities.

Extensive experience of the luciferin/luciferase method indicates that the false positive rate is between 0.2 and 0.06 per cent, and may even be less (Scheuerbrandt *et al.* 1984, 1986). With the fluorimetric/electrophoretic method we have found a false positive rate of at most 0.2 per cent, and this will no doubt be reduced further with more experience. Furthermore, none of the false positives in our series was found to have a grossly elevated creatine kinase level when a subsequent *serum* sample was tested. When a serum sample also yields a grossly elevated SCK level then the diagnosis has to be confirmed by appropriate investigations (p. 47 *et seq.*). There will always be some false positives with this test because it has to be sufficiently sensitive to detect *all* cases. It seems likely, therefore, that the false negative rate among those tested will be low, if not zero. The problem here is more likely to result from a laboratory or administrative error or failing to test an infant who subsequently develops the disease.

Neonatal screening for Duchenne muscular dystrophy has proved to be feasible, and in the United Kingdom is most conveniently carried out on the fifth day of life along with routine testing for phenylketonuria (Skinner *et al.* 1982). The results of neonatal screening for Duchenne muscular dystrophy have already been discussed (p. 155).

However, the important question remains as to whether such screening is really justified. It can be argued that if an affected boy was detected sufficiently early and his mother proved to be a carrier and was counselled, second cases in the family might be prevented. It has been estimated that up to 15–20 per cent of cases might be prevented in this way. In the present series of patients in which precise information was available, there were 67 families in which an affected boy was born but at the time no one else was affected in the family and the mother subsequently became pregnant. The average time between the birth of this son and the birth of the next child was 2.71 years (s.d. 1.45; range 1.0–7.0 years). Thus the next pregnancy was conceived on average less than two years after the birth of a son who *subsequently proved to be affected*. Since at least 75 per cent of affected boys present suspicious signs *after* this age (p. 27) and the mean age at diagnosis is around 5 years of age with a range of 2 to 8 years (Crisp *et al.* 1982), most parents would have been completely unaware of the risks in the next pregnancy. In fact, 10 sons in the next or a following pregnancy subsequently proved to be affected. Until there is a gene specific probe(s), and the finding of small gene deletions in some affected boys is of interest in this regard (p. 178), it may be difficult to reassure a mother of an isolated case that she is *not* a carrier and prenatal diagnosis in any subsequent pregnancy would be indicated.

Neonatal screening has also been justified on financial grounds, it being argued that the tests are relatively cheap to carry out and prevention compared with management would be cost effective (Zellweger *et al.* 1975; Grimm 1981).

Finally, most parents of affected boys appear to favour such screening when questioned (Firth and Wilkinson 1983) for a number of reasons: it would prevent the anxiety which results from the long delays and unfounded reassurances often experienced between the first symptoms and the establishment of the diagnosis; parents have a 'right' to know as soon as possible; it would help prevent further affected children; it has practical advantages in affording an early opportunity to obtain appropriate housing for example; and, finally, it has emotional advantages. However, those questioned in this study were all parents who had already had an affected son. The concern is of presenting a couple with the devastating news that their newborn son has a serious genetic disorder when they were completely unprepared for this. Furthermore, the parents have to cope with the problem some four or five years sooner than they would otherwise have had to. Some have therefore advocated a compromise, that screening might be restricted to those boys who are not walking by the age of 18 months (Gardner-Medwin *et al.* 1978; O'Brien *et al.* 1983), or when there is a delay in motor and mental development for no obvious reason (Crisp *et al.* 1982). The age of 18 months was selected because by this time almost all normal boys have learned to walk but only about 50 per cent of affected boys (p. 26). It has been reasoned that this more restricted screening would have the advantages of involving fewer tests (and therefore lower costs), and that the results would be easier to interpret and less likely to cause anxiety because the parents' concern is already aroused. Of course, since the screening would be carried out later, fewer secondary cases (less than 10 per cent) could be prevented. It would therefore be less effective. It would also be necessary to establish procedures for informing all family doctors of the requirement for testing and the referral of blood samples to an appropriate centre. This could present organizational difficulties.

Nonetheless, however the subject is viewed, screening for Duchenne muscular dystrophy has so far failed to generate a great deal of enthusiasm either among paediatricians or geneticists. There is little doubt, however, that when an effective treatment eventually becomes available interest will be rekindled. For it seems probable that the sooner any treatment is begun the more likely it is to be effective and arrest the course of the disease. A number of issues will then have to be faced including the economics of screening, the logistics of dealing with false positives, and the need for very careful and sensitive counselling of parents of proven positive cases.

At present most paediatricians and geneticists confine their activities to the family of an affected boy. All his female relatives can be screened in order to assess their carrier status, and records of those found to be at risk can be maintained on a genetic register system for subsequent follow up.

Genetic registers

Viewed at the population level, any approach to prevention must first involve ascertaining all cases in the community. There are essentially three ways in which this may be achieved. First, by population screening which has already been discussed. Secondly, studying families in which an affected individual is known to exist. Thirdly, screening of hospital, public health, and special school records for affected individuals. Having now ascertained cases of the disease, the next step is to determine if there are any female relatives who could be at risk of having an affected son and may require genetic counselling. The procedure we have adopted is that unless a family is already known through an affected boy and his parents, individuals who could be at risk are not contacted directly but only through their family doctor. This provides an opportunity to check that the diagnosis has been well established in the affected family member. It also protects individuals from being contacted who have either already had genetic counselling or where it would be imprudent, for religious reasons for example, or unnecessary if they have already completed their family. In Britain the relative's family doctor can be identified when the relative's name and address is known because each local Executive Council holds a list of patients in its area which shows the family doctor with whom they are registered. However, in small nuclear families such measures are usually not necessary. On average there are about three females at high risk (greater than 1 in 10) of having an affected son in each family with a serious X-linked recessive disorder (Emery and Smith 1970).

For ease of follow-up and recall and to maintain strict confidentiality, personal and genetic data on such females are best held in a computerized register. A number of such registers of genetic disorders have been developed in several countries (Emery and Miller 1976), and a register designed specifically for the prevention of genetic disease was developed in Edinburgh with the acronym RAPID (*R*egister for the *A*scertainment and *P*revention of

*I*nherited *D*isease) in the early 1970s (Emery *et al.* 1974). The system is out-linked in Fig. 11.1. To maintain strict confidentiality a number of security checks have been incorporated into the system. Access is only possible when a valid password 'A' is used. If data are to be retrieved, the request is first checked for its validity, i.e. correct family name and number and disease code, etc. A second password 'B' allows data to be retrieved at various levels depending on the particular operator's password. The clinician or geneticist dealing with the family has access to all the medical and genetic information, but someone concerned with tracing relatives may retrieve only names and pedigree data. Information in the register is released only to other physicians and geneticists directly involved in the management of the patient and his family. Finally, no families are included on the register without their fully informed consent. The British Clinical Genetics Society has published a Working Party Report on genetic registers in which various technical and ethical matters are discussed in detail (Emery *et al.* 1978).

Data which can be stored in such a register include information on DNA polymorphisms (Read *et al.* 1986), for example in an affected boy against the day when he might die and the information is required to counsel a female relative. The register can also be designed to facilitate the later recall of female relatives who, *a priori*, are at risk but who are currently too young for counselling. Information on any aborted fetus (e.g. DNA polymorphisms and that it might have been affected, see p. 141) can also be stored which in future might be of additional help in counselling. However, apart from the prevention of Duchenne muscular dystrophy and other genetic diseases, a computerized genetic register system can also be of value in several other ways. For example, it can facilitate the recall of family members should there be new developments in carrier detection, prenatal diagnosis, and, hopefully one day, treatment. It can also be useful in putting families in contact with various welfare agencies and for informing them of changes in medical and social benefits. The European Alliance of Muscular Dystrophy Associations has recommended the setting up of a register of patients with neuromuscular diseases largely for epidemiological purposes (EAMDA 1984). However, many see the main function of a local genetic register system as facilitating the prevention of genetic disease within the community it serves.

Carrier detection

The whole problem of genetic counselling in Duchenne muscular dystrophy revolves around the detection of female carriers. If, as was suggested (Roses *et al.* 1976b), essentially all mothers of affected boys are carriers, the situation would be much simpler. This now, however, seems unlikely to be the case (p. 161; Nicholson *et al.* 1981), and in any event the carrier status of sisters and daughters of carrier mothers often has to be determined.

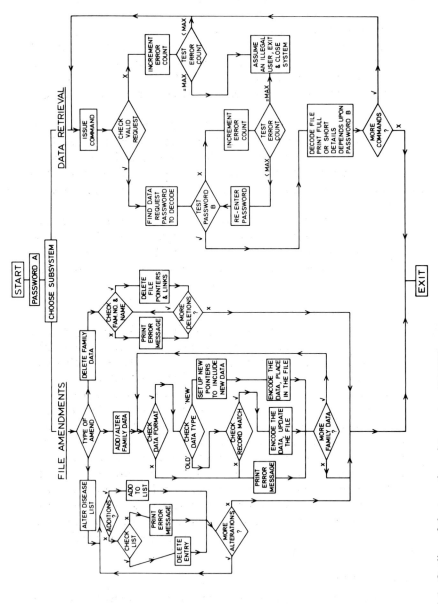

Fig. 11.1. Outline of the genetic register system RAPID.

Definition of carrier status

First it is necessary to consider the definition of a carrier. In the past, confusion on this point has often lead to difficulties in interpreting the results of any proposed tests for detecting carriers. There are three accepted categories of carriers based on genetic considerations.

First, *definite (or obligate) carriers* who are mothers of an affected son but who also have an affected brother, affected nephew by their sister, or an affected maternal uncle or other maternal male relative. Included in this category are also mothers of affected sons by different non-consanguineous fathers.

Secondly, *probable carriers* who are mothers with two or more affected sons but with no other affected relatives. Such women could conceivably be heterozygous for the autosomal recessive limb girdle muscular dystrophy of childhood which clinically resembles Duchenne muscular dystrophy. However, since the latter is comparatively rare these women are usually included with the definite carriers.

Thirdly, *possible carriers* who are mothers of an isolated case as well as their sisters and other female relatives. This category also includes female relatives of definite and probable carriers. The probability of all such women being carriers has to be determined. The term *suspected carrier* is frequently used for any woman who is at risk of being a carrier.

Biological considerations

The evaluation of carrier detection tests has been bedevilled by several factors. Some of these are inherent in that Duchenne muscular dystrophy being an X-linked recessive disorder, there will inevitably be variability in expression in carrier females because of random inactivation of the X-chromosome. This means that a proportion of carriers are unlikely to be detectable by any biochemical method except one employing cloned cells to identify two populations, or based on DNA studies. This problem is further compounded by the fact that the primary biochemical defect is as yet unknown and there is no clear evidence that the disease is unequivocally expressed in myoblasts or fibroblasts in tissue culture. Furthermore, it may be difficult if not impossible to determine the rate of false positives with any test since a potential carrier informed of an abnormal result is unlikely to risk child-bearing. However, if a subsequent pregnancy is terminated it may be possible in some cases to confirm the diagnosis by studying muscle tissue from the aborted fetus (p. 141).

Methodological considerations

Quite apart from these biological factors, confusion has often arisen because of various methodological problems. Sometimes a test has been applied to carriers before its validity has been established in affected boys. Thus, a test which is positive in only a proportion of affected boys, or only in the later stages of the disease, is unlikely to be of much value in detecting healthy carriers. Only in occasional, and mainly early studies, has an attempt been made to compare the results of several different sorts of tests (SCK levels, EMG, muscle histology) on the same individuals (for example, Emery 1965a; Hausmanowa-Petrusewicz *et al.* 1968b; Radu *et al.* 1968; Dubowitz, 1982). However, lack of correlation with SCK levels would not necessarily invalidate a new test. The two might be independent variables and the results of the two tests could then be combined to enhance carrier detection.

Another problem has been that definite carriers have sometimes not been clearly distinguished from possible carriers. For example, the results of a test on mothers of isolated cases have occasionally been reported when the actual carrier status of these mothers is not known. Furthermore, comparisons have often been made with poorly matched or an inadequate number of healthy controls.

Finally, as Harper has emphasized in a thought-provoking essay on the subject (Harper 1982), all too often the results of research investigations have been too hastily applied to service use.

Ideally, any proposed test should be subjected to the following evaluation. First, it should be positive in all affected boys, even from a very early stage in the disease process. There should be no false negatives and false positives should be acceptable only if they occur in conditions unlikely to be confused with Duchenne muscular dystrophy or can be readily distinguished from it. Secondly, its validity in carrier detection should be based on testing a significant number of definite carriers and an equal number of carefully matched healthy female controls. In both controls and carriers the material to be studied (say blood) should be collected and processed in the same way and assayed under identical laboratory conditions. Finally, the results of the test should be compared with an established test, such as the SCK level, carried out on the same individuals. Unfortunately, there have been relatively few reported studies where all these criteria have been met.

It could be argued that the advent of DNA markers for carrier detection has now made other approaches to this problem redundant since they circumvent many of the problems associated with other tests, including mosaicism due to X-inactivation. However, there are still valid reasons for continuing to pursue these studies. It may yet be some time before gene probes specific for each different mutation become available and in some cases this may prove prohibitively expensive. It is quite possible, for example, that since new mutations occur very frequently not exactly the same mutation will occur in every family and either a panel of several different probes or even DNA sequencing may be necessary. Also, information from, say, SCK levels can very usefully be combined with data from linked DNA markers in determining the probability of a woman being a carrier. At present, a suspected carrier may also prove not to be informative for such a marker. Finally, a significant biochemical defect detectable not only in affected boys but also in healthy carriers would confirm its relevance to the basic defect and so throw light on the pathogenesis of the disorder.

Carrier detection tests

Over the years there have been reports of various abnormalities in carriers of Duchenne muscular dystrophy. Some, such as total body potassium and rubidium, have been shown to be valueless in carrier detection. Others of more recent interest are listed in Table 11.1. The references have been selected

Table 11.1 *Some more recent reported abnormalities in female carriers of Duchenne muscular dystrophy*

Abnormality	Reference
Clinical	
Muscle weakness	Reddy *et al.* (1984)
Cardiomyopathy	Wiegand *et al.* (1984)
Muscle pathology	
Histology	Schiffer *et al.* (1984)
Histochemistry	Maunder-Sewry & Dubowitz (1981)
Ultrastructure	Fisher *et al.* (1972); Afifi *et al.* (1973)
Ultrasound	Rott & Rödl (1985)
Computerized tomography	Stern *et al.* (1985)
Muscle biochemistry	
Nuclear calcium	Maunder-Sewry & Dubowitz (1979)
Ribosomal protein synthesis	Ionasescu *et al.* (1980)
Electromyography	Hausmanowa-Petrusewicz *et al.* (1982)
Electrocardiography	Lane *et al.* (1980)
Cell surface membranes	
Erythrocytes morphology/physico-chemistry/biochemistry	Lucy (1980); Rowland (1980)
Lymphocyte capping	Ho *et al.* (1980)
Fibroblasts	Hillier *et al.* (1985)
Serum enzymes & proteins	
Creatine kinase (+ isoenzymes)	–
Pyruvate kinase	Falcão-Conceição *et al.* (1983a)
LDH–5	Somer *et al.* (1980)
Myoglobin	Nicholson (1981); Percy *et al.* (1984)
Haemopexin	Lössner *et al.* (1982)

in order to guide the reader to the related earlier literature.

It should perhaps be emphasized that some of these abnormalities are contentious whereas others have been more convincingly established. For example, there is doubt as to whether significant and consistent abnormalities are found in cell surface membranes (Rowland 1980; Lucy 1980; Nicholson and Sugars 1982). The value of ultrasound has been questioned (Heckmatt and Dubowitz 1983b) and there are doubts as to whether serum levels of LDH–5, myoglobin or haemopexin have any additional value over and above information provided by creatine kinase and pyruvate kinase. With regard to electromyography, some years ago we were unable to find any significant differences between 12 controls and 22 carriers regarding action potential duration and amplitude and the frequency of polyphasic potentials when measurements were made blind (Emery *et al.* 1966), although admittedly some others had a little better success (e.g. Moosa *et al.* 1972). Recently, sophisticated electromyographic techniques involving computer analysis appear to have been more successful but they require considerable expertise in their interpretation and are time consuming.

There is, however, general agreement that a proportion of carriers exhibit some degree of weakness, have abnormalities of muscle pathology, and have significantly raised serum levels of creatine kinase and pyruvate kinase.

Clinically manifesting carriers

It has been long been recognized that females may have a Duchenne-like disorder. Two of Duchenne's original 13 cases were in fact girls and Gowers (1879b) reported a Duchenne-like disorder in a girl with a clearly X-linked pedigree (case 8), in the sister of an affected boy (case 15), and in an isolated case (case 30). There are several reasons for females having a Duchenne-like or Duchenne-related disorder and these have been discussed in Chapter 5, and are summarized in Table 11.2. Some of the conditions listed however are unlikely to cause confusion but are included for the sake of completeness. Manifesting carriers of Becker muscular dystrophy have also been described (p. 75).

It has been estimated that between 5 per cent and 10 per cent of carriers have some degree of weakness (Moser and Emery 1974). But this may be slight and only elicited on careful clinical examination. Calf enlargement has often been emphasized but is in fact an unreliable sign. Actual measurements of calf size reveal no significant difference between controls and definite carriers (Table 11.3 and see Cavanagh and Preece 1981).

Manifesting carriers of Duchenne muscular dystrophy have occasionally been described in the same family (Moser and Emery 1974; Frouhar *et al.* 1975; Falcão-Conceição *et al.* 1983b; Reddy *et al.* 1984), and this has also been observed in other X-linked disorders such as Fabry's disease (Ropers *et al.* 1977) (Fig. 11.2).

Table 11.2 *Possible explanations for a female having a 'limb girdle' type myopathy*

1. *Congenital myopathy*
2. *Spinal muscular atrophy*
3. *Duchenne-related disorder*
   (*a*) Hemizygous
       XO, etc.
   (*b*) Homozygous
       extremely rare
   (*c*) Heterozygous
       'manifesting carrier'
   (*d*) X/autosome translocation
4. *Limb girdle muscular dystrophy*
   (*a*) Childhood
   (*b*) Adult
5. *Polymyositis*
6. *Acquired myopathy*
   Sarcoidosis, thyrotoxic, metabolic bone disease,
   acromegaly, etc.
7. *Drug induced*

Table 11.3 *Calf sizes (mean ± s.d.) in female controls and carriers of Duchenne and Becker muscular dystrophies*

	No.	Calf size (cm)	CS/SA × 1000
Controls	100	34.7 ± 2.4	2.2 ± 0.1
Carriers – Duchenne	21	34.9 ± 2.4	2.1 ± 0.2
Carriers – Becker	30	35.5 ± 3.5	2.2 ± 0.2

Surface area $= (Wt)^{0.425} \times (ht)^{0.725} \times (71.84)$ (Du Bois and Du Bois 1916)

CS, calf size; SA, surface area.

Since such manifestations are a consequence of random X-inactivation (p. 193), their familial occurrence suggests that this process may be under genetic control and might be explained if there were an X-linked gene(s) which controls X-chromosome inactivation. If present on the normal X-chromosome in a female carrier of Duchenne muscular dystrophy it could lead to preferential expression of loci on the X-chromosome bearing the Duchenne locus. With appropriate X-chromosome markers it should be possible to test this hypothesis in the families of manifesting carriers. In the

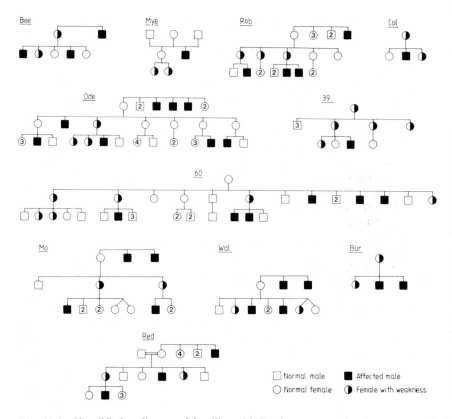

Fig. 11.2. Simplified pedigrees of families with Duchenne muscular dystrophy and several female relatives with weakness. *Bee* (Murphy and Thompson 1969); *Mye*, *Rob*, *Col*, and *Ode* (Moser and Emery 1974); *39* and *60* (Falcão-Conceição *et al.* 1983b); *Mo*, *Wal*, and *Bur* (unpublished); *Red* (Reddy *et al.* 1984).

mouse there is certainly an X-linked locus which controls X-inactivation (X-chromosome controlling element or *Xce*) and can lead to non-random X-inactivation (Cattanach and Williams 1972; Cattanach 1975; Johnston and Cattanach 1981). The idea of an 'X-chromosome controlling element' segregating in families with more than one manifesting carrier is attractive. However, in other families X-inactivation may well be random, which it would have to be in order to reconcile the observation of monozygotic twin girls being *discordant* for manifestations of Duchenne muscular dystrophy (p. 86), unless of course non-random inactivation itself predisposes to monozygotic twinning.

Besides muscle weakness, there is evidence in a proportion of carriers of cardiac involvement. In 4 of 50 carriers the algebraic sum of the R and S waves in the right praecordial lead of the electrocardiogram was found to be outside the normal range, an abnormality similar to that found in affected boys (Emery 1969a). Similar findings have also been reported in a detailed study by Lane *et al.* (1980).

From a practical point of view it may well be that a proportion of carriers have a latent dystrophic cardiomyopathy. This could have important implications since they often have to lift and carry their affected sons. In fact mitral valve prolapse (Biddison *et al.* 1979), and even congestive cardio-myopathy have been described in the occasional carrier (Wiegand *et al.* 1984). However, the proportion of carriers found to have weakness or a relevant ECG abnormality is insufficient to be of general value in carrier detection.

Muscle pathology

Abnormalities in muscle pathology in carriers have been known for some time (Dubowitz 1963b; Emery 1963, 1965b). These abnormalities include increased variation in fibre size, eosinophilic 'hypercontracted fibres', and even fibre necrosis and phagocytosis, although the latter are found only when there is florid muscle weakness. In only about 10 per cent of symptomless carriers is there usually any obvious abnormality on routine histology. However, careful quantitation of muscle fibre size, internal nuclei, and histo-chemical fibre type proportions has been claimed to demonstrate abnormali-ties in around 70 per cent of carriers by Maunder-Sewry and Dubowitz (1981). These investigators believe that significant abnormalities can occa-sionally be detected even when the SCK level is within the normal range. This has yet to be corroborated. What does seem clear however is that two popula-tions of muscle fibres, one normal and the other abnormal, are not found in carriers as was originally suggested by Pearson *et al.* (1963). Instead a wide spectrum of abnormalities can be seen from muscle fibres which appear to be normal through to those which are clearly undergoing necrosis. The explana-tion lies in the way multinucleate muscle fibres originate and develop. If the myotomes were mosaics of nuclei in some of which the active X-chromosome is the one bearing the normal gene and in others the active X-chromosome is the one bearing the Duchenne gene, then fusion between mononucleate myoblasts derived from the myotomes would result in muscle fibres possessing different proportions of the two types of nuclei. The proportion in any one fibre would be determined to some extent by the proportion in the original myotome. The proportion of nuclei in any muscle fibre in which the active X-chromosome is the one bearing the Duchenne gene presumably determines the degree of abnormality in that fibre (Fig. 11.3).

Thompson *et al.* (1974) noted a small (but not significant) decline in SCK levels with increasing age in carriers and interpreted this as perhaps being a reflection of a gradual reduction in the number of affected muscle fibres and

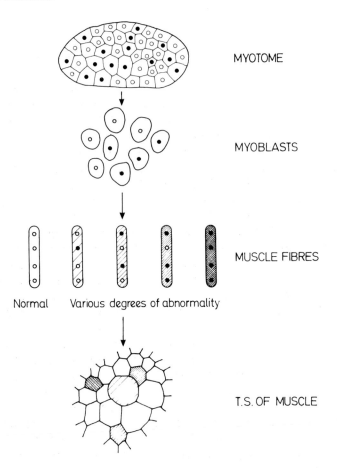

MYOTOME

MYOBLASTS

MUSCLE FIBRES

Normal   Various degrees of abnormality

T.S. OF MUSCLE

Fig. 11.3. Possible explanation for the muscle histological findings in carriers of Duchenne muscular dystrophy. (Nuclei in which the active X-chromosome bears the normal gene, (○), or the Duchenne gene, (● .)

their replacement (from proliferating satellite nuclei) by more normal fibres. However, so far there have been no reported studies of repeated muscle biopsies on carriers which is now feasible with needle biopsy. If anything, muscle weakness in manifesting carriers tends to get worse, not improve, over the years. Presumably, if there is any replacement of dystrophic fibres with age, mosaicism in satellite nuclei would tend to perpetuate the production of variably affected muscle fibres.

Serum creatine kinase

The most widely used single test for detecting carriers is the SCK level (Emery 1969b, 1980). From the very early successful studies of Schapira and colleagues in 1960, the detection rate obtained by a number of investigators in the following 5 years was around 60–70 per cent (Emery 1967b), and has not changed significantly since. Its great advantage is its simplicity and furthermore the results can be combined with data from linked DNA markers to provide valuable additional information for carrier detection. However, in applying the test, possible causes of variation both in female controls and carriers must be considered. This variability is partly technical and partly biological in origin. Considerable variability has been reported in values obtained when the same blood sample has been posted to different laboratories for analysis (Bullock *et al.* 1979). Part of this variability may be due to lack of standardization of the assays used and for this reason recommended methods have been advocated (e.g. Moss *et al.* 1981). However, when different assay methods are carried out in a single laboratory on the same series of controls and carriers, the resulting probability estimates vary very little (Tippett *et al.* 1982). Thus, a laboratory may be able to produce risk estimates of *acceptable precision for genetic counselling purposes* without having to study a series of known carriers provided that the method used has first been standardized on an adequate number of controls and the values obtained are comparable to those in a centre where many carriers have been studied with the same method.

If specimens are stored at 4 °C for no longer than a few days there is little loss of activity. Exposure, however, to extremes of temperature and sunlight can have significant effects. A slight rise in activity over the course of the day (Thomson 1968), and slightly higher levels in summer compared with winter (Smith *et al.* 1979; Percy *et al.* 1982) have been reported. However, both diurnal and seasonal variations are small and from a practical point of view are relatively unimportant.

In our laboratory the coefficient of variation on replicate samples taken at the same time from any one individual is less than 2 per cent. However, in samples obtained from the same individual but at different times, the coefficient of variation ranges from 5–10 per cent. This added variation results from various biological factors. The stage of the menstrual cycle and the use of oral contraception have little effect (Perry and Fraser 1973; Simpson *et al.* 1974), but vigorous exercise may cause significant increases though normal daily activity is without any material effect (Hudgson *et al.* 1967b). Age also has to be considered. After the menarche some reports have indicated a slight increase with increasing age (especially after the menopause) whereas others have found no significant effect (reviewed by Gale and Murphy 1979). It would seem that if there is any effect of age in adult women this is small and can be ignored in estimating the probability of a woman being a carrier. However, since most females are likely to be tested in their teens or in early adult life, it is important to consider the effects of age at these times. Several more recent studies have indicated that levels are significantly *higher* in teenage (especially premenarchal) girls compared with adult women (Bundey *et al.* 1979a; Smith *et al.* 1979; Lane and Roses 1981; Livingstone *et al.* 1982; Passos *et al.* 1985). Pregnancy is also an important factor, levels being significantly lower in the early stages (Blyth and Hughes 1971; Emery and King 1971; King *et al.* 1972; Bundey *et al.* 1979a), and significantly higher *immediately* postpartum (Emery and Pascasio 1965), when the latter is presumably due to the release of enzymes from the involuting myometrium.

Genetic factors also seem to influence SCK levels. Meltzer *et al.* (1978) have presented data on levels in 14 monozygotic and 14 dizygotic twins. Although their method of statistical analysis was not quite appropriate, intrapair variances calculated from their data for monozygotic (1312) and dizygotic (3877) twins differ significantly (F = 2.96, $P < 0.05$), which indicates that variation in identical twins is significantly less than in non-identical twins. Racial factors may also be involved since the mean level in Negro females has been found to be significantly greater than in Caucasian females in the United States (Meltzer 1971; Meltzer and Holy 1974).

All these various factors also have an effect on SCK levels in carriers. *Standardized* exercise (on a walking machine or a bicycle ergometer) has been claimed by some to accentuate SCK levels in carriers more than controls provided that it is strenuous and the effects are followed for several hours afterwards (Emery 1967b; Gaines *et al.* 1982; Herrmann *et al.* 1982; Cordone *et al.* 1984). It has therefore been recommended as a provocative test in suspected carriers with a borderline SCK level. However, as we shall see, an obsession with 'detection rates' is really not justified (p. 200).

We have determined SCK levels by the method of Rosalki (1967), assays being performed at 30 °C and the results expressed in International Units (iu) per litre. After the late teens there is no clear relationship between age and SCK levels in carriers (Fig. 11.4). In 180 measurements on definite carriers tested at different ages, neither the correlation with age ($r = -0.10$), nor the regression on age ($Y = 296 - 2.29X$) were statistically significant. There is also no consistent change in individual adult carriers tested at different ages.

However, a follow-up study by Moser and Vogt (1974) suggested that carrier detection might be better in childhood. Furthermore, Nicholson *et al.* (1979) found that the proportion of 52 daughters (mean age 16) of definite carriers who had raised SCK levels (above the normal 95 per cent confidence limits of 73 iu for girls under 16, and 60 iu for older women) was 45 per cent. Since half the daughters would be expected to be carriers, the detection rate would seem to be around 90 per cent compared with 53 per cent for their adult

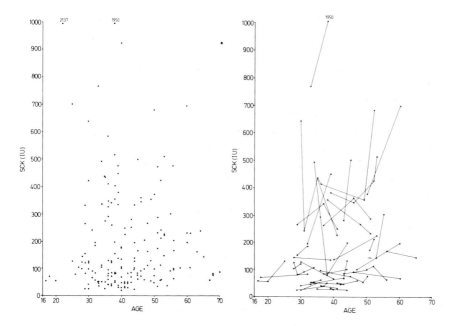

Fig. 11.4. SCK levels and age in definite carriers of Duchenne muscular dystrophy. (*Left*) all values (*N* = 180). (*Right*) values for individual carriers tested at different ages (*N* = 39.) (Unpublished data.)

carriers. However, SCK levels are also higher in normal premenarchal girls, and it has been suggested that these results might be explained if this factor had not been very carefully controlled (Bundey *et al.* 1979b; Carter 1979), and in any event the distribution of SCK levels in premenarchal carriers is unknown.

We have refrained from testing very young girls who are at risk. However, among daughters of definite carriers who are age *15 and over* and who have not yet had any children, the proportion with SCK levels exceeding the normal 95 percentile (86 iu) for adult women is not significantly different from the expected proportion (31.20 per cent) based on the findings in definite carriers (Table 11.4).

SCK levels in carriers may also be affected by genetic factors. Thus Sibert *et al.* (1979) found that the interfamilial variance of SCK levels in carriers was significantly (*P* < 0.05) greater than the intrafamilial variance, suggesting that there might be 'familial clustering' of SCK levels. In the present study this problem has been examined by considering correlations between SCK levels in various female relatives within families of definite carriers (Table 11.5). All the correlations were positive but none was significantly different

Table 11.4   *The proportion of daughters of definite carriers who have SCK levels which exceed the normal 95 percentile (86 iu) for adult women (unpublished data)*

	No.	Age			Proportion	
		Range	Mean	s.d.	No.	%
Controls	200	18–52	27.06	9.10	11	5.50
Carriers	125	17–70	41.69	11.67	78	62.40
Controls	65	15–20	18.72	0.67	3	4.62
Daughters of carriers	49	15–20	17.33	1.84	16	32.65
	72	15–39	19.78	4.64	21	29.17

Table 11.5   *Correlations between SCK levels in females within families of definite carriers. The correlations between sisters (daughters of definite carriers) refer to all sisters (1), or where at least two sisters in a family had SCK levels in excess of 170 iu (2) and therefore likely to be carriers, or less than 86 iu (3) and therefore unlikely to be carriers (unpublished data)*

	Carrier mothers and daughters	Daughters of carriers		
		Sisters (1)	Sisters (2)	Sisters (3)
Number	101	111	20	41
Correlation	0.016	0.138	0.182	0.112
Students 't'	0.158	1.455	0.785	0.704

Table 11.6   *Distribution of SCK levels in controls and carriers (unpublished data)*

SCK	Controls		Carriers		h (Y_1/Y_2)
	No.	% (Y_1)	No.	% (Y_2)	
11–30	26	13.0	5	4.0	3.25
31–50	112	56.0	15	12.0	4.67
51–70	47	23.5	9	7.2	3.26
71–90	6	3.0	20	16.0	0.19
91–110	3	1.5	18	14.4	0.10
111–170	6	3.0	14	11.2	–
>170	0	0.0	44	35.2	–
Total	*200*	*100.0*	*125*	*100.0*	–

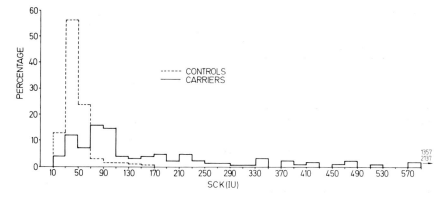

Fig. 11.5. Distribution of SCK levels determined under standardized conditions in 200 normal adult control females and 125 definite carriers.

from zero. If there are any familial similarities in SCK levels these would therefore seem to be relatively unimportant.

In view of the various technical and biological variations which may influence SCK levels, it is therefore not surprising that there is a considerable spread of values in controls, the distribution being positively skewed. In carriers the spread is even greater and the distribution even more skewed, but there is no suggestion of any bimodality (Fig. 11.5). Since the distributions in the two groups are so different results have been expressed as the ratio (h) of normal homozygosity (Y_1) to heterozygosity (Y_2) as in Table 11.6. The normal 95 percentile (based on the cumulative distribution curve) is 86 iu; 78 (62 per cent) of definite carriers had levels which exceeded this, and 44 (35 per cent) had levels outside the upper limit of the normal range of 170 iu.

Because of the variability in SCK levels in carriers our practice, and that of others, has been where possible to take the mean of samples obtained on three separate occasions in the belief that this might provide a better guide to carrier status. However, compared with the values obtained with single determinations in controls, no matter how the upper limit of normal is defined, repeat testing seems to have little overall effect on the discriminatory value of the test (Table 11.7).

Linked DNA markers

There have been many attempts to improve the discriminatory value of the SCK test by combining the results with those of other tests, such as muscle pathology, electromyography, and particularly other serum enzymes and proteins such as haemopexin, myoglobin, and pyruvate kinase. It now seems clear, however, that much more useful information can be gained by combin-

Table 11.7　*Proportion (%) of carriers (N = 94) with SCK levels which exceed the normal upper limit depending on whether the first, mean or highest of three determinations is used (Emery 1982)*

	95 percentile (86 iu)	Median × 2.5 (110 iu)	Median × 3 (132 iu)
First	58	49	40
Mean	64	46	40
Highest	65	52	41
Controls	*5*	*3*	*1*

ing SCK data with information from linked DNA markers. It should be emphasised however that it is entirely incorrect to consider the value of the SCK test purely in terms of 'detection rate'. It is much preferable to consider the probability (odds) of a woman being a carrier based not only on her SCK level but also on pedigree and DNA data. It usually then makes little difference to the final probability estimate in practical terms whether the test result is actually outside the normal range or lies in the upper part of the range.

Calculation of risks

The estimation of genetic risks is usually, although not always (see Bundey 1978), based on Bayes' theorem (Emery and Morton 1968; Murphy and Mutalik 1969). In these calculations four probabilities are considered: *prior, conditional, joint,* and *posterior.* The prior probability is based on knowledge of the individual's antecedents and sibs. The conditional probability is the probability of being a carrier or not depending on the individual's SCK level, data from DNA markers, and the number of normal sons she may have had. The product of the prior and conditional probabilities is the joint probability. The final posterior probability of a woman being a carrier is the joint probability of getting the observed information given she is a carrier, divided by the sum of this probability plus the joint probability of getting the observed information if she is not a carrier. The method of calculation is illustrated in the following examples.

Consider the family in Fig. 11.6 where a daughter III_3 with a normal son seeks genetic counselling. It would appear that the Duchenne gene and RFLP allele-2 are co-inherited in the family (see p. 175). First, we consider the prior probability of III_3 being a carrier or not being a carrier which is 0.5. Let us assume that she has an SCK of 40 iu, that she has inherited RFLP allele-2 from her mother, and the frequency of recombination (θ) between the RFLP and the disease locus is 5 per cent (0.05). Then, if she *is* a carrier the (condi-

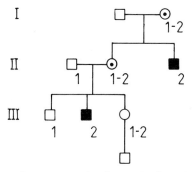

Fig. 11.6. Pedigree of Duchenne muscular dystrophy linked to an RFLP, the alleles of which are represented below the pedigree sybmbols.

tional) probability of her having allele-2 is 0.95 (1 − θ) because crossing-over would *not* have to occur. Since 56 per cent of controls and 12 per cent of definite carriers have an SCK of 31–50 iu (Table 11.6, p. 198), the conditional probability of having an SCK of 40 iu if she is a carrier is 0.12. Finally, the conditional probability of having a normal son if she is a carrier is 0.50. On the other hand if she is *not* a carrier then these conditional probilities are respectively 0.05 (since crossing-over would now have to occur), 0.56 and 1.00. The calculations are set out as follows:

Probability	Carrier	Not a carrier
Prior	0.50	0.50
Conditional		
allele-2	0.95	0.05
SCK 40 iu	0.12	0.56
normal son	0.50	1.00
Joint	0.029	0.014

Posterior
(of being a carrier)

$$= \frac{0.029}{0.029 + 0.014}$$
$$= 0.674$$

i.e. there is a very high probability (67 per cent) that she is a carrier and therefore any son she has would have a 1 in 3 chance of being affected.

However, suppose she had inherited allele-1, and therefore seemed unlikely to be a carrier (unless crossing-over occurred) yet her SCK level was 100 iu (i.e. in the upper part of the normal range), the calculations are then as follows:

Probability	Carrier	Not a carrier
Prior	0.50	0.50
Conditional		
allele-1	0.05	0.95
SCK 100 iu	0.144	0.015
normal son	0.50	1.00
Joint	0.002	0.007

Posterior
(of being a carrier)

$$= \frac{0.002}{0.002 + 0.007}$$
$$= 0.222$$

Thus, the chance of being a carrier remains high and in this case the probability of a son being affected is roughly 1 in 9.

It should be noted that in these calculations for the sake of simplicity the linkage phase in mother (whether allele-2 is coinherited with the Duchenne gene) is assumed and with a closely linked probe ($\theta < 0.10$) this makes no practical difference to the results (Emery 1986). Other worked examples are given in Harper *et al.* (1983) and Pembrey *et al.* (1984).

However, nowadays in many families there is only one affected boy. The affected boy in such a family may represent a new mutation and there is also no certainty as to the linkage phase in the family. Let us first consider for the sake of simplicity that in such a family only data on SCK levels are available. Let us assume that a woman who seeks genetic counselling has an SCK of 80 iu, one normal brother, and a sister with an SCK of 60 iu who has an affected son, there being no one else affected in the family. We first have to go back one generation and consider the *mother* of these two sisters. Like any woman in the population she has a prior probability of being a carrier of 4 μ, where μ is the mutation rate in both males and females. The reason, put simply, is that the chance of a mutation occurring in either of her maternally or paternally derived X-chromosomes is 2 μ and the probability that she might have inherited the mutant gene through her mother is also 2 μ. We then consider the conditional probabilities, firstly of her having had a normal son and secondly of having had a daughter with an SCK of 60 iu and an affected son. In the case of the daughter we first determine the prior probabilities of her being a carrier or not a carrier given her mother is or is not a carrier. Secondly, we determine the conditional probabilities of the daughter having an affected son and a serum level of creatine kinase of 60 iu assuming she is or is not a carrier, and finally we determine her joint probabilities. The final overall joint probabilities are arrived at by multiplying the daughter's joint probabilities by her mother's prior probabilities and her mother's conditional probabilities of having a normal son.

The calculation are set out as follows:

Probability	Carrier		Not a carrier	
Prior	4μ		$1 - 4\mu \simeq 1$	
Conditional				
a normal son	1/2		1	
daughter	Carrier	Not a carrier	Carrier	Not a carrier
Prior	1/2	1/2	2μ	1
Conditional				
affected son	1/2	μ	1/2	μ
SCK 60 iu	0.07	0.24	0.07	0.24
Joint	0.02	$0.12\,\mu$	$0.07\,\mu$	$0.24\,\mu$
Joint	$0.04\,\mu$	$0.24\,\mu^2$ (negligible)	$0.07\,\mu$	$0.24\,\mu$

The final posterior probability of the *mother* being a carrier, taking into account information on her daughter with an affected son, is the sum of the joint probabilities if she is a carrier (columns 1 and 2) divided by the sum of these probabilities plus the sum of the joint probabilities if she is not a carrier (columns 3 and 4) i.e.

$$\frac{0.04\,\mu}{0.04\,\mu + 0.07\,\mu + 0.24\,\mu}$$
$$= 0.11$$

We now consider the sister who came for counselling who now has a prior probability of being a carrier of 0.055, say 0.06:

Probability	Carrier	Not a carrier
Prior	0.06	0.94
Conditional		
SCK 80 iu	0.16	0.03
Joint	0.010	0.028

Her (posterior) probability of being a carrier is therefore:

$$\frac{0.010}{0.010 + 0.028}$$
$$= 0.26$$

Thus, despite the fact that both she and her sister have SCK levels within the normal range, the sister who requested counselling still has a high chance (i.e. about 1 in 4) of being a carrier.

A general formula for a calculating the probability of a woman being a carrier of a *lethal* X-linked disorder, which affects either a brother or a son (*there being no one else affected in the family*) has been derived (Emery and Morton 1968). If h_c and h_m refer respectively to the relative probabilities of normal homozygosity to heterozygosity (Y_1/Y_2 in Table 11.6) in the suspected carrier and her mother, so that if there is no such information $h = 1$,

and if $q =$ number of normal brothers
and $r =$ number of normal sons
and if $s = 1$ where a son is affected and 0 if a brother is affected
and $t = 0$ where a son is affected and 1 if a brother is affected,

then the probability (P) of her being a carrier of a *lethal* X-linked disorder is:

$$P = \frac{1 + sa}{1 + sa + ab + tb}$$

where $a = h_m 2^q$
and $b = h_c 2^r$

It is also helpful to include in these calculations information on SCK levels in all the first degree postpubertal female relatives of a suspected carrier (Emery and Holloway 1977).

Over the years we have tested some 1400 potential carriers in over 400 families, in many of which there was only one affected boy. By using Bayesian statistics and combining both pedigree and SCK data, rather than using pedigree data alone, reduced considerably the proportion of women who fell into the intermediate risk range (Fig. 11.7). Even further separation is possible if DNA data are also included in the calculations.

Finally, even in families with an isolated case of Duchenne muscular dystrophy, carrier detection can be improved by using data from a linked RFLP. The probability of the sister of an affected boy being a carrier (or a subsequent male fetus being affected) depends on whether the individual has the same or a different maternal RFLP from the affected boy. If the sister has a different allele then, barring crossing-over, she is unlikely to be a carrier. The position is improved the closer the DNA marker is to the disease locus. If θ is, say, 0.05 and she has a different allele from her affected brother, her risk becomes about 1 in 16, or less than 1 in 30 if she also has an unaffected brother (Fig. 11.8). The risks could be reduced even further depending on her actual SCK level.

Information on DNA markers lying on either side of the locus (flanking or bridging markers) and from the maternal grandfather's haplotype are also important, and increase the precision (Clayton and Emery 1984; Clark 1985). The likelihood that information from a linked RFLP will be helpful (mother

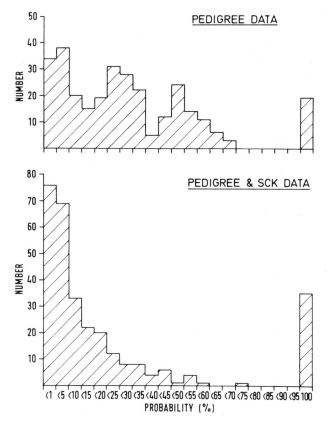

Fig. 11.7. Risks in 300 potential carriers based on: (*above*) pedigree data alone, (*below*) pedigree and SCK data combined.

will be heterozygous and the segregation pattern in the family will be informative) increases as the number of alleles at the RFLP locus increases (Asmussen and Clegg 1985).

The calculations involved in determining the probability of the mother or sister of an isolated case being a carrier, which takes into account both SCK and RFLP data, are detailed in Emery (1986). However, they can be somewhat tedious, especially when more than one DNA marker is involved and there are a number of relatives to be considered. Fortunately there are now computer programs available specifically for these calculations (for example, Clayton 1986; Sarfarazi and Williams 1986). Too much reliance on such programs, however, may lead to problems because serious errors can occur if mistakes are inadvertently made in inserting relevant data. When dealing with straightforward familial cases, and in isolated cases where one is only

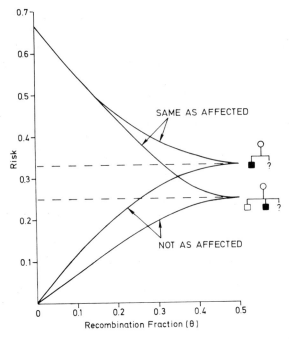

Fig. 11.8. Risks of the sister of an isolated case of Duchenne muscular dystrophy being a carrier (or a subsequent male fetus being affected) depending on whether the individual has the same or a different maternal RFLP allele from the affected boy.

dealing with a single closely linked probe, the calculations can often be performed with a hand calculator.

A guide to the risks of a daughter being a carrier, whose brother is an isolated case, are given in Table 11.8. The risks depend on her SCK level (the relative probability of normal homozygosity to heterozygosity 'h'), whether she has the same or a different RFLP allele as her affected brother, and the frequency of recombination (crossing-over) between the RFLP and the disease locus (0.01–0.50). The risks of the mother having another affected son correspond to the entries in the Table where $h = 1$ (i.e. where in a potential carrier it is assumed there is no information on SCK levels). These risks, however, ignore additional information which might also be available including the number of normal sons and brothers the mother may have, mother's SCK level, information from more than one probe, and the haplotype of the maternal grandfather. Nevertheless, the tabulated risks provide at least a first approximation. Note that until there is more information about subsequent sons and her daughter's status, the risks of the mother being a carrier are *a priori* 2 in 3 and obviously uninfluenced by DNA marker data on her affected son.

Table 11.8 *Risks of the sister of an isolated case of Duchenne muscular dystrophy being a carrier (or of a subsequent male fetus being affected) for different values of* h *and recombination fraction (θ), and whether the sister (or male fetus) has the same* or a different† RFLP allele from the affected boy. (When* θ = 0.50 *there are no data on a DNA marker; when* h = 1.0 *there are no data on SCK)*

	Recombination fraction (θ)							
	0.01	0.05	0.10	0.15	0.20	0.30	0.40	0.50
$h = 0.1$								
Same:	0.950	0.938	0.923	0.908	0.892	0.863	0.841	0.833
Diff:	0.118	0.403	0.577	0.672	0.731	0.795	0.825	0.833
$h = 0.2$								
Same:	0.904	0.884	0.858	0.831	0.806	0.759	0.726	0.714
Diff:	0.063	0.253	0.405	0.506	0.576	0.660	0.702	0.714
$h = 0.5$								
Same:	0.790	0.753	0.707	0.664	0.624	0.558	0.515	0.500
Diff:	0.026	0.119	0.214	0.291	0.352	0.437	0.485	0.500
$h = 1.0$								
Same:	0.653	0.603	0.547	0.497	0.453	0.387	0.347	0.333
Diff:	0.013	0.063	0.120	0.170	0.213	0.280	0.320	0.333
$h = 2.0$								
Same:	0.485	0.432	0.376	0.330	0.293	0.240	0.210	0.200
Diff:	0.007	0.033	0.064	0.093	0.119	0.163	0.190	0.200
$h = 3.0$								
Same:	0.386	0.336	0.287	0.248	0.217	0.174	0.150	0.143
Diff:	0.004	0.022	0.043	0.064	0.083	0.115	0.136	0.143
$h = 4.0$								
Same:	0.320	0.275	0.232	0.198	0.172	0.136	0.117	0.111
Diff:	0.003	0.017	0.033	0.049	0.063	0.089	0.105	0.111
$h = 5.0$								
Same:	0.274	0.233	0.194	0.165	0.142	0.112	0.096	0.091
Diff:	0.003	0.013	0.027	0.039	0.051	0.072	0.086	0.091

$$* \text{ Risk } = \left(1 + \frac{h(1 + 4\theta - 4\theta^2)}{2 - 4\theta + 4\theta^2}\right)^{-1} \qquad \dagger \text{ Risk } = \left(1 + \frac{h(3 - 4\theta + 4\theta^2)}{4\theta - 4\theta^2}\right)^{-1}$$

Prenatal diagnosis

A woman at high risk of having an affected son may chose fetal sexing with selective abortion of any male fetus and in this way be guaranteed a daughter who will not be affected. However, this is unsatisfactory for two reasons.

First, at least half of the aborted fetuses will in fact be normal. Secondly, sons who would not reproduce are replaced by daughters, a proportion of whom will be carriers and may in due course transmit the gene to their offspring. The effect is therefore dysgenic and would be expected to lead eventually to an increase in the incidence of heterozygous carriers. What is therefore required is a reliable test for the *affected* male fetus. At first it seemed that SCK levels in fetal blood obtained at fetoscopy might be valuable, but several false negatives soon invalidated this approach (Ionasescu *et al.* 1978; Emery *et al.* 1979a; Golbus *et al.* 1979). However, the advent of recombinant DNA technology has opened up an entirely different approach to prenatal diagnosis. Fetal DNA can be extracted from amniotic fluid cells obtained by transabdominal amniocentesis at about 16–18 weeks of gestation. Then either using a gene specific probe (p. 178) or a closely linked DNA marker (p. 173) the probability of the fetus being affected can be determined. The use of bridging markers reduces the probability of error due to crossing-over and a prenatal diagnosis has been made on the basis of such markers (Bakker *et al.* 1985). Furthermore, as the number of probes increases so the likelihood that a suspected carrier will be heterozygous, and therefore informative, for at least one marker also increases. Thus in the case of the markers listed in Table 11.9, the probability that a woman would be heterozygous for at least one is 99.7 per cent. However, should she be homozygous for a possibly informative RFLP allele then it will not be clear which of her X-

Table 11.9 *Some DNA probes useful for carrier detection and prenatal diagnosis. The heterozygote frequencies and genetic distances are approximate (data from various sources)*

Probe	Restriction enzyme	Heterozygote frequency	Genetic distance (cM)
Distal (terminal)			
RC8	Taq I	0.25	15
99-6	Pst I	0.50	15
B24	Msp I	0.15	10
C7	Eco RV	0.25	5
PERT 87-8	Bst XI	0.50	
	Taq I	0.40	
PERT 87-1	Xmn I	0.40	<5
	Bst NI	0.50	
XJ-1.1	Taq I	0.30	
754	Pst I	0.45	10
OTC	Msp I	0.30	10
L1.28	Taq I	0.45	15
Proximal (centromere)			

chromosomes is carrying the Duchenne gene. In future this will become less of a problem as more closely linked markers become available.

A more recent development has been the introduction of chorion biopsy for prenatal diagnosis (Rodeck and Morsman 1983; Hogge *et al.* 1985). Essentially the technique consists of inserting a flexible cannula/catheter either through the cervix or transabdominally into the uterine cavity. Chorionic villi (which are of fetal origin) are carefully removed for DNA, cytogenetic, and other studies (Fig. 11.9). Since this procedure can be performed as early as 10 weeks gestation and the material need not be cultured for DNA or chromosome studies, a prenatal diagnosis can be made much earlier than with amniocentesis and if an abortion has to be carried out it is therefore likely to cause less psychological trauma. The risks of chorion biopsy have yet to be fully assessed but it seems already that this is likely to

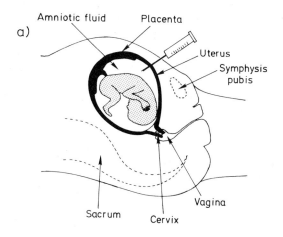

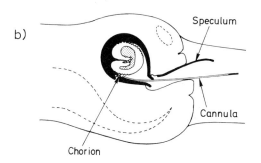

Fig. 11.9. Technique of: (*a*) transabdominal amniocentesis, (*b*) chorion biopsy. (From Emery (1985) reprinted with permission of John Wiley and Sons Ltd.)

become the accepted procedure for the prenatal diagnosis of disorders such as Duchenne muscular dystrophy.

Ova transfer

This procedure might be indicated in the case of a woman who is at high risk of having an affected son but who for various reasons may not be able to face prenatal diagnosis and abortion. Here ova from an unrelàted (non-carrier) female are fertilized *in vitro* by the carrier's husband's sperm. A fertilized ovum is them implanted in the carrier's uterus where it develops normally. Although a theoretical possibility, the author is not aware that this has yet been carried out on a carrier of Duchenne muscular dystrophy.

Finally, a future possibility may be to remove ova by laparoscopy from a carrier female and having fertilized them with her husband's sperm allow them to develop *in vitro* until, say, the early blastocyst stage. It might then prove feasible to remove a single cell without damaging the conceptus and by using appropriate DNA markers determine if it will be affected or a heterozygous carrier. Only unaffected male or non-carrier female conceptuses would be reimplanted in the uterus to undergo further development. However, it will be some time before this procedure becomes technically possible.

Summary and conclusions

Since Duchenne muscular dystrophy is a serious disorder for which at present there is no effective treatment, much emphasis has been given to prevention. This involves the ascertainment of women likely to have an affected son, and the provision of genetic counselling and prenatal diagnosis for such women. The ascertainment of women at risk could be achieved by screening the entire population for affected boys or by screening women within known affected families. Screening for affected boys in the newborn period has the advantage that such early detection might lead to the prevention of second cases in a family. A number of neonatal screening programmes have been developed with some success. There are, however, a number of technical and logistical problems for which reasons some have advocated restricting screening to boys who are, for example, not walking by the age of 18 months. So far, however, there has been little enthusiasm for screening though no doubt interest will be rekindled once an effective treatment is found.

There are merits in recording affected families on a computerized register system with inbuilt safeguards for confidentiality and maintained on a local rather than a national basis. It can ensure that those in need of counselling, welfare services, and therapy can be readily contacted as developments in these various fields occur.

The major problem in prevention is the detection of female carriers. About 5–10 per cent have some degree of muscle involvement but this is rarely serious. The single most reliable test for detecting healthy carriers remains the SCK level, provided due attention is given to the various technical and biological factors which can affect it, including age (before 20) and pregnancy. Particularly valuable information can also be provided from linked DNA markers (Restriction Fragment Length Polymorphisms, RFLPs) which may soon replace other approaches to carrier detection. The probability of a woman being a carrier should be based on combined pedigree, SCK and, when available, DNA data using Bayesian statistics.

Prenatal diagnosis is also possible through the use of DNA probes, and when combined with chorion biopsy a diagnosis can be made as early as 10 weeks gestation which should make the procedure more acceptable.

Finally, as more closely linked DNA markers and gene specific probes become available, so precision will increase and genetic counselling become that much more reliable.

12 Genetic counselling

Much emphasis has so far been placed on the probability of a woman being a carrier and the risks of her having an affected son. In genetic counselling these are important issues, but other matters also have to be considered and discussed.

Nature of genetic counselling

Genetic counselling is essentially a process of communication between the counseller and those who seek counselling. Information to be communicated falls roughly into two main areas. First, information about the nature of the disorder: its severity and prognosis and whether or not there is any effective therapy, what the genetic mechanism is that caused the disease, and what are the risks of its occurring in relatives. Secondly, information on the available options open to a couple who are found to be at risk of transmitting the disease. This latter may include discussions of contraception, sterilization, prenatal diagnosis, and abortion.

When discussing the disease, the genetic counseller has to present an accurate picture, even if depressing and disturbing if the parents are to make a reasoned decision about future children. It seems misleading to offer them encouragement in the hope that any future affected children might be treatable when this possibility, at least at present, appears to be remote. Such discussions require considerable sensitivity and tact when the parents already have a young affected child. It is not uncommon for those involved in both the management of the disease as well as counselling to find themselves in the dilemma of having to maintain an optimistic outlook for the affected child and yet emphasizing the seriousness of the disorder when discussing its possible recurrence in any future children.

Having discussed at length the more medical aspects of the disease, the counsellor then proceeds to explain the genetic mechanism which caused it and the risks of recurrence in terms which are understandable to the individual couple. A preoccupation with risk figures can often be confusing and is best avoided. Often couples merely want to know if there is any chance at all that it could occur again. In many cases genetic mechanisms and recurrence risks need be discussed only in broad terms. In any event the actual interpretation of risks is very subjective (Pearn 1973): what might be an acceptable risk to one couple may be quite unacceptable to another. Nevertheless, risks form a useful basis for further discussions and can be a significant factor in influencing decision making. One important fact which may have to be explained is that being genetic the parents cannot hold themselves in any way responsible and every effort should be made to dispel feelings of guilt and recrimination which they may be harbouring.

If the risks are considered to be unacceptably high, then the options available include family limitation, contraception, prenatal diagnosis, and abortion, and perhaps one day ova transfer. Contraception in this context requires expert advice because the results of failure will be far more devastating than when it is practised for purely social and economic reasons. A deep fear of having an affected child may well generate serious psycho-sexual problems and for this reason some definitive form of contraception may well have to be considered, such as tubal ligation or vasectomy. The effects of sterilization when performed on healthy women whose families are complete are likely to be entirely beneficial (Anon. 1984). But in a young woman in a family with Duchenne muscular dystrophy who either has no children or perhaps only the one affected child, it may have significant psychological sequelae. Counselling is especially important in these cases. To some couples sexual abstinence may be the only acceptable alternative.

Prenatal diagnosis has added a whole new dimension to genetic counselling, and when the result is negative the reassurance it gives is entirely beneficial. However, a proportion of mothers may decide to continue with the pregnancy after fetal sexing and learning that the fetus is male and therefore likely to be affected (Bundey and Ebdy 1982; Thompson 1984), presumably prepared to some extent to cope with the resultant problems (Golbus *et al.* 1974). Certainly therapeutic abortion can cause considerable psychological trauma in many women (Blumberg 1984), and in those genetic disorders where prenatal diagnosis is possible, after pregnancy termination following the diagnosis of an affected fetus, a significant proportion of mothers decline to undergo the procedure again. Sensitive counselling is therefore essential both at the time of prenatal diagnosis and during the period following a therapeutic abortion. However, as Blumberg has stated, although 'Significant psychological trauma may be an unavoidable consequence of selective abortion, the alternative birth of a defective child is usually accompanied by even more intense feelings of guilt and depression' (Blumberg 1984).

As a prelude to genetic counselling it is important to divine a couple's educational and social background, their religious attitudes and, if possible, something of their marital relationships if information is to be presented most effectively and sensitively. The counsellor may sense that for various ethical and other reasons contraception, sterilization or prenatal diagnosis are unacceptable to a couple. These matters should then not be discussed further. The genetic counsellor's role is to inform and guide but not to coerce or impose his own views.

Non-directive counselling

The genetic counsellor's role, until relatively recently, was often seen purely in medical and scientific terms: to establish a precise genetic diagnosis and to communicate factual information about the disease and its genetics. However, more emphasis is now being given to an appreciation of the psychological aspects of counselling. A change from what Kessler (1979) has referred to as *content-oriented* to *person-oriented* counselling. This change has been brought about by several factors. First, a disabling genetic disorder such as Duchenne muscular dystrophy often has profound psychological effects on the immediate family (Buchanan *et al.* 1979; Pullen 1984). Secondly, these effects may have long-term consequences and frequently extend to other relatives. Thirdly, it has been found that couples sometimes opt for a course of action which may well be at variance with what the counsellor might have regarded as 'reasonable'. For example, in a prospective follow-up study of 200 consecutive couples seen in a genetic counselling clinic with various genetic disorders, a proportion of those told that they were at risk of having an affected child were undeterred and actually planned further pregnancies (Emery *et al.* 1979c). At first sight such behaviour might seem irresponsible but on careful questioning in almost all cases the reasons for planning further children were often very understandable when considered from the parents' point of view. In some cases further pregnancies were planned because, after seeing the effects of a disorder in a previous child or in one of the parents, it was not considered sufficiently serious (congenital cataract, congenital deafness, peroneal muscular atrophy), or prenatal diagnosis was available (Sandhoff's disease, X-linked mental retardation), and yet in other cases the parents planned further pregnancies because if a subsequent child were affected it would not survive (renal agenesis), or if it survived it would succumb within a year or so (Werdnig–Hoffmann disease). There was a small but lamentable group of couples who had no living children and dearly wanted a family at whatever cost (Emery *et al.* 1979c).

   Thus a course of action which might seem irresponsible to one person may seem eminently reasonable to another. The choice should be the individual's prerogative, always provided that it is made in the full knowledge of all the facts and possible consequences. Since the genetic counsellor's role is to help couples arrive at decisions which are *the best ones for themselves*, genetic counselling should never be directive. Nevertheless, because Duchenne muscular dystrophy is such a serious ad distressing condition, most counsellors may hope that couples at risk will exercise caution.

Timing of counselling – the coping process

For really successful counselling it is essential to recognize the problems of attempting to communicate information of a personal and delicate nature in a situation when the parents may not yet have recovered from the shock of the diagnosis (Buchanan *et al.* 1979). They may well be harbouring feelings of guilt, recrimination, and lowered self-esteem. They may be angry and tense or just numbed by the situation. But all will be under considerable stress. The psychological sequence of events which follow the initial diagnosis is referred to as the *coping process* and is similar in other stressful situations such as bereavement. Thus parents with a child with Duchenne muscular dystrophy have to face two major stressful events – at the time the diagnosis is first made, and later when the affected boy dies. On both these occasions the family will require considerable support from all those concerned – paediatricians, physicians, geneticists, genetic associates, social workers, and nurses. It should also be remembered that father may be just as affected as mother, but since most men do not express their emotions readily, this may be underestimated or even go unrecognized.

Five sequential stages have been recognized in the coping process (Falek 1977, 1984):

Shock and denial
Anxiety
Anger and guilt
Depression
Psychological homeostasis.

The duration of each stage varies from individual to individual. Very rarely, a parent may never progress beyond the stage of denial, while a few may reach the stage of depression and remain at this stage. The genetic counsellor has to recognise the existence of these stages and to tailor his counselling accordingly. He has to appreciate that the assimilation of information and the process of decision making will be very much influenced by the stage in the coping process that a parent has reached.

At the very beginning, the parent may be unable to accept that the child is affected, and at this stage sympathy and compassion are required until acceptance occurs. Anxiety impairs judgement and reason, and at this stage the counsellor should provide support and encourage the sharing of emotions. Information may have to be repeated on a number of occasions if it is to be fully understood and appreciated. The most difficult stage for the counsellor is when the parent is angry and resentful. Hostility may well be directed towards the counsellor himself. This has to be accepted as being part of the coping process and not taken personally. Gentle persuasion is indicated, although sometimes it may be necessary to withdraw temporarily and make arrangements for a later appointment when the parent's hostility and resentment may have been tempered. At the stage of depression the effects may be such as to necessitate some form of antidepressant therapy but it is probably at this stage that genetic counselling can begin more earnestly. Counselling should not be postponed until homeostasis has been reached, although obviously information will be better received and understood and decisions will be more rational at this last stage.

Genetic counselling is part of the general counselling which parents with an affected child are given, and which calls for special knowledge and skills on the part of the counsellor. These matters are discussed by Freeman and Pearson (1978), Parry (1984), and Maguire (1984) who provide references to the relevant bibliography.

Who should be offered genetic counselling?

Geneticists tend to consider risks greater than one in 10 as being 'high' and less than one in 20 as being 'low'. This is based on early studies which tended to show that, in general, couples are more likely to be deterred from planning a pregnancy when the risk is greater than one in 10, but less so if it is less than one in 20 (e.g. Carter *et al.* 1971; Emery *et al.* 1973b). However, it is difficult to extrapolate from responses to genetic disorders in general to one disease in particular, such as Duchenne muscular dystrophy, because into the equation has to be included the so-called 'burden' of a disorder. By this is meant the psychological, and to a lesser extent the social and economic problems attendant on having a child with a serious genetic disorder. The concept has been discussed in detail by Murphy (1973). In some disorders, such as congenital muscular dystrophy, although the burden is great it is of limited duration and therefore possibly more acceptable than in Duchenne muscular dystrophy where the affected child survives for many years, becoming progressively incapacitated. There is good evidence that couples are often more influenced by the burden of a disease than by the actual risks of recurrence (Carter *et al.* 1971; Leonard *et al.* 1972; Emery *et al.* 1973b; Hsia 1974; Stern and Eldridge 1975). Thus, concern among relatives about the disorder occurring in their children is only partly a reflection of their risk. It is also tempered by their individual views of the 'burden' of the disease.

In part for logistical reasons, it has sometimes been suggested that genetic counselling in Duchenne muscular dystrophy might be restricted to those women whose *a priori* risk is greater than 1 in 10. But this does not seem entirely justified because affected boys have sometimes been born to mothers whose risk had been estimated to be less than 1 in 20 (Hutton and Thompson 1976). However, there can be a serious problem in considering the carrier status of female relatives who are somewhat distantly related to the proband. In such cases it is essential to include the *a priori* risk in the calculations, when it may well be so low as to be little influenced by a slightly elevated SCK level, the result of which taken on its own would be entirely misleading. Apart from this proviso there would seem every reason to offer counselling where appropriate to all first and second degree female relatives of affected boys as well as to any other relative who may be anxious. Some centres with considerable experience in the field offer their services to any woman who is concerned about the problem (Thompson 1984) and this would seem entirely commendable.

Effects of genetic counselling

The effects of genetic counselling and prenatal diagnosis in Duchenne muscular dystrophy can be assessed in various ways: in relation to changes in the incidence of the disorder in a community; the reproductive behaviour of those counselled; and the social and psychological effects on the family.

The effects on population incidence have already been discussed (p. 156) where it was concluded that at best this could be reduced to the occurrence of new mutations which in the past represented about a third of cases.

The effects on the reproductive behaviour of individual women who have been counselled have been assessed in several studies, the results of which are summarized in Table 12.1. The definition of high, moderate and low risks in each of the studies was similar, and only data on those women who were married and of reproductive age are included. Those who were deterred after counselling either avoided pregnancy altogether, or opted for prenatal diagnosis in any future pregnancy. Precise comparisons are difficult because of differences in the religious, cultural, economic, and educational levels of those counselled as well as presumably differences in the counsellors themselves. Nevertheless, it seems clear that those given a high risk are usually deterred from further pregnancies, unless coupled with prenatal diagnosis. In the study of Zatz (1983) from Brazil, the high proportion of those at low risk who were deterred may reflect the use of the information by women to gain priority help from family planning centres.

Follow-up studies have confirmed that the proportion of affected boys among births to mothers considered to be at high risk is significantly greater than among mothers considered to be at low risk (Hutton and Thompson 1976; Dennis *et al.* 1976).

The social and psychological effects of genetic counselling in Duchenne muscular dystrophy are much more difficult to assess. A common complaint from parents is that at the time of diagnosis they were experiencing considerable stress, making it difficult to accept information at all (Buchanan *et al.* 1979). In one extensive study in the United Kingdom, Firth (1983) reported the results of interviews with 53 families. In only 18 were both parents told of the diagnosis together. Many of the parents who had been alone when told,

Table 12.1 *The effects of genetic counselling in Duchenne muscular dystrophy on the reproductive behaviour of married women of reproductive age*

Period	High risk		Moderate risk		Low risk		Reference
	Total No.	% deterred	Total No.	% deterred	Total No.	% deterred	
1965–69	40	95	5	80	6	17	Emery *et al.* (1972)
1965–76	25	88	2	–	46	4	Dennis *et al.* (1976)
1965–74	45	82	33	51	29	24	Hutton & Thompson (1976)
1969–82	126	90	19	84	41	61	Zatz (1983)

described how their distress was heightened by having to break the news to their spouse. A third of the parents were not satisfied with the way the information had been conveyed which was often inadequate and with no follow-up. Although conveying information about a diagnosis is only part of counselling, it is an important part. It is difficult to see that if at this stage a good rapport has not been established with a couple, any meaningful dialogue can follow later. On the basis of her findings Firth made several recommendations: parents should be told of the diagnosis as soon as possible, together and in private, and a series of contacts should be planned not only with the paediatrician but with other health care professionals involved with the disease and who can provide long-term support for the family. Some years ago a Working Party of the National Association for Mental Health concluded:

. . . telling the parents is only a first step in the continuing management of the handicapped child. It is not an end in itself and unless it leads correctly on to the appropriate involvement of other professional workers it would largely have failed in its primary object of securing for the handicapped child the fullest possible developmental goals and an accepted place in the family.   (Carr and Oppé 1971)

Although these sentiments were expressed in regard to handicap in general, they are also relevant to Duchenne muscular dystrophy. Establishing the diagnosis and proffering genetic counselling should only be the beginning of the health professionals' involvement with the parents and the affected child. Their continuing support may well be required for several years to come.

Summary and conclusions

Genetic counselling is essentially a process of communication between the counsellor and those who seek counselling. The information to be communicated concerns first, the disease itself, the genetic mechanism which caused it, and the risks of recurrence; and secondly, the options available if the risks are considered unacceptably high. These include contraception, sterilization, prenatal diagnosis, and abortion, each of which may in itself have important psychological sequelae and require counselling. Some couples, for various ethical and other reasons, may be unable to accept these options. This is their prerogative for genetic counselling should not be directive but help couples reach a decision which is the best one for themselves.

It is particularly important to recognize the psychological aspects of genetic counselling and the sequence of events which follow the initial diagnosis and which are referred to as the *coping process*. This involves five sequential stages: shock and denial, anxiety, anger and guilt, depression, and finally, psychological homeostasis. Each stage requires counselling to be tailored accordingly for only in this way will it be at all affective and rational decisions made.

Concern about the disorder occurring in various relatives is tempered by considerations of the 'burden' of the disease as well as the individual's risks, and counselling should be offered to all those female relatives who are anxious about the problem.

The effects of genetic counselling can be assessed in several ways. There are indications that the population incidence is being reduced to the occurrence of new mutations which in the past represented about a third of cases. Studies of the reproductive behaviour of individual women who have been counselled indicate that those at high risk are very largely deterred from pregnancy unless coupled with prenatal diagnosis. Finally, the social and psychological effects of genetic counselling can be assessed, but so far this has received little attention in the case of Duchenne muscular dystrophy. Indications are that at least in the United Kingdom, there is often some dissatisfaction with the way in which the diagnosis is first made and lack of subsequent follow-up. There is a real need to ensure that parents are told accurately and compassionately as soon as possible. Thereafter a series of contacts can be offered and planned with various health care professionals involved with the disease. The latter can then provide, if need be, long-term support for the family as a whole.

13 Management

Although, at present, Duchenne muscular dystrophy is not curable, it is not untreatable, and a great deal can be done to improve the quality of life of affected boys. This involves maintaining their general well-being, preserving respiratory function, and preventing the development of deformities. Because of its unrelenting course, in the past there was a tendency among health care professionals to take a rather indifferent attitude to management. This view is no longer justified, however, as a great deal can be achieved by taking a positive approach, largely pioneered by Vignos in Cleveland, and Siegel in Chicago, which has now been adopted by most centres throughout the world. Much has been written on the subject and there are several helpful and detailed reviews (Walton 1969; Siegel 1977a, 1978; Bossingham *et al.* 1977; Rideau 1979; Vignos 1979; Dubowitz and Heckmatt 1980). Gardner-Medwin (1984) has written a particularly valuable guide to management for parents.

General management

Whatever stage the disease has reached there are certain general principles to be considered. It would seem hardly necessary to emphasize the need to maintain good health in general. There is no evidence that 'megavitamin therapy' is of any value in the disease, and in any event it may have serious side-effects (Evans and Lacey 1986), and could actually be harmful. Adequate intake of dietary fibre is important because of frequent problems with constipation. Excess weight gain should be avoided since it will overburden the already compromised musculature, and also add to the problems of lifting and carrying the patient when he is no longer able to walk. Oral hygiene is essential.

In the early stages of the disease, and up to the time walking becomes difficult, parents should be encouraged to let their son lead as normal a life as possible. Prolonged bed rest for any intercurrent infection should be avoided, particularly after early childhood when it can precipitate loss of ambulation. Some of the more important aspects of physical management are summarized in Table 13.1.

Active exercise

A question often asked is whether the parents should encourage active exercise in the belief that this might improve muscle strength or perhaps help preserve what strength remains. Muscle exercise has complex physiological and

Table 13.1 *Physical management in
                Duchenne muscular dystrophy*

1. *Promotion of ambulation*
   Weight control
   Exercise: active/passive
   Tenotomies
   Orthoses
2. *Prevention of deformities*
   Posture/support/orthoses
   Passive exercise/stretching
   Surgery
3. *Preservation of respiratory function*

structural effects which vary from person to person, and in different forms of physical handicap (Basmajian 1973).

Early studies of the possible beneficial effects of exercise in Duchenne muscular dystrophy are difficult to interpret for various methodological reasons (reviewed by Vignos 1984). However, in a study of the effects of a one year programme of active exercise against weight resistance in 14 affected boys (Vignos and Watkins 1966) some improvement in muscle strength at the beginning was noted, but this eventually levelled off. Any apparent beneficial effect was more marked in the less severely affected boys. An important general point emerges from this study. An apparent improvement is often detected at the beginning of such studies as the patients learn and become familiar with the methods involved. This we observed (Emery *et al.* 1982) in a double blind study of a calcium blocker in Duchenne muscular dystrophy (Fig. 13.1), which incidentally was not recommended for treatment.

In another more recent study of 18 affected boys who were all still ambulant, there appeared to be no significant effect of resisted exercise on muscle strength (Dubowitz *et al.* 1984). However, the study period was only 6 months, and it would be valuable to know if a prolonged programme of resisted exercise would eventually have a beneficial effect on muscle strength.

Quite apart from any possible improvement in strength, such a regime has a beneficial psychological effect. Certainly these studies showed that active forms of exercise are not deleterious. However, such a regime requires a considerable commitment in time since patients and their families may have to attend a special centre where such exercises can be performed, although, Scott *et al.* (1981) have shown that parents rapidly become competent to give such treatment at home.

Although it is not yet clear whether moderate exercise can actually increase muscle strength, an overly aggressive approach to physical activity could well be counterproductive and possibly aggravate the cardiomyopathy which is a

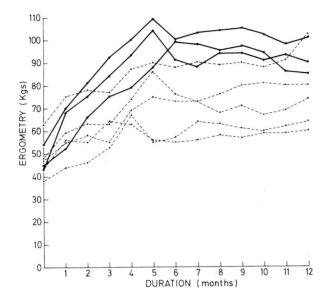

Fig. 13.1. Results of ergometry in patients taking a placebo (---), and those taking the active drug (—). Note the apparent increase in strength in all boys at the beginning as a result of 'training'.

concomitant of the disease (p. 93). In any event as Vignos (1979) has stated '. . . Activities involving recreational sports are generally more likely to win long-term adherence'. Swimming is particularly valuable as the buoyancy of the water makes exercises easier to perform. Cycling can also be beneficial although quite early on boys with Duchenne muscular dystrophy often find this difficult. The best advice would be to encourage normal physical activities as far as they are possible.

Passive exercise and physiotherapy

There seems little doubt that passive, stretching exercises can be valuable in preventing or at least delaying the development of muscle contractures, which are especially likely to develop once the child becomes chairbound. Such exercises include stretching of the Achilles tendon and the knee, hip, shoulder, elbow, and wrist joints. Sylvia Hyde (1984) has produced a helpful guide to such exercises for parents to use in the home, though it is advisable to have a professional physiotherapist explain and demonstrate the procedures at the beginning (Fig. 13.2). The emphasis is on firmness and kindness and the aim is to prevent contractures developing. Once they have developed then such passive stretching exercises are ineffective and the use of force can cause serious trauma. There is no doubt that a routine of passive exercises each day,

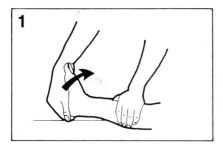 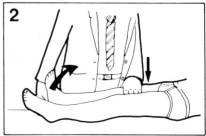

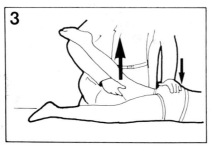 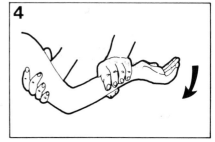

Fig. 13.2. Some of the passive stretching exercises to prevent contractures of the (1) tendo Achilles, and (2) knee, (3) hip, and (4) elbow joints. (After Hyde (1984) with permission.)

say after a nightly bath, will help prevent contractures. However, it is difficult and time consuming, but on the other hand it offers one of the few opportunities where parents can feel involved in doing something for their son.

Coupled with such exercises, the parents can also encourage deep breathing exercises and later postural drainage and assisted coughing. This will be discussed in more detail later (p. 235).

There are those who propose the use of night splints in order to help prevent the development of contractures of the ankle and knee joints. But while a boy is still ambulant it is doubtful if such measures have any real value, and in any event many children find them uncomfortable and, in our experience, compliance is not high.

Because of the growing awareness of the importance of physiotherapy in muscular dystrophy, an International Congress on the subject was held in Italy in 1984, the Proceedings of which have now been published in detail (*Cardiomyology* Vol 3, nos 2–3, 1984) where the reader will find helpful information including some useful guidelines proposed by the European Alliance of Muscular Dystrophy Associations.

Finally, it should be mentioned that in the early stages of the disease there is no place for Achilles tenotomy. Later, when the boy is chairbound, tenotomy and the wearing of light-weight below knee orthoses and normal shoes helps maintain the feet in a satisfactory position, makes dressing easier, and although purely cosmetic, many find it worthwhile (Gardner-Medwin, 1984).

Scoliosis

Once an affected boy has lost the ability to walk, joint contractures and scoliosis soon follow. Although contractures are not a serious problem, their development does limit whatever limb movement remains and can also make dressing difficult. Scoliosis on the other hand is a serious complication (James *et al.* 1976). Sitting becomes difficult and uncomfortable but more importantly, the progressive thoracic deformity restricts adequate pulmonary ventilation and aggravates respiratory problems resulting from weakness of the intercostal muscles. Respiratory impairment becomes a major threat to life (p. 235) and increases once the child is chairbound (Fig. 13.3). It should be noted however that not all boys develop scoliosis. A small proportion develop hyper-lordosis and a very few retain more or less normal spinal curvatures.

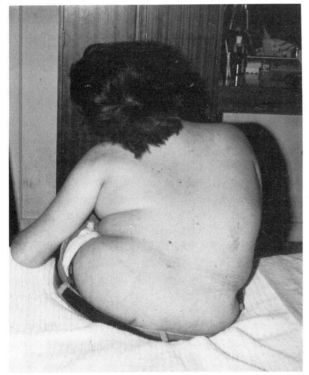

Fig. 13.3. Untreated scoliosis.

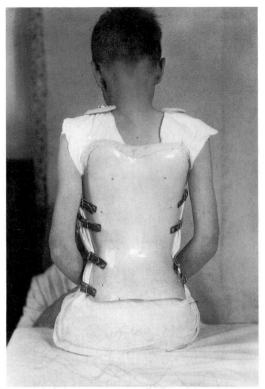

Fig. 13.4. Moulded and fitted back support.

There are several ways in which the development of scoliosis can be limited: the adoption of a correct sitting posture; the fitting of an orthosis; prolongation of ambulation; and surgical intervention. From early on, even before ambulation is lost, it is important to emphasize a habit of adopting a correct sitting position. Once confined to a wheelchair this becomes especially important. A firm back support and special seating (for example, the Toronto seat) will help (Moseley 1984), but such measures on their own are likely to have only a limited effect. Individually designed body jackets or braces (Figs 13.4 and 13.5) fitted when a boy first becomes confined to a wheelchair and before the onset of scoliosis may be more helpful (Miller and Dunn 1982; Shapira and Bresnan 1982; Falewski de Leon 1984; Seeger *et al.* 1984; Young *et al.* 1984). Such measures, however, although they may possibly impede the development of scoliosis, cannot prevent it (Robin 1976; Moseley 1984; Rideau *et al.* 1984; Seeger *et al.* 1984), and are not practical when once it has progressed beyond about 40 degrees from the vertical.

The only real solution is to prolong ambulation or resort to surgery.

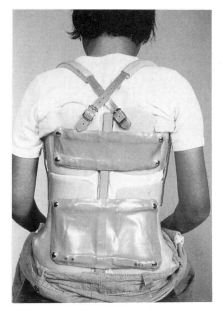
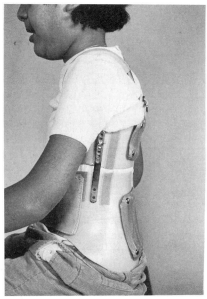
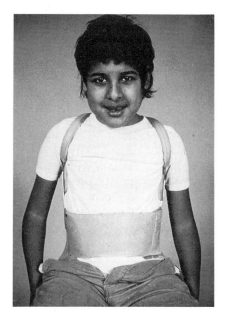

Fig. 13.5. Fitted spinal brace. (Reproduced by kind permission of Dr G. M. Cochrane and the Mary Marlborough Lodge.)

Prolongation of ambulation

There is no doubt that the development of contractures and spinal deformities is impeded by prolonging ambulation beyond the stage when this is normally lost (Swinyard grade 5: Vignos grade 7 – see Appendices C and D). This can be achieved by the application of light plastic or polypropylene long-leg fitted orthoses with an ischial supporting lip. This approach to management was first introduced by Vignos and Siegel in the 1960s (Spencer and Vignos 1962; Vignos *et al.* 1963; Siegel *et al.* 1968). If an equino varus deformity is already present, an Achilles tenotomy may be necessary in order to fit the orthoses. This can be performed percutaneously (Granata *et al.* 1984; Heckmatt *et al.* 1985), although others prefer open operation (Williams *et al.* 1984). Boys not requiring tenotomy at first and walking regularly in their orthoses may subsequently have problems with Achilles tendon tightening and require a tenotomy later. It may also be necessary for tenotomy of the hip flexors and tensor fascia lata (Siegel 1980; Rideau *et al.* 1983a). This can be combined with Achilles tenotomy in the one operation, which is relatively quick, requires brief anaesthesia, and entails minimal blood loss (Siegel 1980). If operation is necessary, long-leg plasters are fitted while the patient is under anaesthesia. A few days later these are replaced by fitted orthoses which are then regularly adjusted as the boy grows. The orthoses should have a knee-flexion device which permits sitting and also gives stability to the knee joint (Allard *et al.* 1981). Such orthoses can be worn with everyday shoes and beneath trousers (Fig. 13.6).

In a study of 57 affected boys (Heckmatt *et al.* 1985), all but 10 achieved useful independent walking by these measures. Among these 10, seven had problems because of delays in providing their orthoses and as a result had to spend several months in plaster, one had severe asymmetrical hip and knee contractures, another lost confidence following a fall at home, and one regained the ability to walk independently without orthoses following tenotomy. It would therefore seem that provided orthoses are available at the time of operation, most boys will do well and retain the ability to walk. These measures prolong walking by about two years on average, but in some cases as long as five years (Hsu 1976; Siegel 1980; Miller and Dunn 1982; Heckmatt *et al.* 1985). However, success depends on several factors, and is most likely in those boys who are not obese or mentally handicapped, have good motivation, and where there is parental compliance. Timing is also particularly important. It should be commenced at the time ambulation is just beginning to be a serious problem. Once a child has been confined to a wheelchair for only a few months, rehabilitation becomes difficult, partly because of the severe loss of power, but also because marked contractures soon develop.

The application of orthoses does *not* accelerate the deterioration in muscle power, and in fact there may be a slight increase for a time (Hyde *et al.* 1982). The advantages include continued independence, easier management by the

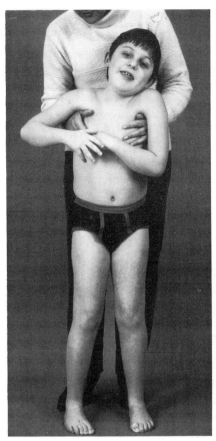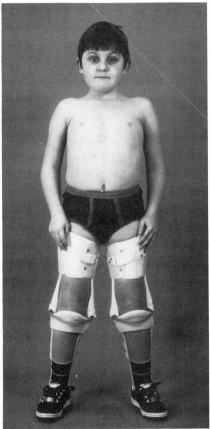

Fig. 13.6. Before (*left*), and after (*right*) fitting of long-leg orthoses to prolong ambulation. (Reproduced by kind permission of Professor V. Dubowitz.)

parents, slowing the development of contractures and spinal deformity, and psychological benefits. However, although there appear to be many benefits in such a regime, there is no evidence as yet that it prolongs life but some data from Western Australia indicate that this might be so (Miller and Dunn 1982).

Some, however, remain a little sceptical. Gardner-Medwin (1984) for example has stated:

. . . that although these boys are able to walk a few steps and maintain an upright posture, they are actually less usefully mobile than they would be in a wheelchair. In our experience the stage of walking precariously and slowly with a risk of heavy falls is a distressing one and boys often accept the chair with relief. Furthermore, the time and energy which are required for physiotherapy might in many cases more profitably be devoted to schooling.

Nevertheless, where the boy and his parents are sufficiently determined and enthusiastic, this option should be offered for it may well prove to have long-term beneficial effects (Miller and Dunn 1982).

Standing frames

In the last few years there has been much discussion of the value of standing frames/tilt tables. These are devices which allow a boy, who can no longer stand unaided, to achieve and maintain an upright position (Fig. 13.7). Modified wheelchairs have also been designed for the same purpose. The place of such equipment would be after a year or two in walking orthoses and the maintenance of an upright position after this stage could be both physiologically and psychologically beneficial. However, these aids in

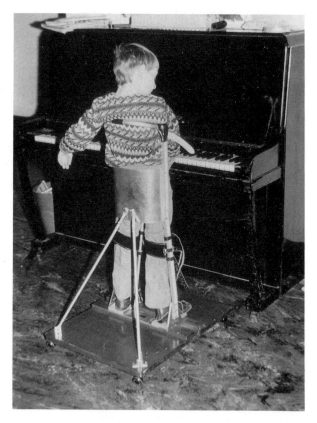

Fig. 13.7. A simple standing frame. (Reproduced by kind permission of Dr G. M. Cochrane and the Mary Marlborough Lodge.)

general have limited manoeuverability and are expensive. They seem likely to find use in adults with more slowly progressive forms of muscular dystrophy.

Surgical correction

Surgical correction of scoliosis using Harrington rods (Aprin *et al.* 1982) has the disadvantages of frequent post-operative pulmonary and other complications, and necessitates immobilization in a cast or brace for some time post-operatively. This approach has now been superseded by the Luque operation in which internal fixation is achieved by each vertebra being individually wired to two stainless steel rods (Luque 1982; Drennan 1984). The rigid stabilization obtained with this technique eliminates the need for post-operative immobilization and therefore reduces the loss of strength and function which follows such immobilization. Post-operative complications are also less (Fig. 13.8).

Some have recommended the operation as a prophylactic measure before the development of scoliosis (Rideau *et al.* 1984), whereas others offer the operation only when scoliosis is approaching 30 degrees (Moseley 1984; Sussman 1984, 1985). The most important points when considering surgery are that spinal deformity is limited and that respiratory function is good. Surgery is indicated when the curve is less than 50 degrees and the forced vital capacity (FVC) is greater than 50 per cent of the expected value, and according to Sussman (1985):

. . . There is a 'window' of time between the point when the curve develops, but prior to a decrease in FVC below 50 per cent, during which the spinal surgery should be performed. If a patient is treated with an orthosis the 'window' will be narrowed, since the progression of the scoliosis will be temporarily slowed while pulmonary function continues to deteriorate.

Because of the resultant spinal rigidity and limited spinal movement, boys treated in this way often have to acquire new trick movements for everyday living, and may need more frequent turning in bed at night. However, boys with stable spines as a result of surgery can be confident that spinal deformity will not increase and often have an enhanced quality of life during the teenage period (Sussman 1984). Over the next few years it will be important to compare the effects of surgery with other forms of therapy on the quality of life and survival of treated boys. In the more benign forms of muscular dystrophy there is no doubt that many years of useful and productive life are possible after various surgical procedures (tendon lengthening, arthrodeses, etc.) and with appropriate orthoses (Fig. 13.9). But although surgery would seem to benefit boys with Duchenne muscular dystrophy, this has yet to be weighed against the risks of surgery in these boys.

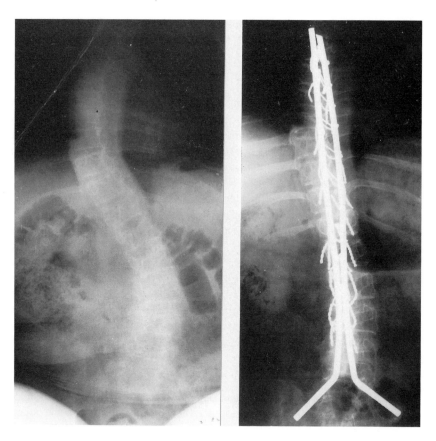

Fig. 13.8. Chest X-rays before (*left*), and (*right*) after surgical correction of scoliosis by the Luque operation. (Reproduced by kind permission of Mr G. R. Houghton.)

Surgical–anaesthetic risks

Many children with Duchenne muscular dystrophy tolerate surgery and general anaesthesis well, but there are recognized dangers. During anaesthesia sinus tachycardia, atrial and ventricular fibrillation and cardiac arrest may occur, even in very young boys aged 3–5 in whom there is no evidence pre-operatively of cardiomyopathy (Seay *et al.* 1978; Boltshauser *et al.* 1980).

Post-operatively other complications may occur, including gastric dilatation and myoglobinuria (rhabdomyolysis). Myoglobinuria does not normally occur in Duchenne muscular dystrophy (p. 124). However, it is frequently found post-operatively (Table 13.2), and reflects enhanced muscle breakdown. Some patients with myoglobinuria post-operatively have been noted

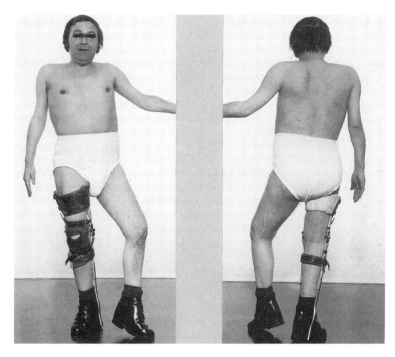

Fig. 13.9. Patient with Becker muscular dystrophy who, despite marked weakness of proximal lower limb girdle musculature, is sufficiently ambulant as a result of surgery and orthoses as to be gainfully employed.

subsequently to be somewhat weaker. In one case (Boltshauser *et al.* 1980) SCK levels were repeatedly normal for 8–12 days after operation, and the authors suggested that this might have been due to a temporary depletion of muscle enzyme as a result of excessive 'leakage' during the acute stage of rhabdomyolysis. An important danger with acute rhabdomyolysis and myoglobinuria is the possible development of renal impairment and even acute renal failure post-operatively (McKishnie *et al.* 1983).

The myoglobinuria (and myoglobinaemia) is probably a direct effect of the anaesthetic agents. Succinylcholine for example is known to occasionally cause myoglobinuria in normal children (Ellis and Heffron, 1985), and the apparent increased incidence of myoglobinuria in patients with Duchenne muscular dystrophy is probably related to the pathophysiology of the disease.

Much has been made of the possible dangers of malignant hyperpyrexia in Duchenne muscular dystrophy (Siegel 1978). However, there are problems in

Table 13.2   *Occurrence of myoglobinuria (rhabdomyolysis) post-operatively in patients with Duchenne muscular dystrophy*

Age	Surgical procedure	Anaesthetic agents	Reference
NR	Adenoidectomy	Succinylcholine, halothane	Watters *et al.* (1977)
NR	Adenoidectomy	Succinylcholine, halothane	Watters *et al.* (1977)
NR	Strabismus correction	Succinylcholine, halothane	Watters *et al.* (1977)
4 yrs	Calcaneal osteotomy	Succinylcholine, N_2O, halothane	Miller *et al.* (1978)
3 yrs	Tonsillectomy	Succinylcholine, nembutal, cyclopropane	Seay *et al.* (1978)
4 yrs	Tonsillectomy	Succinylcholine, nembutal, N_2O, halothane	Seay *et al.* (1978)
5 yrs	Adenoidectomy	Succinylcholine, N_2O, halothane	Boltshauser *et al.* (1980)
21 mths	Ankyloglossia	Succinylcholine, N_2O, halothane	Oka *et al.* (1982)
5 yrs	Dental extraction	Succinylcholine, N_2O, halothane	Brownell *et al.* (1983)
3 yrs	Orchiopexy	Succinylcholine, N_2O, halothane	McKishnie *et al.* (1983)
4 yrs	Muscle biopsy	Protoxide/halothane	Fiacchino *et al.* (1984)

NR, not recorded.

defining this condition purely on the basis of clinical features (Rowland 1984). Evidence of a possible association with Duchenne muscular dystrophy has been critically reviewed by Ellis and Heffron (1985) who conclude that any association is far from proved. Ellis (1985) states that the diagnosis has never been convincingly established on the basis of the now accepted *in vitro* tests in any case of Duchenne muscular dystrophy.

Finally, hyperkalaemia may result from increased muscle breakdown, and succinylcholine and other depolarizing agents are inadvisable due to their intrinsic ability to further raise the serum level of potassium (Ellis 1981).

Respiratory problems are also likely post-operatively, especially in boys whose respiratory function is already reduced. Retention of bronchial secretions, resulting from weakness of the respiratory muscles and associated weak cough, may lead to pneumonitis. Drugs likely to exaggerate respiratory depression, such as barbiturates, have therefore to be used with caution, and post-operative respiratory care and appropriate physiotherapy are essential.

Most of the operative and post-operative problems described in Duchenne muscular dystrophy have been based on case reports and are therefore somewhat selective. In the majority of patients there are no serious anaesthetic problems (Richards 1972), and in a series of patients under-going major surgery for the correction of thoracic deformities, most responded favourably. There were no cases of hyperpyrexia, hyperkalaemia or rhabdomyolysis, but succinylcholine was avoided (Milne and Rosales 1982). It is obviously important that the surgeon and anaesthetist appreciate the problems which can occur and be adequately prepared to deal with them should they arise.

Fractures

Fractures occur not infrequently, usually as a result of falls sustained while the boy is still walking but unsteadily, or due to various accidents later on in the course of the disease when the long bones undergo rarefaction as a result of disuse (p. 104). In the first group immobilization may well result in loss of ambulation, and for this reason fractures should be treated with minimal splintage so as to encourage activity and continued independent mobility. Fractures heal normally and the special orthopaedic problems of fractures of the long bones in Duchenne muscular dystrophy have been reviewed in detail (Siegel 1977b; Hsu 1979).

Respiratory problems

Impaired pulmonary function is the major factor in morbidity and mortality in Duchenne muscular dystrophy. Over 90 per cent of deaths result from pulmonary infection and respiratory failure (Vignos 1977b). Preservation of respiratory function and adequate treatment of respiratory infections are therefore essential elements of patient management.

At the simplest level parents and relatives should be dissuaded from smoking in the same rooms used by the affected boy. Many advocate vaccination against influenza at the beginning of the winter months although the value, even in healthy individuals, is not certain. The adoption of a correct sitting position should be encouraged. Well-designed respiratory exercises are valuable in helping to maintain good pulmonary function (Di Marco *et al.* 1985). However, these measures alone will not prevent the progressive decrease in pulmonary function. It is doubtful if prophylactic antibiotics have any significant effect and are best reserved for use in treating respiratory infections as they occur.

Regular pulmonary function tests, the simplest being the assessment of vital capacity using a spirometer (Macklem 1986), will indicate the development of significant impairment even before problems arise, and can be a good prognostic indicator (Inkley *et al.* 1974; Vignos 1977b; Rideau 1979; Ortaggio *et al.* 1984). Deterioration begins around the time the boy becomes confined to a wheelchair, and measures of pulmonary function (vital capacity, maximum inspiratory, and expiratory pressures), instead of increasing with age as they do normally, remain more or less the same for some time and then in the later stages actually decrease. Differences between predicted and observed values therefore become more marked as the disease progresses. However, only in the very late stages does actual respiratory failure occur with changes in blood gases.

Attempts to impede the development of scoliosis have already been discussed, and will certainly have a beneficial effect on respiratory function. Parents can also be instructed in breathing exercises, postural drainage, percussion, and even pharyngeal suction. A 10 minute programme of breathing exercises should become a part of the daily routine, but respiratory muscle training *per se* seems to have little effect on respiratory function (Martin *et al.* 1986).

Any chest infection must be treated vigorously with antibiotics and physiotherapy. If there is any suggestion that respiratory function is already impaired, then hospitalization is indicated. Since deaths from respiratory problems usually occur only in the most advanced stages and not in those less severely affected, Vignos (1977b) recommends that physicians should be encouraged to attempt energetic treatment of all patients who are at a grade less than Vignos 9.

In the very late stages of the disease some have advocated a rocking bed, abdominal pneumobelt or cuirass, with assisted ventilation especially at night, or a portable ventilator employing a mouth adaptor or even tracheostomy. It has been maintained that such measures may increase the quality of life and prolong survival (Alexander *et al.* 1979; Bach *et al.* 1981; Rideau *et al.* 1983b). However, the long-term management of patients in this way raises many problems, not least being the eventual dependency on assisted respiration which may develop.

Practical considerations in the respiratory care of patients with Duchenne muscular dystrophy have recently been reviewed in considerable detail by Smith *et al.* (1986b) who provide an extensive and helpful bibliography on the subject.

Cardiac problems

In less than 10 per cent of patients death occurs suddenly, presumably as a consequence of the associated cardiomyopathy. Congestive heart failure however is uncommon, and treatment for this is rarely indicated. The enforced immobility probably helps to protect the heart. Long-term prophylactic treatment with cardiac glycosides (digitoxin) although once considered efficacious, has since been shown to have no therapeutic value (Fowler *et al.* 1965).

Verapamil is often used to control a variety of arrhythmias in otherwise normal individuals but is contra-indicated in Duchenne muscular dystrophy because it may precipitate respiratory failure (Zalman *et al.* 1983), and heart block (Emery and Skinner 1983).

Psychological problems

Most boys give every impression of being well adapted and of having come to terms with their disability. In fact one expert has said:

> . . . it is worthwhile to emphasise that the Duchenne muscular dystrophy patient, after some initial frustration, is really not suffering, has above all no pain, and is on the contrary often quite content or at least acceptingly resigned after he becomes wheelchair-bound.   (Zellweger, 1975)

It would, however, be entirely wrong to assume that affected boys are emotionally and psychologically unscathed by their disease. In reviewing the rather scant older literature, as well as the results of her own studies, Staples (1977) concluded that emotional problems do occur and that, not unexpectedly, affected boys tend to be more introverted than normal children. In-depth assessment, however, may require some very careful and direct questioning in order to elicit feelings on matters such as isolation, dependency, lack of privacy, and sexual needs (Taft 1973). Two more recent studies have looked at these matters in some detail (Buchanan *et al.* 1979; Pullen 1984).

The emotional reaction of a boy to his disease varies from individual to individual and from family to family. Paramount may be a feeling of isolation because of his physical disability and perhaps also intellectual impairment. Recognition that his peers are physically and perhaps sometimes intellectually superior may well lead to withdrawal and depression. As the disease advances his dependency on others, and lack of personal privacy will cause more stress. A proportion may feel physically unattractive. Although some apparently deny that their inability to find sexual satisfaction is a cause of distress (Morgan 1975), others no doubt do, particularly because their physical disability may preclude any relief they might obtain from masturbation. Later, they have to face the imminence of premature death. According to Staples (1977) many accept the concept of premature death without disquiet. However, some develop a major depressive disorder (Fitzpatrick *et al.* 1986) or serious behavioural problems as a reaction to their illness (Buchanan *et al.* 1979). The more emotionally disturbed tend to come from families with marked conflicts and the behaviour of the parents and normal sibs will influence that of the affected boy. The problems are made worse if he is also ill-informed about the disease. He is more likely to be emotionally stable and better adapted to his problems if the home environment is stable, there is marital harmony, and the parents are perceived as being close to each other, and there are open and frequent discussions about his problems with a frank expression of feelings. All too often there is little communication within families about the disorder (Fitzpatrick and Barry 1986).

The parents also have to face a great many problems, and again frank discussions between themselves as well as with health professionals can only be beneficial. Quite apart from the emotional problems associated with coping (p. 215), there are others of a more social nature which will also produce psychological reactions. Physical handicap, especially when associated with mental handicap, may be viewed as a social stigma and source of embarrassment. As the physical incapacity increases, there will be a restriction on the family's freedom and activities. The parents might find little time or opportunity to be together or to have a holiday. The husband may feel neglected or rejected because of the mother's necessary involvement with their affected son. Coupled with the fear of also having another affected child, serious psycho-sexual problems may arise. In one survey of 25 families (Buchanan *et al.* 1979), over half had serious marital problems and a quarter had become divorced. On the other hand, in some families the affected child has the effect of actually bringing the parents closer together.

Finally, unaffected sibs are not excluded from the emotional problems which may arise within the family. Overprotection and pampering of an affected boy may result in jealousy and resentment among sibs. Older sisters may adopt a maternal or protective role, yet at the same time harbour increasing concern about their possibly having an affected son.

Pullen (1984) recognizes seven stages in the evolution of a genetic disease within a family, each being associated with different emotional and psychological responses in different members of the family:

   (*i*) Positive family history
  (*ii*) Abnormality noticed by parents
 (*iii*) Abnormality confirmed by family practitioner
 (*iv*) Diagnosis first made/coping process begins
  (*v*) Resolution/adaptation
 (*vi*) Chronic handicap/progression
(*vii*) Death/grieving.

At stage (*i*) (when there is a family history of Duchenne muscular dystrophy), those who see themselves as being at risk of having an affected son are likely to be anxious and concerned. With improved methods of carrier detection in some cases reassurance will be possible. Otherwise the medical and genetic aspects of the problem will need to be discussed in detail, perhaps on several occasions, until an acceptable course of action is reached. All-too-often there is a considerable delay between when the parents first noticed that something appeared to be wrong with their son and this is agreed by the family practitioner and then the diagnosis is established. Most couples interviewed find this period of uncertainty one of the most trying and upsetting (Firth 1983). Increased awareness by family practitioners of the possibility of muscular dystrophy should help reduce this problem in future. Stage (*iv*) involves the emotional reaction to the diagnosis and the beginning of the coping process (p. 215). Stages (*v*) and (*vi*) involve the reactions of the patient and his parents and sibs to the disease. Parents must be encouraged to take time off and have regular times set aside for themselves. Organizations, such as the Muscular Dystrophy Group in Britain, through local set-ups, can provide support and advice and help to reduce feelings of isolation. Open and frank discussions between all members of the family should be encouraged, including the affected boy himself. As Pullen, a psychiatrist experienced in this field, has stated

. . . The physically handicapped child must be allowed to talk about his frustrations, disappointments, depression and anxieties for the future. Many people, including parents, do not allow the child to talk about these areas for fear of putting ideas into his head. The ideas certainly are there already but most children are denied the opportunity of communicating them to others. This may make them feel more isolated and abnormal because it prevents others from empathizing accurately with their position. (Pullen, 1984, p. 122)

About a third of parents we have interviewed had great difficulty in talking to each other about the disease.

Finally, at stage (*vii*) parents again should be encouraged to talk honestly about their emotional reactions: their distress, despair, and perhaps anger. The problems of bereavement in muscular dystrophy are discussed in detail in Charash *et al.* (1983). Ideally, counselling should not end with the death of the patient but should be available to close relatives until grieving has passed. It is doubtful if the sense of loss and the attendant grief will ever completely pass away. With time, however, there is often a sense of relief after all the years of anxiety and concern. This is natural and not a reason for feeling guilty.

Educational and social needs

The first question to be answered is whether an affected boy may require special schooling? In a few cases associated with severe mental handicap this may be indicated when the parents find management difficult. In most cases, however, boys can derive considerable benefit by attending a normal school where the teachers can be very helpful once the problem has been explained. Cohen (1977) has listed many of the problems which may affect a boy's educational ability: progressive motor difficulties make acquisition of new skills more difficult; frequent absence from school often occurs with declining physical condition; and affected boys tire easily and may lack initiative and motivation.

Attention should focus on a boy's positive abilities. A proportion will be academically orientated. But their physical incapacity by the time they reach senior school can present a serious problem, and further education and employment prospects are severely limited. In Britain the Open University Courses on television have been a boon to many highly intelligent boys. But others will be more artistically inclined. Over the years I have made a collection of drawings and paintings by my patients, and their skill and ability is frequently a source of admiration.

As the disease progresses and boys become confined to a wheelchair, day schools which cater specially for the physically handicapped can be an attractive proposition. In such an environment they will feel less isolated and more able to share feelings and expressions with fellow sufferers. Most parents prefer to have their child in a day school with other handicapped children rather than in an institution away from home (Zellweger 1975).

At home consideration should be given to the time when he will be unable to walk unaided and appropriate plans made. Ramps to take a wheelchair may be required. A ground floor bedroom/study is ideal, with TV, hi-fi, and other devices of his choosing. In this way he will have a place which he can consider his private sanctum to entertain friends and be on his own if he chooses.

There are a vast array of aids, including wheelchairs, available for the physically handicapped. In Britain some of these can be obtained through the National Health Service at no cost to the family. It would not be appropriate to deal with these matters here. However, there are several publications which are of considerable practical value and provide information not only on aids but also addresses of where to seek help and advice:

With a little help by Philippa Harpin. A series of detailed guides concerned with such matters as clothing, home adaptations, wheelchairs, etc. Addresses of suppliers and helpful organizations are included. Published by the Muscular Dystrophy Group of Great Britain, 35 Macaulay Road, London SW4 0QP.

The muscular dystrophy handbook. This includes useful information about professional services (including education, leisure, holidays, transport, etc.). Published by the Muscular Dystrophy Group of Great Britain.

Sign post. A directory of where to go for help, advice and information, and *Powered wheelchairs*, a buyer's guide. Published by the Research Institute for Consumer Affairs, 14 Buckingham Street, London WC2N 6DS.

Drug therapy

No drug has yet been found to be therapeutically effective in Duchenne muscular dystrophy. Furthermore, the design of a drug trial in this disease and the assessment of any possible beneficial effects present a number of problems.

Early drug trials

Over the last 50 years there have been many drug trials in Duchenne muscular dystrophy. Some of the drugs which have been tried and the basis for their use are summarized in Table 13.3. Many of the early studies were ill designed and often an initial study claiming benefits for a particular drug was subsequently refuted by a better designed and better controlled study.

Table 13.3 *Drugs used in various therapeutic trials in Duchenne muscular dystrophy*

Drug	Basis for use	First reported trial
Allopurinol	Increases nucleotide formation believed to be depleted in dystrophic muscle	1976
Amino acids	Deficiency of muscle proteins	1953
Anabolic steroids	Anabolic effect	1955
Aspirin, propranolol, etc.	Counteract proposed defect in biogenic amine metabolism	1977
Calcium blockers	Reduce muscle intracellular calcium	1982
Catecholamines	Counteract proposed defect in muscle sympathetic innervation	1930
Coenzyme Q	Possible benefit in murine dystrophy	1974
Dantrolene	Inhibit release of calcium from sarcoplasmic reticulum	1983
Digitalis and other cardiac glycosides	Prevent progressive cardiomyopathy	1963
Glycine	Believed to stimulate muscle creatine synthesis	1932
Growth hormone	Anabolic effect	1973
Growth hormone inhibitor	Growth hormone deficiency ameliorates disease	1984
Ketoacids	Reduce muscle protein degradation	1982
Leucine	Increases protein synthesis	1984
Nucleotides (e.g. Laevadosin)	Replacement of nucleotides believed to be depleted in dystrophic muscle	1960

Table 13.3 *Cont'd*

Drug	Basis for use	First reported trial
Oestrogens	Anabolic effect	1972
Pancreatic extract	Possible benefit in murine dystrophy	1976
Penicillamine	Possible benefit in avian dystrophy	1977
Prednisolone	Anabolic effect	1974
Protease inhibitors	Possible benefit in murine dystrophy	1984
Superoxide dismutase	Removal of superoxide radicals associated with membrane damage	1980
Thyroxine	Thyroxine depresses SCK	1964
Vasodilators	Counteract proposed defect in muscle microcirculation	1963
Vitamins		
B6	Vitamin B6 deficient rats develop a myopathy	1940
E	Vitamin E deficient animals develop a myopathy	1940
Zinc	Membrane 'stabilizer'	1986

Evaluation of drug trials

Dubowitz and Heckmatt (1980) have presented a detailed and critical review of the many therapeutic trials in Duchenne muscular dystropy. They derived a system of awarding a 'quality score' for each report, with a point for each of the following criteria: careful selection and definition of cases; adequate controls; objective ('blind') study; assessment other than by simple clinical ratings; and for a trial lasting longer than two years. Of 34 published trials they analysed, not one was awarded five points, and in half there was no score at all, which means that even the definition of the cases studied was not clear (Table 13.4). Dubowitz and Heckmatt consider that no trial with a score of less than three should be taken seriously otherwise there is the danger of raising false hopes in both the patient and his family.

Design of drug trials

There are a number of general points to be considered in designing a drug trial in Duchenne muscular dystrophy. Patients must be *carefully selected* on the basis of accepted clinical, biochemical, and histological diagnostic criteria

Table 13.4 *Scoring of 34 drug trials in Duchenne muscular dystrophy (1940–79), (data from Dubowitz and Heckmatt (1980))*

Score	Number of trials
0	17
1	7
2	3
3	3
4	4
5	0

for the disease. The inclusion of patients with Becker muscular dystrophy, for example, might give the mistaken impression of slowing the course of the disease. The patients should also be óld enough and intelligent enough to cooperate and yet still be ambulant. Ideally they should therefore be aged between 5 and 10 years. The trial should be 'blind', unless the nature of the treatment (e.g. surgery), or the occurrence of unusual side-effects makes this impossible. Ideally it should be *double-blind* with neither the patient and his family, nor the investigator, knowing who is taking the drug and who is taking a placebo. It may be difficult to convince parents of the value of this method because if they already believe the drug could be effective it would mean in some cases denying the possible benefits of treatment for the duration of the trial. For this reason a *cross-over* double-blind study has an advantage, and also requires fewer patients. The placebo must have the same appearance, texture, and taste as the drug. Boys become adept at recognizing the one from the other on the basis of slight differences in taste or texture. Furthermore the effects of the drug may take some time to wear off (the so-called 'wash-out' effect) and so vitiate the results of a cross-over study.

If there are likely to be clear side-effects this would invalidate a double-blind study, and if they could be serious then a very carefully monitored *pilot study* should be carried out initially.

The possible beneficial effects may be *assessed* in regard to prolonged survival, prolonged ambulation, or the slowed or arrested progression of muscle weakness. Since changes in muscle strength will be evident first, most emphasis has been placed on this aspect of the problem (Table 13.5). Details of the scoring and grading systems are given in Appendices B–F (pp. 255–9). Because there is a subjective element in determining muscle strength, and to some extent functional ability, these are best assessed by one examiner. There is also value in using an ergometer (myometer, dynamometer). One which we favoured is a hand-held, sensitive, dead-beat electronic device produced by Penny and Giles Transducers Limited (Christchurch, Dorset, England). The

Table 13.5   *Methods for assessing the possible beneficial effects of a drug in Duchenne muscular dystrophy*

1. *Muscle strength*
   MRC grading (0–5)
   Ergometry (kg)
2. *Functional ability*
   Swinyard grade (1–8)
   Vignos grade (1–10)
   Hammersmith motor ability score (0–40)
   'CIDD' grade for upper limbs (1–6)
3. *Biochemical*
   SCK
   Urinary creatine/creatinine, 3-methylhistidine, dimethylarginines
4. *Muscle pathology*

unit has a pressure pad and a digital read-out display which indicates the maximum force applied by the examiner in resisting the actual contraction of the patient's muscles. The operating range is 0.1 to 30 kg and has a repeatability error of less than 1 per cent (Fig. 13.10). The power of each of the major muscle groups is measured and summed for both sides of the body. Other similar instruments are also available (Edwards and McDonnell 1974).

In recent years several investigators have measured various biochemical parameters as a means of assessing any possible improvement. Urinary excretion studies are obviously more acceptable than repeated blood sampling though the former require to be very carefully controlled for age, sex, and diet. There is little value in repeated muscle biopsies though at the end of a trial of a drug which seemed beneficial, muscle pathology could be compared with the findings before the trial was commenced.

Statistical considerations

A drug trial should be designed in such a way as to avoid errors of suggesting a beneficial effect when none exists, or alternatively concluding there is no effect when in fact the drug arrests or slows the disease process. To detect a therapeutic effect which is small, such as a gradual slowing of the disease process, requires a prolonged trial involving a large number of patients. Conversely, a marked therapeutic effect would be detectable in a shorter time and would need fewer individuals. In this regard a helpful parameter to be determined is the so-called *power* of the trial. If the rate of decline in untreated boys is r_1 (with a standard deviation of s.d.), and in treated boys is r_2 then the *standard difference* (delta, Δ) is:

$$\frac{r_1 - r_2}{\text{s.d.}}$$

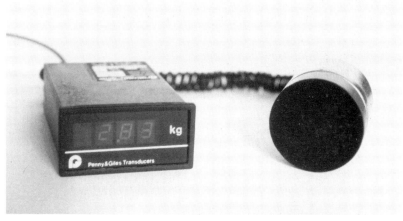

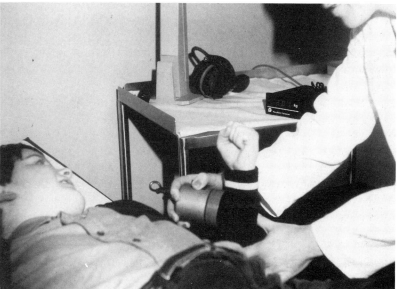

Fig. 13.10. Hand-held ergometer (*above*), and being used to assess the strength of the elbow flexors in an affected boy (*below*).

The power of a trial is the probability of detecting a difference in the two rates which is statistically significant ($P < 0.05$) and can be calculated for different numbers of individuals and for trials of different durations. Based on data from 114 untreated boys with Duchenne muscular dystrophy followed for a year, power curves have been derived by Brooke *et al.* (1983). These investigators found that the rate of decline in untreated boys was 0.4 units (of

muscle strength) per year (s.d. 0.39). If after a year a drug slowed the disease
to 25 per cent of its original rate of progression, then:

$$\Delta = \frac{0.4 - 0.1}{0.39}$$
$$= 0.77$$

To detect such a difference with a 95 per cent probability would require a
study involving at least 40 individuals in each group. On the other hand if a
drug actually arrested the progression of the disease then about 25 individuals
in each group would be required (Fig. 13.11).

The 'power' of therapeutic trials in Duchenne muscular dystrophy is discussed further by Stern (1984). By using more than one set of measurements,
the power of a trial study can be increased, thereby decreasing the number of
individuals needed and/or the duration of the trial. However, the rate of progression is clearly *not* the same in all boys (Ziter *et al.* 1977; Cohen *et al.*
1982). It might therefore be best to consider each boy as being his own control
by comparing rates of progression before and after treatment. Alternatively
groups of boys may be compared who, prior to a trial, showed similar rates of
progression.

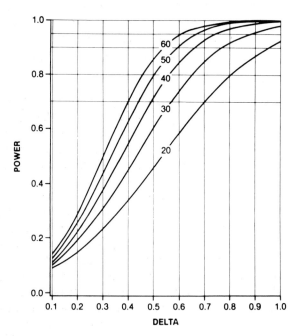

Fig. 13.11. Power curves ($P < 0.05$, one-tail) for drug trials lasting a year for various
values of the standard difference (Delta). (From Brooke *et al.* (1983) with
permission.)

Taking into account the 'power' of a study, the criteria of a good trial in Duchenne muscular dystrophy should be:

Inclusion only of patients with a clearly established diagnosis of the disease
Carefully matched control group
'Blind' study
Assessment by several different methods
Determination of an acceptable 'power' level and therefore the number of individuals to be studied and the duration of the trial.

The assumption underlying the discussion so far is that quite a large number of patients will be involved in a study. Each individual investigator, however, is unlikely to have access to many patients and therefore collaboration between different centres is necessary, to produce data for a so-called 'multi-centre trial'. Uniformity is then essential, both in the design and execution of the trial, particularly with regard to clinical assessment of the possible effects of a drug. The alternative is to study smaller groups of patients but then, as we have seen, only a comparatively large effect would be detected (Table 13.6).

In 1984 a colloquium was held in Bangor, Pennsylvania, sponsored by the Muscular Dystrophy Association of America which addressed many of the problems involved in drug trials in Duchenne muscular dystrophy. The proceedings have been published in full (*Muscle and Nerve* Vol. 8, pp. 451–92, 1985) and provide varied and useful insights into these problems.

Novel approaches to treatment

The emphasis so far has been on the possible benefits of *drug* therapy. But there may well prove to be other approaches to the problem. In 1981 Zatz and her colleagues in Brazil reported a case of Duchenne muscular dystrophy with normal intelligence but who also suffered from growth hormone deficiency (Zatz et al. 1981b; Zatz and Frota-Pessoa 1981). SCK was grossly elevated and the electromyographic and histological findings were consistent with the diagnosis of Duchenne muscular dystrophy. There were two other sibs and seven maternal relatives all affected with classical Duchenne muscular dystrophy and all with normal growth. However, the proband was much more mildly affected than is usual. At 13 he had about the same functional impairment as his 5-year-old affected brother, and at 18 he was still walking unaided although he now had some difficulty in climbing stairs (Fig. 13.12). Thus it would seem that growth hormone deficiency in some way mitigated the effects of the Duchenne gene. This hypothesis is supported to some extent by Chyatte et al. (1973) who found that exogenous growth hormone given to patients with Duchenne muscular dystrophy had a catabolic effect instead of the usual anabolic response. Interestingly, the muscular dystrophy gene is not expressed in genotypic dwarf-dystrophic mice (Totsuka et al. 1981, 1983).

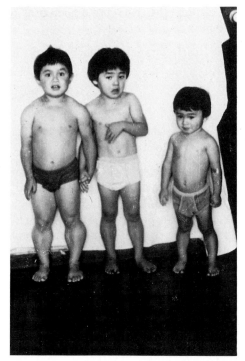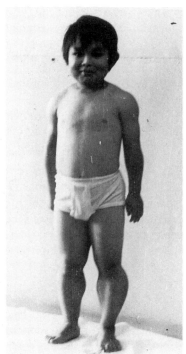

Fig. 13.12. (*Left*) a boy with Duchenne muscular dystrophy and growth hormone deficiency aged 13, and his 2 younger affected brothers aged 5 and 3. (*Right*) proband aged *18*. (Reproduced by kind permission of Dr Mayana Zatz.)

These observations raise a number of interesting questions, notably why growth hormone should have a catabolic effect in dystrophy, and why its deficiency has an ameliorating effect. There is also the possibility that a long-acting somatostatin analogue, or other growth hormone inhibitor, might be of some therapeutic value in the disease (Collipp *et al.* 1984; Zatz *et al.* 1986).

Another observation which may be of relevance in understanding more of pathogenesis is that of an isolated case of apparent Duchenne muscular dystrophy who developed renal failure for which he underwent bilateral nephrectomy with a renal transplant at age 12 (Démos *et al.* 1976). Four months after the operation he was unable to stand upright by himself. However, from then until the age of reporting at 16 there was a progressive amelioration, and two years after the transplant '. . . he was able to walk several hundred yards without help, to climb stairs, and get up from the sitting position'. The question arises as to whether (assuming he had Duchenne and not Becker muscular dystrophy) this effect was a result of the

Table 13.6 *Numbers (rounded off) of individuals (controls and treated) required in a randomized trial where there is a 95 per cent probability ('power') of detecting a significant difference ($P < 0.05$; $P < 0.01$) for various values of Δ, and in each case are roughly four times the required number for a cross-over trial*

	One-tail		Two-tail	
Δ	$P<0.05$	$P<0.01$	$P<0.05$	$P<0.01$
0.1	2165	3154	2599	3563
0.2	541	788	650	891
0.4	135	197	162	223
0.6	60	88	72	99
0.8	34	49	41	56
1.0	22	31	26	36
1.2	15	22	18	25
1.4	11	16	13	18
1.6	8	12	10	14
1.8	7	10	8	11
2.0	5	8	6	9

transplant, the donated normal kidney providing some missing peptide or enzyme, or could it have been the result of the drugs he was taking to prevent graft rejection (azathioprine and prednisolone). The authors themselves think the latter explanation is unlikely, but in view of current ideas on pathogenesis (p. 146) it may well be pertinent.

It could be that an effective treatment may result from a chance observation, and the history of medicine is replete with many such examples. Furthermore, we may not have to wait until the biochemical basis of the disease is known in detail before finding an effective treatment. As Sir Andrew Huxley (1980) has said:

. . . it seems to me that the common assertion that there is no possibility of finding effective treatment until the nature of the genetic defect is known is totally untrue. Myasthenia gravis provides two examples: effective anti-cholinesterase therapy was introduced long before the autoimmune basis of the failure of neuromuscular transmission was known, and at the present time treatment designed to combat the autoimmune attack on the end-plates is used without knowing the original reason for the disturbance of the immune system. . . . Rational therapy can just as well be based on an understanding of intermediate steps in the disease process as on a discovery of the nature of the fundamental defect.

Comprehensive management

Duchenne muscular dystrophy is a relatively rare condition, only about a hundred new cases being born each year in the United Kingdom. For this reason, if for no other, family practitioners may not be fully conversant with the disease. Since family practitioners provide primary care for such children it is essential that they be aware of the existence of the disease so that patients and their families are referred to appropriate specialists as soon as possible and delays in reaching the correct diagnosis are reduced to a minimum. Such awareness may be increased by providing instruction on genetic disorders in medical schools and later in postgraduate refresher courses. In Britain many services for the physically handicapped are provided by Statute. However, for the individual case these services are often inadequate because of poor organization and lack of coordination and communication between health and welfare services (Thomas *et al.* 1985). The problem is particularly acute at the period of transition from childhood to adolescence at the time when affected boys are beginning to require increased medical, social, and educational services. Voluntary agencies can provide help in the form of information on what services are available and how they can be obtained. The Muscular Dystrophy Group of Great Britain and Northern Ireland finances several Family Care Officers, each being attached to a unit with particular interests in muscular dystrophy and related disorders. They are often trained nurses or social workers whose function is to maintain contact with patients and their families, to provide advice on welfare, social and educational services, and in general help families cope with their various problems.

The value of total comprehensive management in Duchenne muscular dystrophy has been argued strongly in Krog (1982), and in order to provide such comprehensive care for the patient and his family there is a need for regional centres for muscular dystrophy in large population areas. Here a team specializing in the disease is able to provide, or have local access to, all the medical and surgical expertise as well as genetic and welfare services needed for comprehensive management. The emphasis is therefore on a team approach (Russman 1984). Patient care could be shared between the centre and local paediatricians, and joint clinics could be held in peripheral hospitals. However, all patients should be notified to, and preferably be assessed at regular intervals by the regional centre. There are a number of arguments to support this idea. A regional centre would concentrate expertise and so reduce the need for patients and families to travel to different hospitals for medical and other services. The members of the centre would also benefit from close relationships with other professionals with related interests. The inclusion of laboratory facilities for enzyme assays and DNA studies would enhance the value of such centres. The inclusion of research facilities as well would ensure that investigators do not work in isolation. But perhaps the most cogent argument is that patients are more likely to benefit from the coordinated efforts of a team with particular expertise in the disease. This could lead to patients with Duchenne muscular dystrophy having an improved quality of life and it has even been suggested they may have increased longevity (Miller and Dunn 1982), which also seems to be the effect in another genetic disorder, namely cystic fibrosis (Anon. 1986). Only by the concerted and coordinated efforts of everyone concerned, will effective management be possible, the prevention of further cases be achieved, and one day an effective treatment be found.

Summary and conclusions

Although Duchenne muscular dystrophy is not yet curable, it is not untreatable and there are many ways to improve the quality of life of affected boys. Paramount is the maintenance of good general health with emphasis on good nutrition and weight control, the prevention of deformities, and the preservation of respiratory function. The development of deformities can be delayed by passive exercises and various orthoses. Scoliosis is a particularly serious problem because the progressive thoracic deformity restricts adequate pulmonary ventilation and aggravates respiratory problems resulting from weakness of the intercostal muscles. The development of scoliosis can be limited by fitting appropriate moulded back supports, but more effectively by prolonging ambulation and surgical fixation of the spine. However, there can be serious operative risks associated with this disorder which include occasionally cardiac arrest and, more commonly, increased muscle breakdown with myoglobinuria. However, these dangers have been mostly based on case reports and are therefore somewhat selective. In the majority of patients there are few serious anaesthetic or post-operative problems though the anaesthetist and surgeon need to be prepared against these eventualities.

Impaired pulmonary function is the major factor in morbidity and mortality, over 90 per cent of deaths being due to pulmonary infection and respiratory failure. The preservation of respiratory function can be achieved to an extent by impeding the development of scoliosis and regular breathing exercises with postural drainage. All respiratory infections must be treated vigorously and often will need brief hospitalization.

The psychological effects of the disease on the patient himself as well as on his parents and unaffected sibs cannot be ignored. Open and frequent discussions between all those concerned, including the health care professionals, should be encouraged. The educational needs of affected boys can also raise problems – for those who are severely handicapped and may require special care, and for those who are highly intelligent and may aspire to further education at a time when they are severely physically handicapped. At the beginning most boys will attend normal schools but later special day schools catering for the physically handicapped may have to be considered.

There is at present no effective treatment. However, in recent years there has been considerable interest in the design of drug trials in this disease, the criteria for a good trial being: the inclusion of patients in whom the diagnosis has been fully established; a carefully matched control group; 'blind' assessment by several different methods; and consideration of the number of individuals required and the duration of the study to demonstrate a significant effect ('power' of the trial).

Finally, comprehensive management through a team approach is advocated. The team should ideally be concentrated in a regional centre for muscular dystrophy where all aspects of management can be coordinated for the benefit of the patient and his family.

Appendices

Appendix A. Duchenne's obituary (*Lancet* 1875)

DUCHENNE (DE BOULOGNE).
(From our Paris Correspondent.)

DUCHENNE (DE BOULOGNE), whose death you noticed in your last issue, was born in 1806, and consequently died at the age of about seventy. After having graduated he began practice in Boulogne-sur-Mer, his native place, but soon found this field too narrow for his restless and inventive mind, and for the experiments which he was already conducting, and so he left for Paris, where, during thirty-three years, he led a life of incessant scientific labour.

In 1847 he presented his first memoir to the Academy of Sciences, and up to within a month previous to his death he continued to publish, either in the Transactions of the two Academies or in the *Archives de Médecine*, the results of his experiments and observations. Amongst the most important of his researches are those on the muscular system; the isolated action and synergy of muscles. His studies on the muscles of the face, and on their office in the mechanism and expression of the human visage, are remarkable, and are familiar in France to artists as well as to medical men. But it was especially in his researches on the nervous centres, on the various forms of paralysis, on congenital or developed deformities, that his great qualities of observation manifested themselves. His name will ever be coupled with the history of progressive muscular atrophy, locomotor ataxy (to which Trousseau proposed that the name of 'Duchenne's disease' should be given), glosso-labio-laryngeal paralysis, and, generally, the microscopical anatomy and pathology of the nervous system. His right of priority to the description of certain forms of nervous diseases has been disputed, and with justice; as, for instance, in the case of locomotor ataxy, where Romberg certainly had the precedence. But at the same time, it may be stated that all Duchenne's descriptions and discoveries were original, and the result of his own labours. The writings of Romberg and other foreign *savants* were at the time unknown in France, not only to Duchenne, but even to the best men having a knowledge of foreign languages.

A great many of his researches were carried on by means of electricity, and in turn they threw light on the uses of this powerful agent, and to Duchenne will redound the honour of having methodically applied electricity to physiological and pathological investigations, and of having scientifically used it for the treatment of disease.

His features were familiar to all who visited habitually the wards of the Paris hospitals. Every morning Duchenne was to be seen in one or other of the hospitals, studying cases, examining specimens, drawing his photographs of microscopical appearances, in which he was extraordinarily skilful. For a long time Duchenne's invariable presence in the wards, his incessant moving about, his ardent interrogation of patients, caused him to be looked upon with a somewhat suspicious and anxious eye by many of the hospital physicians. But his consummate experience of disease, his wonderful keenness and ability in making out a diagnosis in cases of paralysis, the sincerity and earnestness of his manner, the honesty of his proceedings, the authority which he gained by the publication of his original researches, the services which he rendered daily in the wards of the hospitals, brought him the esteem and appreciation of all, and made him a welcome guest everywhere.

He was no orator, and could never have given a lecture on any subject, but he was wonderful at the patient's bedside. Dexterous and nimble in handling his patient, sharp and sensible in his questioning, most striking in the way he got up his data, made out the disease, and gave practical demonstrations of the surety of his diagnosis. Amongst the various instances of this last quality which were related in the hospitals about Duchenne was the fact of his taking patients accounted to be paraplegic out of their beds, and of causing a man to get on their shoulders without their giving way in the slightest.

His patience was extraordinary. He would pursue the investigation of a case for years, never losing sight of it, and following the patient in his peregrinations from hospital to hospital and from house to house, often affording help and means of subsistence.

It may be said of Duchenne that under many adverse circumstances – the suspicions of *confrères*, the disputes as to priority, the difficulty of finding a field of study and experiment, as he had no hospital appointment – his reputation has come out clear and bright, as an honest, hardworking, acute, and ingenious observer, an original discoverer, a skilful professional man, and a kind-hearted, benevolent gentleman.

His various writings have been gathered, and are included in the following important works: – 'Traité de l'Electrisation Localisée' (third edition); 'Le Mécanisme de la Physionomie Humaine'; 'La Physiologie des Mouvements Démontrée à l'aide de l'Expérimentation Electrique'; 'Anatomie du Système Nerveux', 'Orthopédie Physiologique.'

Appendix B. MRC grading of muscle strength (MRC, 1943)

	Grade
No contraction	0
Flicker or trace of contraction only	1
Active movement with gravity eliminated	2
Active movement against gravity	3
Active movement against gravity and resistance	4
Normal power	5

Appendix C. Swinyard grade (Swinyard *et al.* 1957)

	Grade
Walks with waddling gait and marked lordosis. Elevation activities adequate (climbs stairs and curbs without assistance).	1
Walks with waddling gait and marked lordosis. Elevation activities deficient (needs support for curbs and stairs).	2
Walks with waddling gait and marked lordosis. Cannot negotiate curbs or stairs but can achieve erect posture from standard height chair.	3
Walks with waddling gait and marked lordosis. Unable to rise from a standard height chair.	4
Wheelchair independence. Good posture in the chair; can perform all activities of daily living from chair.	5
Wheelchair with dependence. Can roll chair but needs assistance in bed and wheelchair activities.	6
Wheelchair with dependence and back support. Can roll the chair only a short distance; needs back support for good chair position.	7
Bed patient. Can do no activities of daily living without maximum assistance.	8

Appendix D. Vignos grade (Archibald and Vignos 1959)

	Grade
Walks and climbs stairs without assistance.	1
Walks and climbs stairs with aid of railing.	2
Walks and climbs stairs slowly with aid of railing (over 25 seconds for eight standard steps).	3
Walks but cannot climb stairs.	4
Walks unassisted but cannot climb stairs or get out of chair.	5
Walks only with assistance or with braces.	6
In wheelchair. Sits erect, can roll chair and perform bed and wheelchair activities of daily living.	7
In wheelchair. Sits erect. Unable to perform bed and chair activities without assistance.	8
In wheelchair. Sits erect only with support. Able to do only minimal activities of daily living.	9
In bed. Can do no activities of daily living without assistance.	10

Appendix E. Hammersmith motor ability score (Scott *et al.* 1982)

All movements are attempted and scored:
   2 for every completed movement
   1 for help and/or reinforcement
   0 if unable to achieve the movement
   Total possible score = 40

1. Lifts head.
2. Supine to prone over right.
3. Supine to prone over left.
4. Prone to supine over right.
5. Prone to supine over left.
6. Gets to sitting.
7. Sitting.
8. Gets to standing.
9. Standing.
10. Standing on heels.
11. Standing on toes.
12. Stands on right leg.
13. Stands on left leg.
14. Hops on right leg.
15. Hops on left leg.
16. Gets off chair.
17. Climbing step right leg.
18. Descending step right leg.
19. Climbing step left leg.
20. Descending step left leg.

Appendix F. Clinical investigation of Duchenne dystrophy (CIDD) group. Grade for upper limb function (Brooke *et al.* 1983)

	Grade
Starting with arms at the sides, patient can abduct the arms in a full circle until they touch above the head.	1
Can raise arms above head only by flexing the elbow (i.e. shortening the circumference of the movement), or by using accessory muscles.	2
Cannot raise hands above head but can raise an 8 oz glass of water to mouth (using both hands if necessary).	3
Can raise hands to mouth but cannot raise an 8 oz glass of water to mouth.	4
Cannot raise hand to mouth but can use hands to hold pen or pick up pennies from table.	5
Cannot raise hands to mouth and has no useful function of hands.	6

Appendix G. Muscular dystrophy associations and groups in various countries

Argentina
CIDIM
Zapiola 740 CP 1426
Buenos Aires
Argentina

Australia
Muscular Dystrophy Research
  Association of Western Australia
  (Inc)
Box 328
West Perth
WA 6005
Australia

Austria
Österreichische Gesellschaft zur
  Bekämpfung der Muskelkrankheiten
  Neurologischen Universitätsklinik
Lazarettgasse 14
Postfach 23
A–1097 Wien
Austria

Brazil
Associação Brasileira de Distrofia
  Muscular
Rua do Matão 277
Edificio da Biologia
Cidade Universitária
CEP 05499
São Paulo
Brazil

Canada
Society for Muscular Dystrophy
  Information (International)
PO Box 479
Bridgewater NS
B4V 2X6
Canada

Cyprus
Muscular Dystrophy Association
28 Niktariou Street
Limassol
Cyprus

Denmark
Muskelsvindfonden
Vestervang 41
DK 8000 Aarhus–C
Denmark

Finland
Lihastautiliitto R.Y. de
  Muskelhandikappades Forbund R.F.
Mariankatu 4C
20111–Turku 11
Finland

France
Association des Myopathes de France
138 Avenue Felix Faure
75015 Paris
France

Germany
Deutsche Gesellschaft zur Bekämpfung
  der Muskelkrankheiten e.V.
Hohenzollernstrasse 11
D–7800 Freiburg
Germany

India
IMDA
21–136 Batchupet
Machilipatnam–521 001
India

Israel
Muscle Disease Association
52 Shlomo Hamelech Street
Tel Aviv
Israel

Italy
Unione Italiana Lotta Alla Distrofia
  Muscolare
Via PP Vergerio 17
1–35126 Padova
Italy

Japan
Muscular Dystrophy Association of
 Japan
2-2-8, Nishi-waseda
Shinjuku-ku
Tokyo 162
Japan

Malta
Muscular Dystrophy Group of Malta
52 Main Street
Zebbug
Malta

The Netherlands
Vereniging Spierziekten Nederland
Lt.Gen. v. Heutszlaan 6
3743 JN Baarn
The Netherlands

New Zealand
Muscular Dystrophy Association of
 New Zealand Inc
PO Box 56-123
Auckland 3
New Zealand

Norway
Foreningen for Muskelsyke
Sporveisgaten 10
N-0354 Oslo 3
Norway

South Africa
Muscular Dystrophy Research
 Foundation of South Africa
PO Box 5446
Johannesburg 2000
South Africa

Spain
Asociación Española de Enfermedades
 Musculares
Apartado de Correos 14170
08080-Barcelona
Spain

Sweden
R.B.U. Arbetsgruppen for Muskelsjuka
David Bagares Gata 3
S-111 38 Stockholm
Sweden

Neurologiskt Handikappades
 Riksforbund
Kungsgatan 32
111 35 Stockholm
Sweden

Switzerland
Schweiz Gesellschaft für
 Muskelkrankheiten
Feldeggstrasse 71
Postfach 129
CH-8032 Zurich
Switzerland

United Kingdom
Muscular Dystrophy Group of Great
 Britain and Northern Ireland
 Nattrass House
35 Macaulay Road
Clapham
London SW4 0QP
England

United States of America
Muscular Dystrophy Association
810 Seventh Avenue
New York
NY 10019
USA

Uruguay
Asociacion Uruguaya de Aldeas
 Infantiles SOS
Montevideo
Uruguay

Yugoslavia
Savez Distroficara Jugoslavije
Ul. Radomira Vujovica br. 3
11000 Beograd
Yugoslavia

References

Adams, R. D. (1975). *Diseases of muscle – a study in pathology*, 3rd edn. Harper and Row, Hagerstown, Maryland.

Adriaenssens, K. and Vermeiren, G. (1980). Simple electrophoretic technique for creatine kinase MM isozyme in neonatal Duchenne muscular disease screening using dried blood samples. *Clin. Chim. Acta*. **105**, 99–103.

Afifi, A. K., Bergman, R. A., and Zellweger, H. (1973). A possible role for electron microscopy in detection of carriers of Duchenne type muscular dystrophy. *J. Neurol. Neurosurg. Psychiat*. **36**, 643–50.

Aguilar, L., Lisker, R., and Ramos, G. G. (1978). Unusual inheritance of Becker type muscular dystrophy. *J. Med. Genet*. **15**, 116–18.

Alexander, M. A., Johnson, E. W., Petty, J., and Stauch, D. (1979). Mechanical ventilation of patients with late stage of Duchenne muscular dystrophy: management in the home. *Arch. Phys. Med. Rehab*. **60**, 289–92.

Allard, P., Duhaime, M., Thiry, P. S., and Drouin, G. (1981) Use of gait simulation in the evaluation of a spring-loaded knee joint orthosis for Duchenne muscular dystrophy patients. *Med. & Biol. Eng. & Comput*. **19**, 165–70.

Allen, J. E. and Rodgin, D. W. (1960). Mental retardation in association with progressive muscular dystrophy. *Amer. J. Dis. Child*. **100**, 208–11.

Allen, N. R. (1973). Hearing acuity in patients with muscular dystrophy. *Develop. Med. Child. Neurol*. **15**, 500–5.

Allsop, K. G. and Ziter, F. A. (1981). Loss of strength and functional decline in Duchenne's dystrophy. *Arch. Neurol*. **38**, 406–11.

Anand, R. and Emery, A. E. H. (1980). Calcium stimulated enzyme efflux from human skeletal muscle. *Res. Commun. Chem. Path. Pharmacol*. **28**, 541–50.

Anon. (1984). Psychological sequelae of female sterilization. *Lancet* **ii**, 144–5.

—— (1986). Regional centres for cystic fibrosis. *Lancet* **i**, 514.

Appleyard, S. T., Dunn, M. J., Dubowitz, V., and Rose, M. L. (1985). Increased expression of HLA ABC class I antigens by muscle fibres in Duchenne muscular dystrophy, inflammatory myopathy and other neuromuscular disorders. *Lancet* **i**, 361–33.

Aprin, H., Bowen, J. R., MacEwen, G. D., and Hall, J. E. (1982). Spine fusion in patients with spinal muscular atrophy. *J. Bone Joint Surg*. **64A**, 1179–87.

Arahata, K. and Engel, A. G. (1982). Monoclonal antibody analysis of the mononuclear cell in muscle biopsy. *Ann. Neurol*. **12**, 79 (Abstract).

Archibald, K. C. and Vignos, P. J. (1959) A study of contractures in muscular dystrophy. *Arch. Phys. Med. Rehab*. **40**, 150–7.

Armstrong, R. M. and Appel, S. H. (1981). Neuromuscular disorders. *Current Neurol*. **3**, 17–42.

Askanas, V., Engel, W. K., and Kobayashi, T. (1985). Thyrotropin-releasing hormone enhances motor neuron-evoked contractions of cultured human muscle. *Ann. Neurol*. **18**, 716–19.

Asmussen, M. A. and Clegg, M. T. (1985). Multiallelic restriction fragment polymorphisms in genetic counseling: population genetic considerations. *Hum. Hered.* **35**, 129–42.

Averill, D. R. (1980). Diseases of the muscle. *Vet. Clin. North Amer.* **10**, 223–34.

Averyanov, Y. N., Bogomazov, E. A., and Logunova, L. V. (1977). Duchenne muscular dystrophy in a girl with chromosomal mosaicism 45, X/46, XX. (Russian). *Zh. Neuropat. Psikhiat. Korsokova.* **77**, 1449–52.

Aymé S., Pelissier, J. F., Garnier, J. M., Mattei, J. F., and Giraud, F. (1979). Duchenne type muscular dystrophy and consanguinity: difficulties in pedigree analysis. *J. Med. Genet.* **16**, 393–5.

Bach, J., Alba, A., Pilkington, L. A., and Lee, M. (1981). Long-term rehabilitation in advanced stage of childhood onset, rapidly progressive muscular dystrophy. *Arch. Phys. Med. Rehab.* **62**, 328–31.

Bakker, E., Hofker, M. H., Goor, N., Mandel, J. L., Wrogemann, K., Davies K. E., Kunkel, L. M., Willard, H.F., Fenton, W.A., Sandkuyl, L., Majoor-Krakauer, D., Van Essen, A. J., Jahoda, M. G. J., Sachs, E. S., Van Ommen, G. J. B., and Pearson, P. L. (1985). Prenatal diagnosis and carrier detection of Duchenne muscular dystrophy with closely linked RFLPs. *Lancet* **i**, 655–8.

Ballard, F. J., Tomas, F. M., and Stern, L. M. (1979). Increased turnover of muscle contractile proteins in Duchenne muscular dystrophy as assessed by 3-methyl-histidine and creatinine excretion. *Clin. Sci.* **56**, 347–52.

Bank, W. J., Rowland, L. P., and Ipsen, J. (1971). Amino acids of plasma and urine in diseases of muscle. *Arch. Neurol.* **24**, 176–86.

Baraitser, M. (1985). *The genetics of neurological disorders*, 2nd edn. Oxford University Press, Oxford.

Bartley, J. A., Miller, D. K., Hayford, J. T., and McCabe, E. R. B. (1982). Concordance of X-linked glycerol kinase deficiency with X-linked congenital adrenal hypoplasia. *Lancet* **ii**, 733–6.

——, Patil, S., Davenport, S., Goldstein, D., and Pickens, J. (1986). Duchenne muscular dystrophy, glycerol kinase deficiency and adrenal insufficiency associated with Xp21 interstitial deletion. *J. Pediat.* **108**, 189–92.

Barwick, D. D., Osselton, J. W., and Walton, J. N. (1965). Electroencephalographic studies in hereditary myopathy. *J. Neurol. Neurosurg. Psychiat.* **28**, 109–14.

Basmajian, J. V. (editor). (1973). *Therapeutic exercise*, 3rd edn. Williams and Wilkins, Baltimore.

Bassöe, H. H. (1956). Familial congenital muscular dystrophy with gonadal dysgenesis. *J. Clin. Endocrin.* **16**, 1614–21.

Bawle, E., Tyrkus, M., Lipman, S., and Bozimowski, D. (1984). Aarskog syndrome: full male and female expression associated with an X-autosome translocation. *Amer. J. Med. Genet.* **17**, 595–602.

Beam, K. G., Knudson, C. M., and Powell, J. A. (1986). A lethal mutation in mice eliminates the slow calcium current in skeletal muscle cells. *Nature, London*, **320**, 168–70.

Becker, P. E. (1953). *Dystrophia Musculorum Progressiva*. Thieme-Verlag, Stuttgart.

—— (1957). Neue Ergebnisse der Genetik der Muskeldystrophien. *Acta Genet* **7**, 303–10.

—— (1962). Two new families of benign sex-linked recessive muscular dystrophy. *Rev. Canad. Biol.* **21**, 551–66.

—— (1964). Myopathien. In *Humangenetik: Ein kurzes Handbuch in fünf Bänden.* (ed. P. E. Becker) Vol. 3, Pt. 1. Thieme-Verlag, Stuttgart.

—— (1972). Neues zur Genetik und Klassifikation der Muskeldystrophien. *Humangenetik* **17**, 1–22.

—— (1980). Epidemiology of Duchenne muscular dystrophy in South-West Germany. In *Muscular dystrophy research: advances and new trends* (ed. C. Angelini, G. A. Danieli, and D. Fontanari) pp. 149–56. Excerpta Medica, Amsterdam.

—— and Kiener, F. (1955). Eine neue X-chromosomale Muskeldystrophie. *Arch. Psychiat. Zeitschr. Neurol.* **193**, 427–48.

Beckmann, R. and Scheuerbrandt, G. (1976). Screening auf erhöhte CK-aktivitäten. *Der Kinderarzt.* **7**, 1267–72.

Bell, C. (1830). *The nervous system of the human body: as explained in a series of papers read before the Royal Society of London.* Adam and Charles Black, Edinburgh.

Bell, J. (1943). On pseudohypertrophic and allied types of progressive muscular dystrophy. In *Treasury of human inheritance* Vol. 4, Pt. 4. Cambridge University Press, London.

Ben Hamida, M., Fardeau, M., and Attia, N. (1983). Severe childhood muscular dystrophy affecting both sexes and frequent in Tunisia. *Muscle and Nerve* **6**, 469–80.

Benjamin, R. J. and Waldmann, H. (1986). Induction of tolerance by monoclonal antibody therapy. *Nature* **320**, 449–51.

Berg, B. O. and Conte, F. (1974) Duchenne muscular dystrophy in a female with a structurally abnormal X-chromosome. *Neurology* **24**, 356 (Abstract).

Berthillier, G., Eichenberger, D., Carrier, H. N., Guibaud, P., and Got, R. (1982). Carnitine metabolism in early stages of Duchenne muscular dystrophy. *Clin. Chim. Acta.* **122**, 369–75.

Bertorini, T. E. Bhattacharya, S. K., Palmieri, G. M. A., Chesney, C. M., Pifer, D., and Baker, B. (1982). Muscle calcium and magnesium content in Duchenne muscular dystrophy. *Neurology* **32**, 1088–92.

——, Cornelio, F., Bhattacharya, S. K., Palmieri, G. M. A., Dones, I., Dworzak, F., and Brambati, B. (1984). Calcium and magnesium content in fetuses at risk and prenecrotic Duchenne muscular dystrophy. *Neurology* **34**, 1436–40.

—— and Igarashi, M. (1985). Postpoliomyelitis muscle pseudohypertrophy. *Muscle and Nerve* **8**, 644–9.

Bethlem, J. (1970). *Muscle pathology – introduction and atlas* Elsevier/North-Holland, Amsterdam.

Bevans, M. (1945). Changes in the musculature of the gastrointestinal tract and in the myocardium in progressive muscular dystrophy. *Arch. Path.* **40**, 225–38.

Biddison, J. H., Dembo, D. H., Spalt, H., Hayes, M. G., and LeDoux, C. W. (1979). Familial occurence of mitral valve prolapse in X-linked muscular dystrophy. *Circulation* **59**, 1299–1304.

Bjerglund Nielsen, L., Jacobsen, B. B., Nielsen, I. M., and Tabor, A. (1983). X; autosome translocation in a girl with muscular dystrophy. *Clin. Genet.* **23**, 242 (Abstract).

—— and Nielsen, I. M. (1984). Turner's syndrome and Duchenne muscular dystrophy in a girl with an X; autosome translocation. *Ann. Génét.* **27**, 173–7.

Black, F. W. (1973). Intellectual ability as related to age and stage of disease in muscular dystrophy: a brief note. *J. Psychol.* **84**, 333–4.

Blau, H. M., Webster, C., and Pavlath, G. K. (1983). Defective myoblasts identified in Duchenne muscular dystrophy. *Proc. Natl. Acad. Sci.* **80**, 4856–60.

Blum, D., and Brauman, J. (1975). Serum enzymes in the neonatal period. *Biol. Neonate* **26**, 53–7.

Blumberg, B. (1984). The emotional implications of prenatal diagnosis. In *Psychological aspects of genetic counselling* (ed. A. E. H. Emery and I. M. Pullen) pp. 201–17. Academic Press, London, New York.

Blyth, H., Carter, C. O., Dubowitz, V., Emery, A. E. H., Gavin, J., Johnston, H. A., McKusick, V. A., Race, R. R., Sanger, R., and Tippett, P. (1965). Duchenne's muscular dystrophy and the Xg blood groups: a search for linkage. *J. Med. Genet.* **2**, 157–60.

—— and Hughes, B. P. (1971). Pregnancy and serum CPK levels in potential carriers of 'severe' X-linked muscular dystrophy. *Lancet* **i**, 855–6.

—— and Pugh, R. J. (1959). Muscular dystrophy in childhood; the genetic aspect. *Ann. Hum. Genet.* **23**, 127–63.

Bodensteiner, J. B. and Engel, A. G. (1978). Intracellular calcium accumulation in Duchenne dystrophy and other myopathies: a study of 567,000 muscle fibres in 114 biopsies. *Neurology* **28**, 439–46.

Boltshauser, E., Steinmann, B., Meyer, A., and Jerusalem, F. (1980). Anaesthesia-induced rhabdomyolysis in Duchenne muscular dystrophy. *Brit. J. Anaesth.* **52**, 559.

Bonsett, C. A. (1969). *Studies of pseudohypertrophic muscular dystrophy.* Charles C. Thomas, Springfield, Illinois.

Bortolini, E. R. and Zatz, M. (1986). Investigation on genetic heterogeneity in Duchenne muscular dystrophy. *Amer. J. Med. Genet.* **24**, 111–17.

Bossingham, D. H., Williams, E., and Nichols, P. J. R. (1977). *Severe childhood neuromuscular disease – the management of Duchenne muscular dystrophy and spinal muscular atrophy.* Muscular Dystrophy Group of Great Britain, London.

Boyd, Y. and Buckle, V. J. (1986). Cytogenetic heterogeneity of translocations associated with Duchenne muscular dystrophy. *Clin. Genet.* **29**, 108–15.

Bradley, R., McKerrell, R. E., and Barnard, E. A. (1987). Neuromuscular diseases in animals. In *Disorders of voluntary muscle*, 5th edn (ed. J. N. Walton). Churchill Livingstone, Edinburgh. (in press)

Bradley, W. G. and Fulthorpe, J. J. (1978). Studies of sarcolemmal integrity in myopathic muscle. *Neurology* **28**, 670–7.

——, Hudgson, P., Larson, P. F., Papapetropoulos, T. A., and Jenkison, M. (1972). Structural changes in the early stages of Duchenne muscular dystrophy. *J. Neurol. Neurosurg. Psychiat.* **35**, 451–5.

——, Jenkison, M., and Montgomery, A. (1975). The significance of neural abnormalities in muscular dystrophy. In *Recent advances in myology* (ed. W. G. Bradley, D. Gardner–Medwin, and J. N. Walton) pp. 116–24. Excerpta Medica, Amsterdam.

——, Jones, M. Z., Mussini, J. M., and Fawcett, P. R. W. (1978). Becker-type muscular dystrophy. *Muscle and Nerve* **1**, 111–32.

——, O'Brien, M. D., Walder, D. N., Murchison, D., Johnson, M., and Newell, D. J. (1975). Failure to confirm a vascular cause of muscular dystrophy. *Arch. Neurol.* **32**, 466–73.

Brooke, M. H., Carroll, J. E., and Ringel, S. P. (1979). Congenital hypotonia revisited. *Muscle and Nerve* **2**, 84–100.

——, Fenichel, G. M., Griggs, R. C., Mendell, J. R., Moxley, R., Miller, J. P., Province, M. A., and the CIDD Group. (1983). Clinical investigation in Duchenne dystrophy: 2. Determination of the 'power' of therapeutic trials based on the natural history. *Muscle and Nerve* **6**, 91–103.

—— and Kaiser, K. K. (1970). Muscle fiber types: how many and what kind? *Arch. Neurol.* **23**, 369–79.

Brooks, A. P. and Emery, A. E. H. (1977). The incidence of Duchenne muscular dystrophy in the South-East of Scotland. *Clin. Genet.* **11**, 290–4.

Brown, C. S., Thomas, N. S. T., Sarfarazi, M., Davies, K. E., Kunkel, L., Pearson, P. L., Kingston, H. M., Shaw, D. J., and Harper, P. S. (1985). Genetic linkage relationships of seven DNA probes with Duchenne and Becker muscular dystrophy. *Hum. Genet.* **71**, 62–74.

Brownell, A. K. W., Paasuke, R. T., Elash, A., Fowlow, S. B., Seagram, C. G. F., Diewold, R. J., and Friesen, C. (1983). Malignant hyperthermia in Duchenne muscular dystrophy. *Anesthesiology* **58**, 180–2.

Brumback, R. A. and Leech, R. W. (1984). *Color atlas of muscle histochemistry*. PSG Publishing Company, Littleton, Mass.

Buchanan, D. C., Labarbera, C. J., Roelofs, R., and Olson, W. (1979). Reactions of families to children with Duchenne muscular dystrophy. *Gen. Hosp. Psychiat.* **1**, 262–9.

Bucher, K., Ionasescu, V., and Hanson, J. (1980). Frequency of new mutants among boys with Duchenne muscular dystrophy. *Amer. J. Med. Genet.* **7**, 27–34.

Buchthal, F. (1957). *An introduction to electromyography*. Gyldendal, Copenhagen.

—— and Clemmesen, S. (1941). On the differentiation of muscle atrophy by electromyography. *Acta Psych. Neurol.* **16**, 143–81.

——, Guld, C., and Rosenfalck, P. (1954a). Action potential parameters in normal human muscle and their dependence on physical variables. *Acta Physiol. Scand.* **32**, 200–18.

—— and Olsen, P. Z. (1970). Electromyography and muscle biopsy in infantile spinal muscular atrophy. *Brain* **93**, 15–30.

—— and Pinelli, P. (1951). Analysis of motor action potentials as a diagnostic aid in neuro-muscular disorders. *Acta Med. Scand.* **142** (Suppl. 266), 315–27.

——, and Rosenfalck, P. (1954b). Action potential parameters in normal human muscle and their physiological determinants. *Acta Physiol. Scand.* **32**, 219–29.

—— and Rosenfalck, P. (1963). Electrophysiological aspects of myopathy with particular reference to progressive muscular dystrophy. In *Muscular dystrophy in man and animals* (ed. G. H. Bourne and M. N. Golarz) pp. 193–262. Hafner Pub. Co., New York and S. Karger, Basel, Switzerland.

Bulfield, G., Siller, W. G., Wight, P. A. L., and Moore, K. J. (1984). X chromosome-linked muscular dystrophy (*mdx*) in the mouse. *Proc. Natl. Acad. Sci (USA)* **81**, 1189–92.

Buller, A., Eccles, J. C., and Eccles, R. M. (1960). Interactions between motor neurones and muscles in respect of the characteristic speeds of their responses. *J. Physiol.* **150**, 417–39.

Bullock, D. G., McSweeney, F. M., Whitehead, T. P., and Edwards, J. H. (1979). Serum creatine kinase activity and carrier status for Duchenne muscular dystrophy. *Lancet* **ii**, 1370.

Bundey, S. (1978). Calculation of genetic risks in Duchenne muscular dystrophy by geneticists in the United Kingdom. *J. Med. Genet.* **15**, 249–53.

—— (1981). A genetic study of Duchenne muscular dystrophy in the West Midlands. *J. Med. Genet.* **18**, 1–7.

—— (1985). *Genetics and neurology.* Churchill Livingstone, Edinburgh.

——, Crawley, J. M., Edwards, J. H., and Westhead, R. A. (1979a). Serum creatine kinase levels in pubertal, mature, pregnant, and postmenopausal women. *J. Med. Genet.* **16**, 117–21.

—— and Ebdy, J. (1982). Fetal sexing in possible carriers for Duchenne muscular dystrophy. *Prenatal Diag.* **2**, 1–6.

——, Edwards, J. H., and Insley, J. (1979b). Carrier detection in Duchenne muscular dystrophy. *Lancet* **i**, 881.

Burn, J. Povey, S., Boyd, Y., Munro, E. A., West, L., Thomas, D., and Baraitser, M. (1986). Duchenne muscular dystrophy in one of monozygotic twin girls. (In press)

Call, G. and Ziter, F. A. (1985). Failure to thrive in Duchenne muscular dystrophy. *J. Pediat.* **106**, 939–41.

Cammann, R., Vehreschild, T., and Ernst, K. (1974). Eine neue Sippe von X-chromosomaler benigner Muskeldystrophie mit Frühkontrakturen (Emery–Dreifuss). *Psychiat. Neurol. Med. Psychol., Leipzig* **26**, 431–8.

Canki, N., Dutrillaux, B., and Tivadar, I. (1979). Dystrophie musculaire de Duchenne chez une petite fille porteuse d'une translocation t(X; 3) (p21; q13) *de novo. Ann. Génét.* **22**, 35–9.

Capaldi, M. J., Dunn, M. J., Sewry, C. A., and Dubowitz, V. (1985). Lectin blotting of human muscle. Identification of a high molecular weight glycoprotein which is absent or altered in Duchenne muscular dystrophy. *J. Neurol. Sci.* **68**, 225–31.

Carpenter, S. and Karpati, G. (1984). *Pathology of skeletal muscle.* Churchill Livingstone, Edinburgh.

Carr, E. F. and Oppé, T. E. (1971). The birth of an abnormal child: telling the parents. *Lancet* **ii**, 1075–7.

Carroll, J. E., Villadiego, A., and Brooke, M. H. (1983). Increased long chain acyl CoA in Duchenne muscular dystrophy. *Neurology* **33**, 1507–10.

Carry, M. R., Ringel, S. P., and Starcevich, J. M. (1986). Distribution of capillaries in normal and diseased muscle. *Muscle & Nerve* **9**, 445–54.

Carter, C. O. (1979). Carrier detection in Duchenne muscular dystrophy. *Lancet* **i**, 979.

——, Roberts, J. A. F., Evans, K. A., and Buck, A. R. (1971). Genetic clinic: a follow up. *Lancet* **i**, 281–5.

Carter, N., Jeffery, S., Shiels, A., Edwards, Y., Tipler, T., and Hopkinson, D. A. (1979). Characterization of human carbonic anhydrase III from skeletal muscle. *Biochem. Genet.* **17**, 837–54.

Carter, N. D., Heath, R., and Jeffery, S. (1980). Serum carbonic anhydrase III in Duchenne dystrophy. *Lancet* **ii**, 542.

Caskey, C. T., Nussbaum, R. L., Cohan, L. C., and Pollack, L. (1980). Sporadic occurrence of Duchenne muscular dystrophy: evidence for new mutation. *Clin. Genet.* **18**, 329–41.

Caskey, C. T. (1986). Personal communication.

Cattanach, B. M. (1975). Control of chromosome inactivation. *Ann. Rev. Genet.* **9**, 1–18.

—— and Williams, C. E. (1972). Evidence of non-random X chromosome activity in the mouse. *Genet. Res.* **19**, 229–40.

Cavanagh, N. P. C. and Preece, M. A. (1981). Calf hypertrophy and asymmetry in female carriers of X-linked Duchenne muscular dystrophy: an over-diagnosed clinical manifestation. *Clin. Genet.* **20**, 168–72.

Cestan, R. and Lejonne.   (1902). Une myopathie avec rétractions familiales. *Nouvelle Iconographie de la Salpêtrière* **15**, 38–52.

Chakrabarti, A. and Pearce, J. M. S. (1981). Scapuloperoneal syndrome with cardiomyopathy: report of a family with autosomal dominant inheritance and unusual features. *J. Neurol. Neurosurg. Psychiat.* **44**, 1146–52.

Charash L. I., Wolf, S. G., Kutscher A. H., Lovelace, R. E., and Hale M. S. (eds) (1983). *Psychosocial aspects of muscular dystrophy and allied diseases.* Charles C. Thomas, Springfield Ill.

Cheeseman, E. A., Kilpatrick, S. J., Stevenson, A. C., and Smith, C. A. B. (1958). The sex ratio of mutation rates of sex-linked recessive genes in man with particular reference to Duchenne type muscular dystrophy. *Ann. Hum. Genet.* **22**, 235–43.

Chyatte, S. B., Rudman, D., Patterson, J. H., Gerron, G. G., O'Beirne, I., Barlow, J., Jordan, A., and Shavin, J. S. (1973). Human growth hormone and estrogens in boys with Duchenne muscular dystrophy. *Arch. Phys. Med. Rehab.* **54**, 248–53.

Claes, C., Smets, J., and Jacobs, K. (1968). La myopathie précocissime étude électroclinique et pathologique d'une entité clinique particulière. *J. Neurol. Sci.* **6**, 141–54.

Clark, A. G. (1985). The use of multiple restriction fragment length polymorphisms in prenatal risk estimation. *Amer. J. Hum. Genet.* **37**, 60–72.

Clark, J. I., Puite, R. H., Marczynski, R., and Mann, J. D. (1963). Evidence for the absence of detectable linkage between the genes for Duchenne muscular dystrophy and the Xg blood group. *Amer. J. Hum. Genet.* **15**, 292–7.

Clayton, J. and Emery, A. E. H. (1984). DNA probes in Duchenne muscular dystrophy. *Lancet* **ii**, 1151–2.

Clayton, J. F. (1986). A computer programme to calculate risk in X linked disorders using multiple marker loci. *J. Med. Genet.* **23**, 35–9.

Coërs, C. and Woolf, A. L. (1959). *The innervation of muscle – a biopsy study.* Blackwell, Oxford.

Cohen, A. (1977). Education of children with muscular dystrophy. In *Muscular dystrophy 1976* (ed. G. C. Robin and G. Falewski de Leon) pp. 139–41. Karger, Basel.

Cohen, H. J., Molnar, G. E., and Taft, L. T. (1968). The genetic relationship of progressive muscular dystrophy (Duchenne type) and mental retardation. *Develop. Med. Child. Neurol.* **10**, 754–65.

Cohen, L., Morgan, J., Babbs, R., Gilula, Z., Karrison, T., and Meier, P. (1982). A statistical analysis of the loss of muscle strength in Duchenne's muscular dystrophy. *Res. Commun. Chem. Pathol. Pharmacol.* **37**, 123–38.

Collipp, P. J., Kelemen, J., Chen, S. Y., Castro-Magana, M., Angulo, M., and Derenoncourt, A. (1984) Growth hormone inhibition causes increased selenium levels in Duchenne muscular dystrophy: a possible new approach to therapy. *J. Med. Genet.* **21**, 254–6.

Conomy, J. P. (1970). Late-onset slowly progressive sex-linked recessive muscular dystrophy. *Military Med.* **135**, 471–5.

Cordone, G., Venzano, V., Rossi, G., Cavallero, G., and Minetti, C. (1984). Valutazione critica della variazione della CK serica dopo sforzo nell'identificazione delle portatrici di distrofia muscolare di Duchenne. *Pediatr. Med. Chir.* **6**, 819–22.

Cornelio, F. and Dones, I. (1984). Muscle fiber degeneration and necrosis in muscular dystrophy and other muscle diseases: cytochemical and immunocytochemical data. *Ann. Neurol.* **16**, 694–701.

Cosmos, E. and Butler, J. (1980). Animal models of muscle diseases, Part III: Compilation of therapeutic trials for hereditary muscular dystrophy. *Muscle and Nerve* **3**, 427–35.

——, Mazliah, J., and Allard, E. P. (1980). Animal models of muscle diseases, Part II: Murine dystrophy. *Muscle and Nerve* **3**, 350–9.

Cowan, J., Macdessi, J., Stark, A., and Morgan, G. (1980). Incidence of Duchenne muscular dystrophy in New South Wales and the Australian Capital Territory. *J. Med. Genet.* **17**, 245–9.

Crisp, D. E., Ziter, F. A., and Bray, P. F. (1982). Diagnostic delay in Duchenne's muscular dystrophy. *J. Amer. Med. Assoc.* **247**, 478–80.

Critchley, M. (1949). *Sir William Gowers (1845–1915) – biographical appreciation.* Wm. Heinemann, London.

Cullen, M. J. and Mastaglia, F. L. (1980). Morphological changes in dystrophic muscle. *Brit. Med. Bull.* **36**, 145–52.

Cuthbertson, R. A. (1977). *Duchenne de Boulogne, his life, his times and the significance of his work, with special reference to his study of mechanism of human facial expression.* Thesis, University of Melbourne.

Dangain, J. and Vrbova, G. (1984). Muscle development in *mdx* mutant mice. *Muscle and Nerve* **7**, 700–4.

Danieli, G. A. (1984). Studies on the prevalence of the Duchenne muscular dystrophy genotype at birth. In *Research into the origin and treatment of muscular dystrophy* (ed. L. P. ten Kate, P. L. Pearson, and A. M. Stadhouders) pp. 17–32. Excerpta Medica, Amsterdam.

—— and Barbujani, G. (1984). Duchenne muscular dystrophy – frequency of sporadic cases. *Hum. Genet.* **67**, 252–6.

—— Mostacciuolo, M. L., Bonfante, A., and Angelini, C. (1977). Duchenne muscular dystrophy – a population study. *Hum. Genet.* **35**, 225–31.

——, Pilotto, G., Angelini, C., and Bonfante, A. (1980). Duchenne muscular dystropy – data from family studies. *Hum. Genet.* **54**, 63–8.

Danilowicz, D., Rutkowski, M., Myung, D., and Schively, D. (1980). Echocardiography in Duchenne muscular dystrophy. *Muscle and Nerve* **3**, 298–303.

Davidson, R. G. (1970). Application of cell culture techniques to human genetics. In *Modern trends in human genetics* (ed. A. E. H. Emery) Vol. 1, pp. 143–80. Butterworth, London.

Davie, A. M. and Emery, A. E. H. (1978). Estimation of proportion of new mutants among cases of Duchenne muscular dystrophy. *J. Med. Genet.* **15**, 339–45.

Davies, K. E., Briand, P., Ionasescu, V., Ionasescu, G., Williamson, R., Brown, C., Cavard, C., and Cathelineau, L. (1985a). Gene for OTC: characterization and linkage to Duchenne muscular dystrophy. *Nucleic Acids Res.* **13**, 155–65.

——, Forrest, S., Smith, T., Kenwrick, S., Ball, S., Dorkins, H., and Patterson, M. (1986). Molecular analysis of human muscular dystrophies. *Muscle and Nerve* (In press)

——, Pearson, P. L., Harper, P. S., Murray, J. M., O'Brien, T., Sarfarazi, M., and Williamson, R. (1983). Linkage analysis of two cloned DNA sequences flanking the Duchenne muscular dystrophy locus on the short arm of the human X chromosome. *Nucleic Acids Res.* **11**, 2303–12.

——, Speer, A., Herrmann, F., Spiegler, A. W. J., McGlade, S., Hofker, M. H., Briand, P., Hanke, R., Schwartz, M. *et al.* (1985b). Human X chromosome markers and Duchenne muscular dystrophy. *Nucleic Acids Res.* **13**, 3419–26.

——, Young, B. D., Elles, R. G., Hill, M. E., and Williamson, R. (1981). Cloning of a representative genomic library of the human X chromosome after sorting by flow cytometry. *Nature* **293**, 374–6.

Dawson, D. M., Eppenberger, H. M., and Kaplan, N. O. (1965). Creatine kinase: evidence for a dimeric structure. *Biochem. Biophys. Res. Commun.* **21**, 346–53.

—— and Fine, I. H. (1967). Creatine kinase in human tissues. *Arch. Neurol.* **16**, 175–80.

De Coster, W., De Reuck, J., and Thiery, E. (1974). A late autosomal dominant form of limb-girdle muscular dystrophy. A clinical, genetic and morphological study. *Europ. Neurol.* **12**, 159–72.

Dellamonica, C., Collombel, C., Cotte, J., and Addis, P. (1983). Screening for neonatal Duchenne muscular dystrophy by bioluminescence measurement of creatine kinase in a blood sample spotted on paper. *Clin. Chem.* **29**, 161–3.

Demany, M. A. and Zimmerman, H. A. (1969). Progressive muscular dystrophy: haemodynamic, angiographic and pathologic study of a patient with myocardial involvement. *Circulation* **40**, 377–84.

Démos, J. (1961). Un nouveau problème posé par la myopathie humaine; les troubles des temps de circulation et leur liaison avec l'activité enzymatique sérique. *Bull. et Mém. Soc. Méd. Hop. Paris* **77**, 636–46.

——, Dreyfus, J. C., Schapira, F., and Schapira, G. (1962). Anomalies biologiques chez les transmetteurs apparement sains de la myopathie. *Rev. Canad. Biol.* **21**, 587–97.

—— and Maroteaux, P. (1961). Mesure des temps de circulation chez 141 sujets normaux par une technique originale. Rôle de la taille de l'enfant sur les temps de circulation de bras à bras. *Rev. Franç. Etudes Clin. Biol.* **6**, 773–8.

——, Tuil, D., Berthelon, M., Katz, P., Broyer, M., Riberi, P., Testard, R., Rognon, L. M., Pillet, J., and Collin, P. (1976). Progressive muscular dystrophy – functional improvement after a renal allograft. *J. Neurol. Sci.* **30**, 41–53.

Dennis, N. R., Evans, K., Clayton, B., and Carter, C. O. (1976). Use of creatine kinase for detecting severe X-linked muscular dystrophy carriers. *Brit. Med. J.* **2**, 577–9.

Denny-Brown, D. (1949). Interpretation of the electromyogram. *Arch. Neurol. Psychiat.* **61**, 99–128.

Desai, A. D., Jayam, A. V., Banerji, A. P., Kohiyar, F. N., and Ardhapurkar, I. (1969). Study of the central nervous system in Duchenne type of muscular dystrophy. *Neurology, India* **17**, 184–90.

Dickey, R. P., Ziter, F. A., and Smith, R. A. (1984). Emery-Dreifuss muscular dystrophy *J. Pediat.* **104**, 555–9.

DiMarco, A. F., Kelling, J. S., DiMarco, M. S., Jacobs, I., Shields, R., and Altose, M. D. (1985). The effects of inspiratory resistive training on respiratory muscle function in patients with muscular dystrophy. *Muscle and Nerve* **8**, 284–90.

DiMauro, S., Angelini, C., and Catani, C. (1967). Enzymes of the glycogen cycle and glycolysis in various human neuromuscular disorders. *J. Neurol. Neurosurg. Psychiat.* **30**. 411–5.

—— and Rowland, L. P. (1976). Urinary excretion of carnitine in Duchenne muscular dystrophy *Arch. Neurol.* **33**, 204–5.

Dominici, P., Bonfiglioli, S., Merlini, L., and Granata, C. (1984). Implicazioni cardiache nella sindrome di Emery–Dreifuss. *Cardiomyology* 3 (**No. 2–3**), 47–52.

Donner, M., Rapola, J., and Somer, H. (1975). Congenital muscular dystrophy: a clinico-pathological and follow-up study of 15 patients. *Neuropädiatrie* **6**, 239–58.

Drachman, D. B., Murphy, S. R., Nigam, M. P., and Hills, J. R. (1967). 'Myopathic' changes in chronically denervated muscle. *Arch. Neurol.* **16**, 14–24.

Dreifuss, F. E. and Hogan, G. R. (1961). Survival in X-chromosomal muscular dystrophy. *Neurology* **11**, 734–7.

Drennan, J. C. (1984). Surgical management of neuromuscular scoliosis. In *Neuromuscular diseases* (ed. G. Serratrice *et al.*) pp. 551–6. Raven Press, New York.

Dreyfus, J. C., Démos, J., Schapira, F., and Schapira, G. (1962). La lacticodéshydrogénase musculaire chez le myopathie: persistance apparente du type foetal. *Comp. Rend. Acad. Sci.* **254**, 4384–6.

—— Schapira, G., and Démos, J. (1960). Etude de la créatine-kinase sérique chez les myopathes et leurs familles. *Rev. Franç. Etudes Clin. et Biol.* **5**, 384–6.

——, Schapira, F., and Démos, J. (1956). Activités enzymatiques du muscle humain. Recherches sur la biochimie comparée de l'homme normal et myopathique et du rat. *Clin. Chim. Acta.* **1**, 434–49.

Drummond, L. M. (1979). Creatine phosphokinase levels in the newborn and their use in screening for Duchenne muscular dystrophy. *Arch. Dis. Child.* **54**, 362–6.

—— and Veale, A. M. O. (1978). Muscular dystrophy screening. *Lancet* **i**, 1258–9.

Du Bois, D. and Du Bois, E. F. (1916). A formula to estimate the approximate surface area if height and weight be known. *Arch. Intern. Med.* **17**, 863–71.

Dubowitz, V. (1960). Progressive muscular dystrophy of the Duchenne type in females and its mode of inheritance. *Brain* **83**, 432–9.

—— (1963a). Some clinical observations on childhood muscular dystrophy. *Brit. J. Clin. Pract.* **17**, 283–8.

—— (1963b) Myopathic changes in a muscular dystrophy carrier. *J. Neurol. Neurosurg. Psychiat.* **26**, 322–5.

—— (1965). Intellectual impairment in muscular dystrophy. *Arch. Dis. Child.* **40**, 296–301.

—— (1978). *Muscle disorders in childhood*. W. B. Saunders, London, Philadelphia, Toronto.

—— (1982). Carrier detection. In *Disorders of the motor unit* (ed. D. L. Schotland) pp. 858–9. John Wiley, Chichester, New York.

—— (1985). *Muscle biopsy – a practical approach*, 2nd edn. Baillière Tindall, London.

—— (1987). *Muscle disorders in childhood*, 2nd edn. W. B. Saunders, London, Philadelphia, Toronto. In press.

—— and Crome, L. (1969). The central nervous system in Duchenne muscular dystrophy. *Brain* **92**, 805–8.

—— and Heckmatt, J. (1980). Management of muscular dystrophy – pharmacological and physical aspects. *Brit. Med. Bull.* **36**, 139–44.

——, Hyde, S. A., Scott, O. M., and Goddard, C. (1984). Controlled trial of exercise in Duchenne muscular dystrophy. In *Neuromuscular diseases* (ed. G. Serratrice *et al.*) pp. 571–5. Raven Press, New York.

Duchenne, G. B. A. (1861). *De l'electrisation localisée et son application à la pathologie et à la thérapeutique*, 2nd edn. Baillière et fils, Paris.

—— (1868). Recherches sur la paralysie musculaire pseudohypertrophique ou paralysie myo-sclérosique. *Arch. Gén. Méd.* **11**, 5–25; 179–209; 305–21; 421–43; 552–88.

Dudley, M. and Gibson, W. C. (1964). Photomicrographic study on the capillary nail beds of muscular dystrophy patients. *Canad. Med. Ass. J.* **90**, 1226–8.

Duncan, C. J. (1978). Role of intracellular calcium in promoting muscle damage: a strategy for controlling the dystrophic condition. *Experientia* **34**, 1531–5.

Dunger, D. B., Davies, K. E., Pembrey, M., Lake, B., Pearson, P., Williams, D., Whitfield, A., and Dillon, M. J. D. (1986). Deletion on the X chromosome detected by direct DNA analysis in one of two unrelated boys with glycerol kinase deficiency, adrenal hypoplasia, and Duchenne muscular dystrophy. *Lancet* **i**, 585–7.

Durnin, R. E., Ziska, J. H., and Zellweger, H. (1971). Observations on the electrocardiogram in Duchenne's progressive muscular dystrophy. *Helvetica Paed. Acta* **26**, 331–9.

EAMDA. Registration of patients with neuromuscular diseases in Europe. In *Research into the origin and treatment of muscular dystrophy* (ed. L. P. ten Kate, P. L. Pearson, and A. M. Stadhouders) pp. 82–7. Excerpta Medica, Amsterdam.

Ebashi, S., Toyokura, Y., Momoi, H., and Sugita, H. (1959). High creatine phosphokinase activity of sera of progressive muscular dystrophy. *J. Biochem., Tokyo* **46**, 103–4.

Edwards, R. H. T. (1977). Energy metabolism in normal and dystrophic human muscle. In *Pathogenesis of human muscular dystrophies* (ed. L. P. Rowland) pp. 415–428. Excerpta Medica, Amsterdam, Oxford.

—— and McDonnell, M. (1974). Hand–held dynamometer for evaluating voluntary–muscle function. *Lancet* **ii**, 757–8.

—— Young, A., and Wiles, M. (1980). Needle biopsy of skeletal muscle in the diagnosis of myopathy and the clinical study of muscle function and repair. *New Engl. J. Med.* **302**, 261–71.

Edwards, R. J., Watts, D. C., Watts, R. L., and Rodeck, C. H. (1984). Creatine kinase estimation in pure fetal blood samples for the prenatal diagnosis of Duchenne muscular dystrophy *Prenatal Diag.* **4**, 267–77.

Ellis, D. A. (1978). Changes in muscle enzymes in Duchenne dystrophy and their possible relations to functional disturbance. In *The biochemistry of myasthenia gravis and muscular dystrophy* (ed. G. G. Lunt and R. M. Marchbanks) pp. 245–65. Academic Press, London.

—— (1980). Intermediary metabolism of muscle in Duchenne muscular dystrophy. *Brit. Med. Bull.* **36**, 165–71.

Ellis, F. R. (1981). Muscle disease. In *Inherited disease and anaesthesia* (ed. F. R. Ellis) pp. 315–36. Elsevier, North-Holland, Amsterdam.

—— (1985). Personal communication.

—— and Heffron, J. J. A. (1985). Clinical and biochemical aspects of malignant hyperpyrexia. In *Recent advances in anaesthesia and analgesia* (ed. R. S. Atkinson and A. P. Adams) pp. 173–207. Churchill Livingstone, Edinburgh.

Emanuel, B. S., Zackai, E. H., and Tucker, S. H. (1983). Further evidence for Xp21 location of Duchenne muscular dystrophy (DMD) locus: X; 9 translocation in a female with DMD. *J. Med. Genet.* **20**, 461–3.

Emery, A. E. H. (1963). Clinical manifestations in two carriers of Duchene muscular dystrophy. *Lancet* **i**, 1126–8.

—— (1964a). Hereditary myopathies. *Clin. Orthop.* **33**, 164–73.

—— (1964b). Electrophoretic pattern of lactic dehydrogenase in carriers and patients with Duchenne muscular dystrophy. *Nature* **201**, 1044–5.

—— (1965a). Carrier detection in sex-linked muscular dystrophy. *J. Génét. Hum.* **14**, 318–29.

—— (1965b). Muscle histology in carriers of Duchenne muscular dystrophy. *J. Med. Genet.* **2**, 1–7.

—— (1966). Genetic linkage between the loci for colour blindness and Duchenne type muscular dystrophy. *J. Med. Genet.* **3**, 92–5.

—— (1967a). The determination of lactate dehydrogenase isoenzymes in normal human muscle and other tissues. *Biochem. J.* **105**, 599–604.

—— (1967b). The use of serum creatine kinase for detecting carriers of Duchenne muscular dystrophy. In *Exploratory concepts in muscular dystrophy and related disorders* (ed. A. T. Milhorat) pp. 90–7. Excerpta Medica, Amsterdam.

—— (1968). Muscle lactate dehydrogenase isoenzymes in hereditary myopathies. *J. Neurol. Sci.* **7**, 137–48.

—— (1969a) Abnormalities of the electrocardiogram in female carriers of Duchenne muscular dystrophy. *Brit. Med. J.* **2**, 418–20.

—— (1969b). Genetic counselling in X-linked muscular dystrophy. *J. Neurol. Sci.* **8**, 579–87.

—— (1971). The nosology of the spinal muscular atrophies. *J. Med. Genet.* **8**, 481–95.

—— (1972). Abnormalities of the electrocardiogram in hereditary myopathies. *J. Med. Genet.* **9**, 8–12.

—— (1977a). Muscle histology and creatine kinase levels in the foetus in Duchenne muscular dystrophy. *Nature* **266**, 472–3.

—— (1977b). Genetic considerations in the X-linked muscular dystrophies. In *Pathogenesis of human muscular dystrphies* (ed. L. P. Rowland) pp. 42–52. Excerpta Medica, Amsterdam.

—— (1980). Duchenne muscular dystrophy. Genetic aspects, carrier detection and antenatal diagnosis. *Brit. Med. Bull.* **36**, 117–22.

—— (1982). Prevention of Duchenne muscular dystrophy: genetic counselling and prenatal diagnosis. In *New approaches to nerve and muscle disorders: basic and applied contributions* (ed. A. D. Kidman, J. K. Tomkins, and R. A. Westerman) pp. 332–41. Excerpta Medica, Amsterdam.

—— (1983). The muscular dystrophies. In *Principles and practice of medical genetics* (ed. A. E. H. Emery and D. Rimoin) Vol. 1, pp. 392–413. Churchill Livingstone, Edinburgh, London, New York.

—— (1984). Genetic heterogeneity in Duchenne muscular dystrophy. *J. Med. Genet.* **21**, 76–7.

—— (1985). *An introduction to recombinant DNA.* John Wiley, Chichester.

—— (1986). *Methodology in medical genetics – an introduction to statistical methods,* 2nd edn. Churchill Livingstone, Edinburgh.

—— (1987). Genetic aspects of neuromuscular disease In *Disorders of voluntary muscle,* 5th edn (ed. J. N. Walton). Churchill Livingstone, Edinburgh. (In press)

——, Anderson, A. R., and Noronha, M. J. (1973a). Electromyographic studies in parents of children with spinal muscular atrophy. *J. Med. Genet.* **10**, 8–10.

—— Brough, C., Crawfurd, M. D'A., Harper, P., Harris, R., and Oakshott, G. (1978). A report on genetic registers. *J. Med. Genet.* **15**, 435–42.

—— and Burt, D. (1980). Intracellular calcium and pathogenesis and antenatal diagnosis of Duchenne muscular dystrophy. *Brit. Med. J.* **280**, 355-7.

——, Dubowitz, V., Rocker, I., Donnai, D., Harris, R., and Donnai P. (1979a). Antenatal diagnosis of Duchenne muscular dystrophy. *Lancet* **i**, 847-9.

—— Davie, A. M., Holloway, S., and Skinner, R. (1976b). International collaborrative study of the spinal muscular atrophies. Part 2. Analysis of genetic data. *J. Neurol. Sci.* **30**, 375-84.

—— and Dreifuss, F. E. (1966). Unusual type of benign X-linked muscular dystrophy. *J. Neurol. Neurosurg. Psychiat.* **29**, 338-42.

——, Elliott, D., Moores, M., and Smith, C. (1974). A genetic register system (RAPID). *J. Med. Genet.* **11**, 145-51.

——, Hausmanowa-Petrusewicz, I., Davie, A. M., Holloway, S., Skinner, R., and Borkowska, J. (1976a). International collaborative study of the spinal muscular atrophies. Part 1. Analysis of clinical and laboratory data. *J. Neurol. Sci.* **29**, 83-94.

—— and Holloway, S. (1977). Use of normal daughters' and sisters' creatine kinase levels in estimating heterozygosity in Duchenne muscular dystrophy. *Hum. Hered.* **27**, 118-26.

—— (1982). Familial motor neuron diseases. In *Human motor neuron diseases* (ed. L. P. Rowland) pp. 139-45. Raven Press, New York.

—— and King, B. (1971). Pregnancy and serum creatine kinase levels in potential carriers of Duchenne X-linked muscular dystrophy. *Lancet* **i**, 1013.

——, King, B., and Brock, D. J. H. (1971). Leucocyte metabolism in hereditary neuromuscular disorders. *J. Neurol. Sci.* **14**, 463-8.

—— and McGregor, L. (1977). The foetus in Duchenne muscular dystrophy: muscle growth in tissue culture. *Clin. Genet.* **12**, 183-7.

—— and Miller, J. R. (eds) (1976). *Registers for the detection and prevention of genetic disease* Symposia Specialists, Miami, Fla., and Stratton Intercontinental, New York.

—— and Morton, R. (1968). Genetic counselling in lethal X-linked disorders. *Acta Genet., Basel* **18**, 534-42.

—— and Pascasio, F. M. (1965). The effects of pregnancy on the concentration of creatine kinase in serum, skeletal muscle, and myometrium. *Amer. J. Obstet. Gynec.* **91**, 18-22.

——, Raeburn, J. A., Skinner, R., Holloway, S., and Lewis, P. (1979c). Prospective study of genetic counselling. *Brit. Med. J.* **1**, 1253-6.

—— and Schelling, J. L. (1965). Limb blood flow in patients and carriers of Duchenne muscular dystrophy. *Acta Genet., Basel* **15**, 337-44.

—— and Skinner, R. (1976). Clinical studies in benign (Becker type) X-linked muscular dystrophy. *Clin. Genet.* **10**, 189-201.

—— and Skinner, R. (1983). Double-blind controlled trial of a 'calcium blocker' in Duchenne muscular dystrophy. *Cardiomyology* **2**, 13-23.

——, Skinner, R. and Holloway, S. (1979b). A study of possible heterogeneity in Duchenne muscular dystrophy. *Clin. Genet.* **15**, 444-9.

——, Skinner, R. Howden, L. C., and Matthews, M. B. (1982). Verapamil in Duchenne muscular dystrophy. *Lancet* **i**, 559.

—— and Smith, C. (1970). Ascertainment and prevention of genetic disease. *Brit. Med. J.* **3**, 636-7.

—— and Spikesman, A. M. (1970a). The existence of a subclinical form of Duchenne muscular dystrophy? In *Muscle diseases* (ed. J. N. Walton, N. Canal, and G. Scarlato) pp. 424–30. Excerpta Medica, Amsterdam.

—— (1970b). Evidence against the existence of a subclinical form of X-linked Duchenne muscular dystrophy. *J. Neurol. Sci.* **10**, 523–33.

——, Teasdall, R. D., and Coomes, E. N. (1966). Electromyographic studies in carriers of Duchenne muscular dystrophy. *Bull. Johns Hopkins Hosp.* **118**, 439–43.

—— and Walton, J. N. (1967). The genetics of muscular dystrophy. *Prog. Med. Genet.* **5**, 116–45.

——, Watt, M. S., and Clack, E. R. (1972). The effects of genetic counselling in Duchenne muscular dystrophy. *Clin. Genet.* **3**, 147–50.

——, Watt, M. S., and Clack, E. (1973b). Social effects of genetic counselling. *Brit. Med. J.* **1**, 724–6.

Engel, A. G., Arahata, K., and Biesecker, G. (1984). Mechanisms of muscle fiber destruction. In *Neuromuscular diseases* (ed. G. Serratrice *et al.*) pp. 137–41. Raven Press, New York.

—— and Banker, B. Q. (1986). *Myology* (2 vols). McGraw-Hill, New York.

—— and Biesecker, G. (1982). Complement activation in muscle fiber necrosis: demonstration of the membrane attack complex of complement in necrotic fibers. *Ann. Neurol.* **12**, 289–96.

Engel, W. K. (1970). Selective and nonselective susceptibility of muscle fibre types. A new approach to human neuromuscular diseases. *Arch. Neurol.* **22**, 97–117.

—— (1975). The vascular hypothesis. In *Recent advances in myology* (ed. W. G. Bradley, D. Gardner-Medwin, and J. N. Walton) pp. 166–73. Excerpta Medica, Amsterdam.

—— (1977). Integrative histochemical approach to the defect of Duchenne muscular dystrophy. In *Pathogenesis of human muscular dystrophies* (ed. L. P. Rowland) pp. 277–309. Excerpta Medica, Amsterdam, Oxford.

Ennor, A. H. and Rosenberg, H. (1954). Some properties of creatine phosphokinase. *Biochem. J.* **57**, 203–12.

Erb, W. H. (1884). Über die 'juvenile Form' der progressiven Muskelatrophie und ihre Beziehungen zur sogenannten Pseudohypertrophie der Muskeln. *Deutsch. Arch. Klin. Med.* **34**, 467–519.

—— (1891). Dystrophia muscularis progressiva - Klinische und pathologisch-anatomische Studien. *Deutsch. Zeit. Nervenheilk.* **1**, 13–261.

van Essen, A. J. and ten Kate, L. P. (1984). Epidemiologic survey of Duchenne muscular dystrophy in the Netherlands. Preliminary results. In *Research into the origin and treatment of muscular dystrophy* (ed. L. P. ten Kate, P.L. Pearson, and A. M. Stadhouders) pp. 33–40. Excerpta Medica, Amsterdam.

Etiemble, J., Kahn, A., Boivin, P., Bernard, J. F., and Goudemand, M. (1976). Hereditary haemolytic anemia with erythrocyte phosphofructokinase deficiency. Studies of some properties of erythrocytes and muscle enzyme. *Hum. Genet.* **31**, 83–91.

Evans, C. D. H. and Lacey, J. H. (1986). Toxicity of vitamins: Complications of a health movement. *Brit. Med. J.* **292**, 509–10.

Fadda, S., Mochi, M., Roncuzzi, L., Sangiorgi, S., Sbarra, D., Zatz, M., and Romeo, G. (1985). Definitive localization of Becker muscular dystrophy in Xp by linkage to a cluster of DNA polymorphisms (DXS43 and DXS9). *Hum. Genet.* **71**, 33–6.

Falcão-Conceição, D. N., Gonçalves-Pimentel, M. M., Baptista, M. L., and Ubatuba, S. (1983a). Detection of carriers of X-linked gene for Duchenne muscular dystrophy by levels of creatine kinase and pyruvate kinase. *J. Neurol. Sci.* **62**, 171–80.

——, Pereira, M. C. G., Gonçalves, M. M., and Baptista, M. L. (1983b). Familial occurence of heterozygous manifestations in X-linked muscular dystrophies. *Brazil J. Genetics* **6**, 527–38.

Falek, A. (1977). Use of the coping process to achieve psychological homeostasis in genetic counseling. In *Genetic counseling* (ed. H. A. Lubs and F. de la Cruz) pp. 179–88. Raven Press, New York.

—— (1984). Sequential aspects of coping and other issues in decision making in genetic counseling. In *Psychological aspects genetic counselling* (ed. A. E. H. Emery and I. M. Pullen) pp. 23–36. Academic Press, London, New York.

Falewski de Leon, G. H. (1984). Orthotic jackets for scoliosis. In *Neuromuscular diseases* (ed. G. Serratrice *et al.*) pp. 539–43. Raven Press, New York.

Feiling, A. (1958). *A history of the Maida Vale Hospital for nervous diseases* Butterworths, London.

Feingold, J., Feingold, N., and Démos, J. (1971). Gènes majeurs, gènes modificateurs et effets du milieu dans la myopathie de Duchenne de Boulogne. *Ann. Génét.* **14**, 207–11.

Fenichel, G. M., Sul, Y. C., Kilroy, A. W., and Blouin, R. (1982). An autosomal-dominant dystrophy with humeropelvic distribution and cardiomyopathy. *Neurology* **32**, 1399–1401.

Ferrari, E., Intino, M. T., Perniola, T., and Russo, M. G. (1980). Epidemiology of Duchenne dystrophy and carrier detection in Puglia. Preliminary reports. In *Muscular dystrophy research: advances and new trends* (ed. C. Angelini, G. A. Danieli, and D. Fontanari) pp. 264–5. Excerpta Medica, Amsterdam.

Ferrier, P., Bamatter, F., and Klein, D. (1965). Muscular dystrophy (Duchenne) in a girl with Turner's syndrome. *J. Med. Genet.* **2**, 38–46.

Fiacchino, F., Bricchi, M., Balestrini, M. R., Ferrazza, C., Montolivo, M., Daniel, S., Morandi, L., and Ariano, C. (1984). La rabdomiolisi anestesiologica nella distrofia muscolare. Segnalazione di un caso. *Minerva Anestesiol.* **50**, 521–6.

Fidziańska, A., Goebel, H. H., Kosswig, R., and Burck, U. (1984). 'Killer' cells in Duchenne disease: Ultrastructural study. *Neurology* **34**, 295–303.

Filippi, G. and Macciotta, A. (1967). Xg blood groups in muscular dystrophy. *Lancet* **ii**, 565.

Fingerman, E., Campisi, J., and Pardee, A. B. (1984). Defective Ca^{2+} metabolism in Duchenne muscular dystrophy: effects on cellular and viral growth. *Proc. Natl. Acad. Sci. (USA)* **81**, 7617–21.

Firth, M. A. (1983). Diagnosis of Duchenne muscular dystrophy: experiences of parents and sufferers. *Brit. Med. J.* **286**, 700–1.

—— and Wilkinson, E. J. (1983). Screening the newborn for Duchenne muscular dystrophy: parents' views. *Brit. Med. J.* **286**, 1933–4.

Fischbeck, K. H., Ritter, A. W., Tirschwell, D. L., Kunkel, L. M. *et al.* (1986). Recombination with PERT 87 (DXS 164) in families with X-linked muscular dystrophy. *Lancet* **ii**, 104.

Fisher, E. R., Wissinger, A., Gerneth, J. A., and Danowski, T. S. (1972). Ultrastructural changes in skeletal muscle of muscular dystrophy carriers. *Arch. Path.* **94**, 456–60.

Fisher, R. A. and Yates, F. (1967). *Statistical tables for biological, agricultural and medical research*, 6th edn. Oliver and Boyd, Edinburgh.

Fitch, C. D. (1977). Significance of abnormalities of creatine metabolism. In *Pathogenesis of human muscular dystrophies* (ed. L. P. Rowland) pp. 328–36. Excerpta Medica, Amsterdam, Oxford.

Fitzpatrick, C., and Barry, C. (1986). Communication within families about Duchenne muscular dystrophy. *Develop. Med. Child. Neurol.* **28**, 596–9.

—— ——, Garvey, C. (1986). Psychiatric disorder among boys with Duchenne muscular dystrophy. *Develop. Med. Child. Neurol.* **28**, 589–95.

Fitzsimons, R. B. and Hoh, J. F. Y. (1981). Embryonic and foetal myosins in human skeletal muscle. The presence of foetal myosins in Duchenne muscular dystrophy and infantile spinal muscular atrophy. *J. Neurol. Sci.* **52**, 367–84.

Florek, M. and Karolak, S. (1977). Intelligence level of patients with the Duchenne type of progressive muscular dystrophy (PMD-D). *Europ. J. Pediat.* **126**, 275–82.

Fowler, W. M. and Nayak, N. N. (1983). Slowly progressive proximal weakness: limb-girdle syndromes. *Arch. Phys. Med. Rehab.* **64**, 527–38.

——, Pearson, C. M., Egstrom, G. H., and Gardner, G. W. (1965). Ineffective treatment of muscular dystrophy with an anabolic steroid and other measures. *New. Engl. J. Med.* **272**, 875–82.

Francke, U., Ochs, H. D., de Martinville, B., Giacalone, J., Lindgren, V., Distèche, C., Pagon, R. A., Hofker, M. H., van Ommen, G. J. B., Pearson, P. L., and Wedgwood, R. J. (1985). Minor Xp21 chromosome deletion in a male associated with expression of Duchenne muscular dystrophy, chronic granulomatous disease, retinitis pigmentosa and McLeod syndrome. *Amer. J. Hum. Genet.* **37**, 250–67.

Frankel, K. A., and Rosser, R. J. (1976). The pathology of the heart in progressive muscular dystrophy: epimyocardial fibrosis. *Human Pathol.* **7**, 375–86.

Franklin, G. I., Cavanagh, N. P. C., Hughes, B. P., Yasin, R., and Thompson, E. J. (1981). Creatine kinase isoenzymes in altered human muscle cells. I. Comparison of Duchenne muscular dystrophy with other myopathic and neurogenic diseases. *Clin. Chim. Acta* **115**, 179–89.

Fraser, F. C. (1963). Taking the family history. *Amer. J. Med.* **34**, 585–93.

Freeman, R. D. and Pearson, P. H. (1978). Counselling with parents. In *Care of the handicapped child* (Clinics in Developmental Medicine, No. 67), (ed. J. Apley) pp. 35–47. Wm. Heinemann, London.

Frostick, S. P. (1986). Personal communication.

Frouhar, Z. R., Spiro, R., and Lubs, M. L. (1975). Familial carrier manifestations in families with X-linked Duchenne muscular dystrophy. *Amer. J. Hum. Genet.* **27**, 37A (Abstract).

Fukuyama, Y., Kawazura, M., and Haruna, H. (1960). A peculiar form of congenital progressive muscular dystrophy: report of 15 cases. *Paediatria, Tokyo* **4**, 5–8.

Furukawa, T. and Peter, J. B. (1977). X-linked muscular dystrophy. *Ann. Neurol.* **2**, 414–6.

Furukawa, T. and Toyokura, Y. (1977). Congenital, hypotonic-sclerotic muscular dystrophy *J. Med. Genet.* **14**, 426–9.

Gaines, R. F., Pueschel, S. M., Sassaman, E. A., and Driscoll, J. L. (1982). Effect of exercise on serum creatine kinase in carriers of Duchenne muscular dystrophy. *J. Med. Genet.* **19**, 4–7.

Gale, A. N. and Murphy, E. A. (1979). The use of serum creatine phosphokinase in genetic counselling for Duchenne muscular dystrophy. *J. Chron. Dis.* **32**, 639–51.

Gardner-Medwin, D. (1970). Mutation rate in Duchenne type of muscular dystrophy. *J. Med. Genet.* **7**, 334–7.

—— (1975). The effects of genetic counselling in Duchenne muscular dystrophy. In *Recent advances in myology* (ed. W. G. Bradley, D. Gardner-Medwin, and J. N. Walton) pp. 474–6. Exerpta Medica, Amsterdam.

—— (1977). Children with genetic muscular disorders. *Brit. J. Hosp. Med.* (April) 314–40.

—— (1982a). The natural history of Duchenne muscular dystrophy. In *Topics in child neurology* (ed. G. B. Wise, M. E. Blaw, and P. G. Procopis) Vol. 2, pp. 17–29. S. P. Medical and Scientific Books, Spectrum Publications, New York, London.

—— (1982b). Uncertainties in the diagnosis of Duchenne muscular dystrophy. *Cardiomyology* **1**, 15–20.

—— (1984). *Children with neuromuscular disease – a layman's guide to the neuromuscular diseases and their management.* Muscular Dystrophy Group of Great Britain and Northern Ireland, London.

——, Bundey, S., and Greer, S. (1978). Early diagnosis of Duchenne muscular dystrophy. *Lancet* i, 1102.

——, Hudgson, P., and Walton, J. N. (1967). Benign spinal muscular atrophy arising in childhood and adolescence. *J. Neurol. Sci.* **5**, 121–58.

—— and Johnston, H. M. (1984). Severe muscular dystrophy in girls. *J. Neurol. Sci.* **64**, 79–87.

Gerald, P. S. and Brown, J. A. (1974). Report of the Committee on the genetic constitution of the X chromosome. *Birth Defects Orig. Ser.* **10**, 29–34.

Gilgenkrantz, S., Tridon, P., Pinel-Briquel, N., Beurey, J., and Weber, M. (1985). Translocation (X; 9) (p11; q34) in a girl with incontinentia pigmenti (IP): implications for the regional assignment of the IP locus to Xp11. *Ann. Génét.* **28**, 90–2.

Gilliatt, R. W. (1962). Electrodiagnosis and electromyography in clinical practice. *Brit. Med. J.* **2**, 1073–9.

Gilroy, J., Cahalan, J. L., Berman, R., and Newman, M. (1963). Cardiac and pulmonary complications in Duchenne's progressive muscular dystrophy. *Circulation* **27**, 484–93.

Golbus, M. S., Conte, F., Schneider, E., and Epstein, C. (1974). Intrauterine diagnosis of genetic defects: results, problems and follow-up of one hundred cases in a prenatal genetic detection center. *Amer. J. Obstet. Gynec.* **118**, 897–905.

——, Stephens, J. D., Mahoney, M. J., Hobbins J. C., Haseltine, F. P., Caskey, C. T., and Banker, B. Q. (1979). Failure of fetal creatine phosphokinase as a diagnostic indicator of Duchenne muscular dystrophy. *New Engl. J. Med.* **300**, 860–1.

Goldberg, S. J., Stern, L. Z., Feldman, L., Allen, H. D., Sahn, D. J., and Valdes-Cruz, L. M. (1982). Serial two-dimensional echocardiography in Duchenne muscular dystrophy. *Neurology* **32**, 1101–5.

Gomard, E., Begue, B., Sodoyer, S., Maryanski, J. L., Jordan, B. R., and Levy, J. P. (1986). Murine cells expressing an HLA molecule are specifically lysed by HLA-restricted antiviral human T cells. *Nature* **319**, 153–4.

Gomez, M. R., Engel, A. G., Dewald, G., and Peterson, H. A. (1977). Failure of inactivation of Duchenne dystrophy X-chromosome in one of female identical twins. *Neurology* **27**, 537–41.

Gordon-Taylor, G. and Walls, E. W. (1958). *Sir Charles Bell: his life and times.* E. & S. Livingstone, Edinburgh, London.

Gowers, W. R. (1879a). Clinical lecture on pseudo-hypertrophic muscular paralysis. *Lancet* 2, 1-2; 37-9; 73-5; 113-6.

—— (1879b). *Pseudo-hypertrophic muscular paralysis – a clinical lecture* J. and A. Churchill, London.

Granata, C., Merlini, L., Rubbini, L., Bonfiglioli, S., and Mattutini, P. (1984). Tenotomia sottocutanea del tendine di Achille in anestesia locale, nella distrofia musolare di Duchenne. *Cardiomyology* 3 (No. 2-3), 89-96.

Greenstein, R. M., Reardon, M. P., and Chan, T. S. (1977). An X/autosome translocation in a girl with Duchenne muscular dystrophy (DMD): evidence for DMD gene localization. *Pediatr. Res.* 11, 457 (Abstract).

——, Middleton, A. B., Mulivor, R. A., Greene, A. E., and Coriell, L. L. (1980). An (X; 11) translocation in a girl with Duchenne muscular dystrophy. *Cytogenet. Cell Genet.* 27, 268.

Greig, D. N. H. (1977). Family in which Duchenne's muscular dystrophy and protan colour blindness are segregating. *J. Med. Genet.* 14, 130-2.

Griffiths, R. D., Cady, E. B., Edwards, R. H. T., and Wilkie, D. R. (1985). Muscle energy metabolism in Duchenne dystrophy studied by ^{31}P-NMR: controlled trials show no effect of allopurinol or ribose. *Muscle and Nerve* 8, 760-7.

Griggs, R., Mendell, J., Fenichel, G., Brooke, M. *et al.* (1986). Genetic heterogeneity in Duchenne dystrophy. *Muscle and Nerve* 9 (suppl.) p. 227 (Abstract).

Grimm, T. (1981). Neugeborenen-Screening nach Duchennescher Muskeldystrophie. *Monatsschr. Kinderheilkd.* 129, 414-7.

de Grouchy, J., Lamy, M., Frézal, J., and Garcin, R. (1963). Étude d'un couple de jumeaux monozygotes dont un seul est atteint de myopathie (Forme pseudo-hypertrophique). *Acta Genet. Med., Roma* 12, 324-34.

Guggenheim, M. A., McCabe, E. R. B., Roig, M., Goodman, S. I., Lum, G. M., Bullen, W. W., and Ringel, S. P. (1980). Glycerol kinase deficiency with neuromuscular, skeletal, and adrenal abnormalities. *Ann. Neurol.* 7, 441-9.

Guibaud, P., Carrier, H. N., Plauchu, H., Lauras, B., Jolivet, M. J., and Robert, J. M. (1981). Manifestations musculaires précoces cliniques et histopathologiques, chez 14 garçons présentant dans la première année une activité sérique elevée de creatine-phosphokinase. *J. Génét. Hum.* 29, 71-84.

Guilly, P. (1936). *Duchenne de Boulogne.* J. B. Bailliere et fils, Paris.

Haldane, J. B. S. (1935). The rate of spontaneous mutation of a human gene. *J. Genet.* 31, 317-26.

—— (1956). Mutation in the sex-linked recessive type of muscular dystrophy. A possible sex difference. *Ann. Hum. Genet., London* 22, 344-7.

Hammond, J., Howard, N. J., Brookwell, R., Purvis-Smith, S., Wilcken, B., Hoogenraad, N. (1985). Proposed assignment of loci for X-linked adrenal hypoplasia and glycerol kinase genes. *Lancet* i, 54.

Harper, P. S. (1982). Carrier detection in Duchenne muscular dystrophy: a critical assessment. In *Disorders of the motor unit* (ed. D. L. Schotland) pp. 821-44. John Wiley, Chichester, New York.

——, O'Brien, T., Murray, J. M., Davies, K. E., Pearson, P., and Williamson, R. (1983). The use of linked DNA polymorphisms for genotype prediction in families with Duchenne muscular dystrophy. *J. Med. Genet.* 20, 252-4.

Harris, J. B. (ed.) (1979). *Muscular dystrophy and other inherited diseases of skeletal muscle in animals. Ann. N. Y. Acad. Sci.* Vol. 317. Academy of Sciences, New York.

—— and Slater, C. R. (1980). Animal models: what is their relevance to the pathogenesis of human muscular dystrophy? *Brit. Med. Bull.* **36**, 193–7.

Hastings, B. A., Groothuis, D. R., and Vick, N. A. (1980). Dominantly inherited pseudohypertrophic muscular dystrophy with internalized capillaries. *Arch. Neurol.* **37**, 709–14.

Hauschka, S. D. (1982). Muscle cell culture: future goals for facilitating the investigation of human muscle disease. In *Disorders of the motor unit* (ed. D. L. Schotland) pp. 925–36. John Wiley, Chichester, New York.

Hausmanowa-Petrusewicz, I., Askanas, W., Badurska, B., Emeryk, B., Fidzianska, A., Garbalinska, W., Hetnarska, L., Jedrzejowska, H., Kamieniecka, Z., Niebrój-Dobosz, I., Prot, J., and Sawicka, E. (1968a). Infantile and juvenile spinal muscular atrophy. *J. Neurol. Sci.* **6**, 269–87.

—— and Borkowska, J. (1978). Intrafamilial variability of X-linked progressive muscular dystrophy. Mild and acute form of X-linked muscular dystrophy in the same family. *J. Neurol.* **218**, 43–50.

——, Prot, J., Niebrój-Dobosz, I., Hetnarska, L., Emeryk, B., Wasowicz, B., Askanas, W., and Slucka, C. (1968b). Studies of healthy relatives of patients with Duchenne muscular dystrophy. *J. Neurol. Sci.* **7**, 465–80.

——, Spiegler, A., and Borkowska, J. (1986). Atypical and typical cases of X-linked dystrophy. (In press)

——, Wierzbicka, M., Jozwik, A., Szmidt-Salkowska, E., and Borkowska, J. (1982). A nearest neighbour decision rule for EMG detection of carriers of Duchenne muscular dystrophy. *Electromyogr. Clin. Neurophysiol.* **22**, 445–57.

——, Zaremba, J., Borkowska, J., and Szirkowiec, W. (1984). Chronic proximal spinal muscular atrophy of childhood and adolescence: sex influence. *J. Med. Genet.* **21**, 447–50.

Haymond, M. W., Strobel, K. E., and DeVivo, D. C (1978). Muscle wasting and carbohydrate homeostasis in Duchenne muscular dystrophy. *Neurology* **28**, 1224–31.

Hazama, R., Tsujihata, M., Mori, M., and Mori, K. (1979). Muscular dystrophy in six young girls. *Neurology* **29**, 1486–91.

Heckmatt, J. Z. and Dubowitz, V. (1983a). Congenital myopathies. In *Principles and practice of medical genetics* (ed. A. E. H. Emery and D. Rimoin) Vol. 1, pp. 367–91. Churchill Livingstone, Edinburgh.

—— (1983b). Detecting the Duchenne carrier by ultrasound and computerized tomography. *Lancet* **ii**, 1364.

——, Hyde, S. A., Florence, J., Gabain, A. C., and Thompson, N. (1985). Prolongation of walking in Duchenne muscular dystrophy with lightweight orthoses: review of 57 cases. *Develop. Med. Child. Neurol.* **27**, 149–54.

——, Leeman, S., and Dubowitz, V. (1982). Ultrasound imaging in the diagnosis of muscle disease. *J. Pediat.* **101**, 656–60.

Held, F. W., Groothuis, D. R., Salafsky, I. S., and Vick, N. A. (1980). Autosomal recessive pseudohypertrophic muscular dystrophy: a Duchenne phenocopy. *Neurology* **30**, 402 (Abstract).

Henson, T. E., Muller, J., and DeMyer, W. E. (1967). Hereditary myopathy limited to females. *Arch. Neurol.* **17**, 238–47.

Herrmann, F. H. and Spiegler, A. W. J. (1985). *X-linked muscular dystrophies – a bibliography.* University Press, Leipzig.

——, Spiegler, A., and Wiedemann, G. (1982). Muscle provocation test. A sensitive method for discrimination between carriers and non-carriers of Duchenne muscular dystrophy. *Hum. Genet.* **61**, 102–4.

Herva, R., Kaluzewski, B., and de la Chapelle, A. (1979). Inherited interstitial del. (Xp) with minimal clinical consequences: with a note on the location of genes controlling phenotypic features. *Amer. J. Med. Genet.* **3**, 43–58.

Heyck, H. and Laudahn, G. (1969). *Die progressiv-dystrophischen Myopathien.* Springer-Verlag, Berlin.

—— and Lüders, C. J. (1963). Fermentaktivitätsbestimmungen in der gesunden menschlichen Muskulatur und bei Myopathien. II. Enzymaktivitätsveränderungen im Muskel bei Dystrophia musculorum progressiva. *Klin. Woch.* **41**, 500–9.

Hillier, J., Jones, G. E., Statham, H. E., Witkowski, J. A., and Dubowitz, V. (1985). Cell surface abnormality in clones of skin fibroblasts from a carrier of Duchenne muscular dystrophy. *J. Med. Genet.* **22**, 100–3.

Hirano, K., Sakamoto, Y., and Itagaki, Y. (1983). The disability state and urinary excretion of dimethylarginine, glycine and creatine in Duchenne and non-Duchenne muscular dystrophy. *Brain and Develop.* **5**, 242.

Hirsch-Kauffmann, M., Valet, G., Wieser, J., and Schweiger, M. (1985). Progressive muscular dystrophy(Duchenne): biochemical studies by flow-cytometry. *Hum. Genet.* **69**, 332–6.

Ho, A. D., Reitter, B., Stojakowits, S., Fiehn, W., and Weisser, J. (1980). Capping of lymphocytes for carrier detection in Duchenne muscular dystrophy: technical problems and a review of the literature. *Europ. J. Pediatr.* **134**, 211–6.

Hodgson, S. V., Boswinkel, E., Cole, C., Walker, A., Dubowitz, V., Granata, C., Merlini, L., and Bobrow, M. (1986b). A linkage study of Emery–Dreifuss muscular dystrophy. *Hum. Genet.* (In Press)

Hodgson, S. V., Heckmatt, J. Z., Hughes, E., Crolla, J., Dubowitz, V., and Bobrow, M. (1986a). A balanced *de novo* X/autosome translocation in a girl expressing many of the features of Lowe's syndrome. (In Press)

Hodson, A. and Pleasure, D. (1977). Erythrocyte cation-activated adenosine triphosphatases in Duchenne muscular dystrophy. *J. Neurol. Sci.* **32**, 361–9.

Hogge, W. A., Schonberg, S. A., and Golbus, M. S. (1985). Prenatal diagnosis by chorionic villus sampling: lessons of the first 600 cases. *Prenatal Diag.* **5**, 393–400.

Hohlfeld, R. and Toyka, K. V. (1985). Strategies for the modulation of neuro-immunological disease at the level of autoreactive T-lymphocytes. *J. Neuroimmunol.* **9**, 193–204.

Homburger, F., Baker, J. R., Nixon, C. W., and Wilgram, G. (1962). New hereditary disease of Syrian hamsters. Primary, generalized polymyopathy and cardiac necrosis. *Arch. Intern. Med.* **110**, 660–2.

Hopkins, L. C., Jackson, J. A., and Elsas, L. J. (1981). Emery-Dreifuss humeroperoneal muscular dystrophy: an X-linked myopathy with unusual contractures and bradycardia. *Ann. Neurol.* **10**, 230–7.

Horvath, B. and Proctor, J. B. (1960). Muscular dystrophy: quantitative studies on the composition of dystrophic muscle. *Res. Publ. Assoc. Res. Nerv. Ment. Dis.* **38**, 740–66.

Hovstad, L., Løchen, E. A., and Sjaastad, O. (1976). Pneumoencephalographic findings in various primary and secondary muscular disorders. *Acta Neurol. Scand.* **53**, 128–36.

Hsia, D. Y. Y. (1970). Use of white blood cells and cultured somatic cells in clinical genetic disorders. *Clin. Genet.* **1**, 5–14.

Hsia, Y. E. (1974). Choosing my children's genes: genetic counselling. In *Genetic responsibility: on choosing our children's genes* (ed. M. Lipkin and P. T. Rowley) pp. 43–59. Plenum Press, New York.

Hsu, J. D. (1976). Management of foot deformity in Duchenne's pseudohypertrophic muscular dystrophy. *Orthop. Clin. North Amer.* **7**, 979–84.

—— (1979). Extremity fractures in children with neuromuscular disease. *Johns Hopkins Med. J.* **145**, 89–93.

Hudgson, P., Gardner-Medwin, D., Pennington, R. J. T., and Walton, J. N. (1967b). Studies of the carrier state in the Duchenne type of muscular dystrophy. Part 1. Effect of exercise on serum creatine kinase activity. *J. Neurol. Neurosurg. Psychiat.* **30**, 416–9.

——, Mastaglia, F. L., and Cullen, M. J. (1987). Ultrastructural studies of neuromuscular muscle. In *Disorders of voluntary muscle*, 5th edn (ed. J. N. Walton). Churchill Livingstone, Edinburgh. (In Press)

——, Pearce, G. W., and Walton, J. N. (1967a). Preclinical muscular dystrophy: histopathological changes observed on muscle biopsy. *Brain* **90**, 565–76.

Hughes, B. P. (1972). Lipid changes in Duchenne muscular dystrophy. *J. Neurol. Neurosurg. Psychiat.* **35**, 658–63.

Hughes, J. T. (1974). *Pathology of muscle.* Lloyd-Luke, London.

Hunsaker, R. H., Fulkerson, P. K., Barry, F. J., Lewis, R. P., Leier, C. V., and Unverferth, D. V. (1982). Cardiac function in Duchenne's muscular dystrophy. Results of 10-year follow-up study and noninvasive tests. *Amer. J. Med.* **73**, 235–8.

Hunter, S. (1980). The heart in muscular dystrophy. *Brit. Med. Bull.* **36**, 133–4.

Hurse, P. V and Kakulas, B. A. (1974). Genetic counselling in neuromuscular diseases in Western Australia. *Proc. Austral. Assoc. Neurol.* **11**, 145–53.

Hutton, E. M. and Thompson, M. W. (1970). Parental age and mutation rate in Duchenne muscular dystrophy. *Amer. J. Hum. Genet.* **22**, 26A (Abstract).

—— (1976). Carrier detection and genetic counselling in Duchenne muscular dystrophy: a follow up study. *Canad. Med. Assoc. J.* **115**, 749–52.

Huvos, A. G. and Pruzanski, W. (1967). Smooth muscle involvement in primary muscle disease. II. Progressive muscular dystrophy. *Arch. Path.* **83**, 234–40.

Huxley, A. F. (1980). Future prospects. *Brit. Med. Bull.* **36**, 199–200.

Hyde. S. A. (1984). *The parents' guide to the physical management of Duchenne muscular dystrophy.* Muscular Dystrophy Group of Great Britain and Northern Ireland, London.

——, Scott, O. M., Goddard, C. M., and Dubowitz, V. (1982). Prolongation of ambulation in Duchenne muscular dystrophy by appropriate orthoses. *Physiotherapy* **68**, 105–8.

Inkley, S. R., Oldenburg, F. C., and Vignos, P. J. (1974). Pulmonary function in Duchenne muscular dystrophy related to stage of disease. *Amer. J. Med.* **56**, 297–306.

Inoue, R., Miyake, M., Kanazawa, A., Sato, M., and Kakimoto, Y. (1979). Decrease of 3-methylhistidine and increase of N^G, N^G-dimethylarginine in the urine of patients with muscular dystrophy. *Metabolism* **28**, 801–4.

Ionasescu, V., Burmeister, L., and Hanson, J. (1980). Discriminant analysis of ribosomal protein synthesis findings in carrier detection of Duchenne muscular dystrophy. *Amer. J. Med. Genet.* **5**, 5–12.

—— and Ionasescu, R. (1982). Increased collagen synthesis by Duchenne myogenic clones. *J. Neurol. Sci.* **54**, 79–87.

—— and Zellweger, H. (1974). Duchenne muscular dystrophy in young girls? *Acta Neurol. Scand.* **50**, 619–30.

——, and Cancilla, P. (1978). Fetal serum creatine phosphokinase not a valid predictor of Duchenne muscular dystrophy. *Lancet* **ii**, 1251.

——, Zellweger, H., Ionasescu, R., and Lara-Braud, C. (1977). Protein synthesis in human muscular dystrophies. In *Pathogenesis of human muscular dystrophies* (ed. L. P. Rowland) pp. 362–73. Excerpta Medica, Amsterdam, Oxford.

Ishikawa, K., Shirato, C., Yotsukura, M., Ishihara, T., Tamura, T., and Inoue, M. (1982). Sequential changes in high frequency notches on QRS complexes in progressive muscular dystrophy of the Duchenne type – a 3-year follow-up study. *J. Electrocardiol.* **15**, 23–30.

Jackson, C. E. and Strehler, D. A. (1968). Limb-girdle muscular dystrophy: clinical manifestations and detection of preclinical disease. *Pediatrics* **41**, 495–502.

Jackson, R. C., Taylor, B. D., Zellweger, H., and Bianchine, J. W. (1974). Muscular dystrophy: Duchenne type and Becker type within a kindred. *Amer. J. Hum. Genet.* **26**, 44A (Abstract).

Jacobs, P. A., Hunt, P. A., Mayer, M., and Bart, R. D. (1981). Duchenne muscular dystrophy (DMD) in a female with an X/autosome translocation: further evidence that the DMD locus is at Xp21. *Amer. J. Hum. Genet.* **33**, 513–8.

Jalbert, P., Mouriquand, C., Beaudoing, A., and Jaillard, M. (1966). Myopathie progressive de type Duchenne et mosaique XO/XX/XXX: consideration sur la genèse de la fibre musculaire striée. *Ann. Génét.* **9**, 104–8.

James, J. I. P., Zorab, P. A., and Wynne-Davies, R. (1976). *Scoliosis*, 2nd edn. Churchill Livingstone, Edinburgh.

Jedrzejowska-Kulakowska, H., Hausmanowa-Petrusewicz, I., Gawlik, Z., Rafalowska, J., and Slucka, C. (1968). Zweryfikowany sekcyjnie przypadek postępującej dystrofii mięśniowej typu Duchenne'a. *Neuropatologia Polska* **6**, 71–85.

Jellett, L. B., Kennedy, M. C., and Goldblatt, E. (1974). Duchenne pseudohypertrophic muscular dystrophy: a clinical and electrocardiographic study of patients and female carriers. *Aust. N.Z. J. Med.* **4**, 41–7.

Jerusalem, F., Engel, A. G., and Gomez, M. R. (1974). Duchenne dystrophy. I. Morphometric study of the muscle microvasculature. *Brain* **97**, 115–22.

Johnson, E. W., Reynolds, H. T., and Stauch, D. (1985). Duchenne muscular dystrophy: a case with prolonged survival. *Arch. Phys. Med. Rehab.* **66**, 260–1.

Johnson, M. A., Polgar, J., Weightman, D., and Appelton, D. (1973). Data on the distribution of fibre types in thirty-six human muscles – an autopsy study. *J. Neurol. Sci.* **18**, 111–29.

Johnston, A. W., and McKay, E. (1986). X-linked muscular dystrophy with contractures *J. Med. Genet.* (In press).

Johnston, P. G. and Cattanach, B. M. (1981). Controlling elements in the mouse. IV. Evidence of non-random X-inactivation. *Genet. Res.* **37**, 151–60.

Jones, G. E. and Witkowski, J. A. (1983). A cell surface abnormality in Duchenne muscular dystrophy: intercellular adhesiveness of skin fibroblasts from patients and carriers. *Hum. Genet.* **63**, 232–7.

Julian, L. M. and Asmundson, V. S. (1963). Muscular dystrophy of the chicken. In *Muscular dystrophy in man and animals* (ed. G. H. Bourne and M. N. Golarz) pp. 457–98. Hafner, New York.

Kaeser, H. E. (1965). Scapuloperoneal muscular atrophy. *Brain* **88**, 407–18.

Kagen, L. J. (1984). Dermatomyositis and polymyositis: clinical aspects. *Clin. Exper. Rheumatol.* **2**, 271-7.

Kakulas, B. A. and Adams, R. D. (1985). *Diseases of Muscle. Pathological foundations of clinical myology*, 4th edn. Harper and Row, Philadelphia.

Kamoshita, S., Konishi, Y., Segawa, M., and Fukuyama, Y. (1976). Congenital muscular dystrophy as a disease of the central nervous system. *Arch. Neurol.* **33**, 513-6.

Kaplan, L. C. and Elias, E. R. (1986). Diagnosis of muscular dystrophy in patients referred for evaluation of language delay. *Develop. Med. Child Neurol.* **28**, 110 (Abstract).

Kar, N. C. and Pearson, C. M. (1972a). Acyl phosphatase in normal and diseased human muscle. *Clin. Chim. Acta* **40**, 262-5.

—— (1972b). Acid, neutral and alkaline cathepsins in normal and diseased human muscle. *Enzyme* **13**, 188-96.

—— (1973). Muscle adenylic acid deaminase activity. Selective decrease in early-onset Duchenne muscular dystrophy. *Neurology* **23**, 478-82.

—— (1977). Hydrolytic enzymes and human muscular dystrophy. In *Pathogenesis of human muscular dystrophies* (ed. L. P. Rowland) pp. 387-94. Excerpta Medica, Amsterdam.

—— (1980). Methylthioadenosine nucleosidase in normal and dystrophic human muscle. *Clin. Chim. Acta.* **108**, 465-8.

Karagan, N. J., Richman, L. C., and Sorensen, J. P. (1980). Analysis of verbal disability in Duchenne muscular dystrophy. *J. Nerv. Ment. Dis.* **168**, 419-23.

—— and Sorensen, J. P. (1981). Intellectual functioning in non-Duchenne muscular dystrophy. *Neurology* **31**, 448-52.

—— and Zellweger, H. U. (1978). Early verbal disability in children with Duchenne muscular dystrophy. *Develop. Med. Child Neurol.* **20**, 435-41.

Kark, R. A. P. and Becker, D. M. (1981). Multiple genotypes, multiple phenotypes, and partial defects. *Muscle and Nerve* **4**, 31-40.

Kawai, M., Kunimoto, M., Motoyoshi, Y., Kuwata, T., and Nakano, I. (1985). Computed tomography in Duchenne type muscular dystrophy – morphological stages based on the computed tomographical findings. *Clin. Neurol.* **25**, 578-90. (Japanese with detailed abstract in English.)

Kazakov, V. M., Bogorodinsky, D. K., and Skorometz, A. A. (1976). The myogenic scapulo-peroneal syndrome. Muscular dystrophy in the K kindred: clinical study and genetics. *Clin. Genet.* **10**, 41-50.

Kessler, S. (1979). The psychological foundations of genetic counseling. In *Genetic counseling – psychological dimensions* (ed. S. Kessler) pp. 17-33. Academic Press, New York.

Ketelsen, U. P., Freund-Mölbert, E., and Beckmann, R. (1971). Klinische und ultrastrukturelle Befunde bei kongenitaler Muskeldystrophie. *Monatsschrift. Kinderheilk.* **119**, 586-92.

King, B. and Emery, A. E. H. (1973). Leucocyte fatty acid oxidation in hereditary neuromuscular disorders. *J. Neurol. Sci.* **20**, 297-302.

——, Spikesman, A., and Emery, A. E. H. (1972). The effect of pregnancy on serum levels of creatine kinase. *Clin. Chim. Acta* **36**, 267-9.

Kingston, H. M., Sarfarazi, M., Thomas, N. S. T., and Harper, P. S. (1984). Localisation of the Becker muscular dystrophy gene on the short arm of the X chromosome by linkage to cloned DNA sequences. *Hum. Genet.* **67**, 6-17.

——, Thomas, N. S. T., Pearson, P. L., Sarfarazi, M., and Harper, P. S. (1983). Genetic linkage between Becker muscular dystrophy and a polymorphic DNA sequence on the short arm of the X chromosome. *J. Med. Genet.* **20**, 255–8.

Kleine, T. O. (1970). Evidence for the release of enzymes from different organs in Duchenne's muscular dystrophy. *Clin. Chim. Acta* **29**, 227–31.

Klip, A., Elder, B., Ruiz-Funes, H. P., Buchwald, M., and Grinstein, S. (1985). The free cytoplasmic Ca^{2+} levels in Duchenne muscular dystrophy lymphocytes. *Muscle & Nerve* **8**, 317–20.

Kloepfer, H. W. and Emery, A. E. H. (1969). Genetic aspects of neuromuscular disease. In *Disorders of voluntary muscle*, 2nd edn (ed. J. N. Walton) pp. 683–712. Churchill Livingstone, Edinburgh.

Koehler, J. (1977). Blood vessel structure in Duchenne muscular dystrophy. I. Light and electron microscopic observations in resting muscle. *Neurology* **27**, 861–8.

Konagaya, M., Takayanagi, T., Kamiya, T., and Takamatsu, S. (1982). Genetic linkage study of Duchenne muscular dystrophy and haemophilia A. *Neurology* **32**, 1046–9.

Kott, E., Golan, A., Don, R., and Bornstein, B. (1973). Muscular dystrophy: the relative frequency in the different ethnic groups in Israel. *Confin. Neurol.* **35**, 177–85.

Kousseff, B. (1981). Linkage between chronic granulomatous disease and Duchenne's muscular dystrophy *Amer. J. Dis. Child.* **135**, 1149.

Kozicka, A., Prot, J., and Wasilewski, R. (1971). Mental retardation in patients with Duchenne progressive muscular dystrophy. *J. Neurol. Sci.* **14**, 209–13.

Krog, E. (ed.) (1982). *Total management in muscular dystrophy.* Muskelsvind-fonden, Copenhagen.

Krstić, R. V. (1978). *Die Gewebe des Menschen und der Säugetiere.* Springer-Verlag, Berlin.

Kryschowa, N. and Abowjan, W. (1934). Zur Frage der Heredität der Pseudohyper-trophie Duchenne. *Zeitschr. ges. Neurol.* **150**, 421–6.

Kuby, S. A., Noda, L., and Lardy, H. A. (1954). Adenosinetriphosphate-creatine transphosphorylase. *J. Biol. Chem.* **209**, 191–201.

Kugelberg, E. (1947). Electromyograms in muscular disorders. *J. Neurol. Neurosurg. Psychiat.* **10**(NS), 122–33.

—— and Welander, L. (1956). Heredofamilial juvenile muscular atrophy simulating muscular dystrophy. *Arch. Neurol. Psychiat.* **75**, 500–9.

Kuhn, E., Fiehn, W., Schröder, J. M., Assmus, H. A., and Wagner, A. (1979). Early myocardial disease and cramping myalgia in Becker-type muscular dystrophy: a kindred. *Neurology* **29**, 1144–9.

Kunkel, L. M., Monaco, A. P., Middlesworth, W., Ochs, H. D., and Latt, S. A. (1985). Specific cloning of DNA fragments absent from the DNA of a male patient with an X chromosome deletion. *Proc. Natl. Acad. Sci. (USA)* **82**, 4778–82.

—— *et al.* (1986). Analysis of deletions in DNA from patients with Becker and Duchenne muscular dystrophy. *Nature (Lond).* **322**, 73–7.

Kuroiwa, Y. and Miyazaki, T. (1967). Epidemiological study of myopathy in Japan. In *Exploratory concepts in muscular dystrophy and related disorders* (ed. A. T. Milhorat) pp. 98–102. Excerpta Medica. Amsterdam.

Lamy, M. and de Grouchy, J. (1954), L'hérédité de la myopathie (formes basses). *J. Génét. Hum.* **3**, 219–61.

Landon, D. N. (1982). Skeletal muscle – normal morphology, development and innervation. In *Skeletal muscle pathology* (ed. F. L. Mastaglia and J. N. Walton) pp. 1–87. Churchill Livingstone, Edinburgh.

Lane, R. J. M., Gardner-Medwin, D., and Roses, A. D. (1980). Electrocardiographic abnormalities in carriers of Duchenne muscular dystrophy. *Neurology* **30**, 497–501.

——, Robinow, M., and Roses, A. D. (1983). The genetic status of mothers of isolated cases of Duchenne muscular dystrophy. *J. Med. Genet.* **20**, 1–11.

—— and Roses, A. D. (1981). Variations of serum creatine kinase levels with age in normal females: implications for genetic counselling in Duchenne muscular dystrophy. *Clin. Chim. Acta* **113**, 75–86.

Lathrop, G. M. and Lalouel, J. M. (1984). Easy calculations of lod scores and genetic risks on small computers. *Amer. J. Hum. Genet.* **36**, 460–5.

Laurent, C., Biemont, M. C., and Dutrillaux, B. (1975). Sur quatre nouveaux cas de translocation du chromosome X chez l'homme. *Humangenetik* **26**, 35–46.

Lawrence, E. F., Brown, B., and Hopkins, I. J. (1973). Pseudohypertrophic muscular dystrophy of childhood: an epidemiological survey in Victoria. *Aust. N.Z. J. Med.* **3**, 142–51.

Lazaro, R. P., Fenichel, G. M., and Kilroy, A. W. (1979). Congenital muscular dystrophy: case reports and reappraisal. *Muscle and Nerve* **2**, 349–55.

Lebenthal, E., Shochet, S. B., Adam, A., Seelenfreund, M., Fried, A., Najenson, T., Sandbank, U., and Matoth, Y. (1970). Arthrogryposis multiplex congenita: twenty-three cases in an Arab kindred. *Pediatrics* **46**, 891–9.

Leibowitz, D. and Dubowitz, V. (1981). Intellect and behaviour in Duchenne muscular dystrophy. *Develop. Med. Child. Neurol.* **23**, 577–90.

Lenman, J. A. R. and Ritchie, A. E. (1970). *Clinical eletromyography.* Pitman Medical and Scientific, London.

Leon, S. H., Schuffler, M. D., Kettler, M., and Rohrmann, C. A. (1986). Chronic intestinal pseudoobstruction as a complication of Duchenne's muscular dystrophy. *Gastroenterology* **90**, 455–9.

Leonard, C. O., Chase, G. A., and Childs, B. (1972). Genetic counseling: a consumer's view. *New Engl. J. Med.* **287**, 433–9.

Levene, P. A and Kristeller, L. (1909). Factors regulating the creatinin output in man. *Amer. J. Physiol.* **24**, 45–65.

Levison, H. (1951). *Dystrophia musculorum progressiva.* Munksgaard, Copenhagen.

Lewis, A. J. and Besant, D. F. (1962). Muscular dystrophy in infancy. Report of 2 cases in siblings with diaphragmatic weakness. *J. Pediat.* **60**, 376–84.

Lilienthal, J. L., Zierler, K. L., Folk, B. P., Buka, R., and Riley, M. J. (1950). A reference base and system for analysis of muscle constituents. *J. Biol. Chem.* **182**, 501–8.

Lindenbaum, R. H., Clarke, G., Patel, C., Moncrieff, M., and Hughes, J. T. (1979). Muscular dystrophy in an X;1 translocation female suggests that Duchenne locus is on X chromosome short arm. *J. Med. Genet.* **16**, 389–92.

Lindgren, V., de Martinville, B., Horwich, A. L., Rosenberg, L. E., and Francke, U. (1984). Human ornithine transcarbamylase locus mapped to band Xp21.1 near the Duchenne muscular dystrophy locus. *Science* **226**, 698–700.

Little, W. J. (1853). *On the nature and treatment of the deformities of the human frame: being a course of lectures delivered at the Royal Orthopaedic Hospital in 1843*, pp. 14–6. Longman, Brown, Green and Longmans, London.

Livingstone, I. R., Gardner-Medwin, D., Pennington, R. J. T., and Walton, J. N.

(1982). Serum creatine kinase and pyruvate kinase activities in normal adolescent females. *J. Neurol. Sci.* **54**, 349–52.

Lloyd, S. J. and Emery, A. E. H. (1981). A possible circulating plasma factor in Duchenne muscular dystrophy. *Clin. Chim. Acta* **112**, 85–90.

—— and Brown, J. N. (1981) Erythrocyte membrane studies. *Neurology* **31**, 1371.

——, Skinner, R., and Emery, A. E. H. (1982) Neonatal screening for Duchenne muscular dystrophy (DMD) using a fluorimetric electrophoretic assay for creatine kinase (CK) in dried blood samples. *Proc. Vth Internat. Congr. Neuromuscular Diseases* Abstract No. 34. Marseilles.

Lössner, J., Kühn, H. J., and Ruchholtz, U. (1982). Hämopexin und Muskeldystrophis. Zur Carrierdiagnostik der Duchenne-Form. *Psychiatr. Neurol. Med. Psychol.* **34**, 53–9.

Lou, M. F. (1979). Human muscular dystrophy: elevation of urinary dimethylarginines. *Science* **203**, 668–70.

Lowenstein, A. S., Arbeit, S. R., and Rubin, I. L. (1962). Cardiac involvement in progressive muscular dystrophy. An electrocardiographic and ballistocardiographic study. *Amer. J. Cardiol* **9**, 528–33.

Lubs. M. L. (1974). Hemophilia A and Duchenne muscular dystrophy in Colorado. *Amer. J. Hum. Genet.* **26**, 56A (Abstract).

Lucci, B. (1980). Incidence, prevalence and mutation rate of Duchenne muscular dystrophy in the province of Reggio Emilia. In *Muscular dystrophy research: advances and new trends* (ed. C. Angelini, G. A. Danieli, and D. Fontanari) pp. 289–90. Excerpta Medica, Amsterdam.

Lucy, J. A. (1980). Is there a membrane defect in muscle and other cells? *Brit. Med. Bull.* **36**, 187–92.

Luque, E. R. (1982). Segmental spinal instrumentation for correction of scoliosis. *Clin. Orthop.* **163**, 192–8.

Luthra, M. G., Stern, L. Z., and Kim, H. D. (1979). $(Ca^{++} + Mg^{++})$-ATPase of red cells in Duchenne and myotonic dystrophy: effect of soluble cytoplasmic activator. *Neurology* **29**, 835–41.

Mabry, C. C., Roeckel, I. E., Munich, R. L., and Robertson, D. (1965). X-linked pseudohypertrophic muscular dystrophy with a late onset and slow progression. *New Engl. J. Med.* **273**, 1062–70.

McComas, A. J., Sica, R. E. P., and Currie, S. (1970). Muscular dystrophy: evidence for a neural factor. *Nature* **226**, 1263–4.

McKeran, R. O., Halliday, D., and Purkiss, P. (1977). Increased myofibrillar protein catabolism in Duchenne muscular dystrophy measured by 3-methylhistidine excretion in the urine. *J. Neurol. Neurosurg. Psychiat.* **40**, 979–81.

McKishnie, J. D., Muir, J. M., and Girvan, D. P. (1983). Anaesthesia induced rhabdomyolysis – a case report. *Can. Anaesth. Soc. J.* **30**, 295–8.

Macklem, P. T. (1986). Muscular weakness and respiratory function. *New Engl. J. Med.* **314**, 775–6.

McKusick, V. A. (1964). *On the X chromosome of man.* American Institute of Biological Sciences, Washington.

MacLeod, P. M., Holden, J., and Masotti, R. (1983). Duchenne muscular dystrophy in a female with an X-autosome translocation. *Amer. J. Hum. Genet.* **35**, 104A (Abstract).

McMenamin, J. B., Becker, L. E., and Murphy, E. G. (1982). Congenital muscular dystrophy: a clinicopathologic report of 24 cases. *J. Pediat.* **100**, 692–7.

Maguire, P. (1984). Training in genetic counselling. In *Psychological aspects of genetic counselling*. (ed. A. E. H. Emery and I. M. Pullen) pp. 219-28. Academic Press, London, New York.

Mair, W. G. P. and Tomé, F. M. S. (1972). *Atlas of the ultrastructure of diseased human muscle*. Churchill Livingstone, Edinburgh.

Marandian, M. H., Ramine, M., Djafarian, M., Farian, H., Behvad, A., Lessani, M., and Mahchid, M. (1977). Association de rétinopathie pigmentaire et de maladie de Duchenne dans une famille. *Ann. Pediat.* **24**, 789-95.

Markand, O. N., North, R. R., D'Agostino, A. N., and Daly, D. D. (1969). Benign sex-linked muscular dystrophy: clinical and pathological features. *Neurology* **19**, 617-33.

Marsh, G. G. and Munsat, T. L. (1974). Evidence for early impairment of verbal intelligence in Duchenne muscular dystrophy. *Arch. Dis. Child.* **49**, 118-22.

Marsh, W. L. (1978). Chronic granulomatous disease, the McLeod syndrome, and the Kell blood groups. *Birth Defects Orig. Art. Ser.* **XIV (No. 6A)**, 9-25.

——, Marsh, N. J. Moore, A., Symmans, W. A., Johnson, C. L., and Redman, C. M. (1981). Elevated serum creatine phosphokinase in subjects with McLeod syndrome. *Vox Sang.* **40**, 403-11.

Martin, A. J., Stern, L., Yeates, J., Lepp, D., and Little, J. (1986). Respiratory muscle training in Duchenne muscular dystrophy. *Develop. Med. Child. Neurol.* **28**, 314-18.

Mastaglia, F. L. and Walton, J. (eds) (1982). *Skeletal muscle pathology*. Churchill Livingstone, Edinburgh.

Maunder, C. A., Yarom. R., and Dubowitz, V. (1977). Electron-microscopic X-ray microanalysis of normal and diseased human muscle. *J. Neurol. Sci.* **33**, 323-34.

Maunder-Sewry, C. A. and Dubowitz, V. (1979). Myonuclear calcium in carriers of Duchenne muscular dystrophy. An X-ray microanalysis study. *J. Neurol. Sci.* **42**, 337-47.

—— (1981). Needle muscle biopsy for carrier detection in Duchenne muscular dystrophy. Part 1. Light microscopy-histology, histochemistry and quantitation. *J. Neurol. Sci.* **49**, 305-24.

——, Gorodetsky, R., Yarom, R., and Dubowitz, V. (1980). Element analysis of skeletal muscle in Duchenne muscular dystrophy using X-ray fluorescence spectrometry. *Muscle and Nerve* **3**, 502-8.

Mauro A (ed.) (1979). *Muscle Regeneration*. Raven Press, New York.

Mawatari, S. and Katayama, K. (1973). Scapuloperoneal muscular atrophy with cardiopathy. An X-linked recessive trait. *Arch. Neurol.* **28**, 55-9.

Meadows, J. C., Marsden, C. D., and Harriman, D. G. F. (1969). Chronic spinal muscular atrophy in adults. Part 1, The Kugelberg–Welander syndrome. *J. Neurol. Sci.* **9**, 527-50.

Mechler, F., Mastaglia, F. L., Haggith, J., and Gardner-Medwin, D. (1980). Adrenergic receptor responses of vascular smooth muscle in Becker muscular dystrophy. A muscle blood flow study using the ^{133}Xe clearance method. *J. Neurol. Sci.* **46**, 291-302.

Meltzer, H. Y. (1971). Factors affecting serum creatine phosphokinase levels in the general population: the role of race, activity and age. *Clin. Chim. Acta* **33**, 165-72.

——, Dorus, E., Grunhaus, L., Davis, J. M., and Belmaker, R. (1978). Genetic control of human plasma creatine phosphokinase activity. *Clin. Genet.* **13**, 321-6.

—— and Holy, P. A. (1974). Black-white differences in serum creatine phosphokinase (CPK) activity. *Clin. Chim. Acta* **54**, 215-24.

Mendell, J. R., Higgins, R., Sahenk, Z., and Cosmos, E. (1979). Relevance of genetic animal models of muscular dystrophy to human muscular dystrophies. *Ann. N.Y. Acad. Sci.* **317**, 409-30.

Merlini, L., Granata, C., Dominici, P., and Bonfiglioli, S. (1986). Emery–Dreifuss muscular dystrophy: Report of five cases in a family and review of the literature. *Muscle and Nerve* **9**, 481-5

Meryon, E. (1852). On granular and fatty degeneration of the voluntary muscles. *Med. Chir. Trans.* **35**, 73-84.

—— (1864). *Practical and pathological researches on the various forms of paralysis.* Churchill, London.

Michal, V. (1972). Psychika ditete s progresivni svalovou dystrofi. *Ceskoslovenska Psychiatrie* **68**, 226-30.

Michelson, A. M., Russell, E. S., and Harman, P. J. (1955). Dystrophia muscularis: a hereditary primary myopathy in the house mouse. *Proc. Natl. Acad. Sci. (USA)* **41**, 1079-84.

Milhorat, A. T. and Wolff, H. G. (1943). Studies in diseases of muscle. *Arch. Neurol. and Psychiat.* **49**, 641-54.

Miller, E. D., Sanders, D. B., Rowlingson, J. C., Berry, F. A., Sussman, M. D., and Epstein, R. M. (1978). Anaesthesia-induced rhabdomyolysis in a patient with Duchenne's muscular dystrophy. *Anesthesiology* **48**, 146-8.

Miller, G. and Dunn, N. (1982). An outline of the management and prognosis of Duchenne muscular dystrophy in Western Australia. *Aust. Paediatr. J.* **18**, 277-82.

——, Tunnecliffe, M., and Douglas, P. S. (1985). IQ, prognosis and Duchenne muscular dystrophy. *Brain and Development* **7**, 7-9.

Miller, R. G., Layzer, R. B., Mellenthin, M. A., Golabi, M., Francoz, R. A., and Mall, J. C. (1985). Emery-Dreifuss muscular dystrophy with autosomal dominant transmission. *Neurology* **35**, 1230-3.

Milne, B. and Rosales, J. K. (1982). Anaesthetic considerations in patients with muscular dystrophy undergoing spinal fusion and Harrington rod insertion. *Can. Anaesth. Soc. J.* **29**, 250-3.

Miranda, A. F. and Mongini, T. (1984). Duchenne muscle culture: current status and future trends. In *Neuromuscular diseases* (ed. G. Serratrice *et al.*) pp. 365-71. Raven Press, New York.

Mokri, B. and Engel, A. G. (1975). Duchenne dystrophy: electron microscopic findings pointing to a basic defect or early abnormality in the plasma membrane of the muscle fiber. *Neurology* **25**, 1111-20.

Mokuno, K., Riku, S., Matsuoka, Y., Sobue, I., and Kato, K. (1984). Serum muscle-specific enolase in progressive muscular dystrophy and other neuromuscular diseases. *J. Neurol. Sci.* **63**, 345-52.

Monaco, A. P., Bertelson, C. J., Middlesworth, W., Colletti, C-A., Aldridge, J., Fischbeck, K. H., Bartlett, R., Pericak-Vance, M. A., Roses, A. D. and Kunkel, L. M. (1985). Detection of deletions spanning the Duchenne muscular dystrophy locus using a tightly linked DNA segment. *Nature* **316**, 842-5.

Monaco, A. P., Neve, R. L., Colletti-Feener, C., Bertelson, C. J., Kurnit, D. M. and Kunkel, L. M. (1986). Isolation of candidate cDNAs for portions of the Duchenne muscular dystrophy gene. *Nature* **323**, 646-50.

Monckton, G., Hoskin, V., and Warren, S. (1982). Prevalence and incidence of muscular dystrophy in Alberta, Canada. *Clin. Genet.* **21**, 19–24.

Moosa, A., Brown, B. H., and Dubowitz, V. (1972). Quantitative electromyography – carrier detection in Duchenne type muscular dystrophy using a new automatic technique. *J. Neurol. Neurosurg. Psychiat.* **35**, 841–4.

Morgan, G. (1975). Effects of genetic counselling in Duchenne muscular dystrophy. In *Recent advances in myology* (ed. W. G. Bradley, D. Gardner-Medwin, and J. N. Walton) pp. 477–8. Excerpta Medica, Amsterdam.

Morrell, R. M. (1959). Abnormal hepatic tests in muscular disease. *Arch. Intern. Med.* **104**, 83–90.

Morton, N. E. (1959). Genetic tests under incomplete ascertainment. *Amer. J. Hum. Genet.* **11**, 1–16.

—— (1969). Segregation analysis. In *Computer applications in genetics* (ed. N. E. Morton) pp. 129–39. University of Hawaii Press, Honolulu.

—— and Chung, C. S. (1959). Formal genetics of muscular dystrophy. *Amer. J. Hum. Genet.* **11**, 360–79.

Moseley, C. F. (1984). Natural history and management of scoliosis in Duchenne muscular dystrophy. In *Neuromuscular diseases* (ed. G. Serratrice *et al.*) pp. 545–9. Raven Press, New York.

Moser, H. (1971). Trisomie 21 bei einem Knaben mit progressiver Muskeldystrophie Duchenne. *Z. Kinderheilk.* **109**, 318–25.

—— (1977). Heterozygotenerfassung und genetische Beratung bei der progressiven Muskeldystrophie Duchenne. *Schweiz. Rundschau. Med. (PRAXIS)* **66**, 814–22.

—— (1984). Duchenne muscular dystrophy: pathogenetic aspects and genetic prevention. *Hum. Genet.* **66**, 17–40.

—— (1986). Personal communication.

—— and Emery, A. E. H. (1974). The manifesting carrier in Duchenne muscular dystrophy. *Clin. Genet.* **5**, 271–84.

—— and Vogt, J. (1974). Follow-up study of serum creatine kinase in carriers of Duchenne muscular dystrophy. *Lancet* ii, 661–2.

—— and Wiesmann, U. (1971). Serum-Creatin-Kinase und Sulfhydril-Konzentration nach ischämischer Arbeitsbelastung der Vorderarmmuskulatur bei Patienten und Konduktorinnen der progressiven Muskeldystrophie Duchenne. *Klin. Woch.* **49**, 488–94.

——, Richterich, R., and Rossi, E. (1964). Progressive Muskeldystrophie. VI. Häufigkeit, Klinik, und Genetik der Duchenne-form, *Schweiz. Med. Woch.* **94**, 1610–21.

—— (1966). Progressive Muskeldystrophie. VII. Häufigkeit, Klinik und Genetik der Typen I and II. *Schweiz. Med. Woch.* **96**, 169–74, 205–11.

Moss, D. W., Whitaker, K. B., Parmar, C., Heckmatt, J., Witkowski, J., Sewry, C., and Dubowitz, V. (1981). Activity of creatine kinase in sera from healthy women, carriers of Duchenne muscular dystrophy and cord blood, determined by the "European" recommended method with NAC-EDTA activation. *Clin. Chim. Acta* **116**, 209–16.

Mossman, J., Blunt, S., Stephens, R., Jones, E. E., and Pembrey, M. (1983). Hunter's disease in a girl: association with X:5 chromosome translocation disrupting the Hunter gene. *Arch. Dis. Child.* **58**, 911–5.

Moxley, R. T. (1984). Skeletal muscle blood flow and exercise. In *Neuromuscular diseases* (ed. G. Serratrice *et al.*) pp. 51–6. Raven Press, New York.

MRC (1943). *Aids to the investigation of peripheral nerve injuries* MRC War Memorandum No. 7, 2nd edn. London, HMSO.

Mumenthaler, M. (1970). Myopathy in neuropathy. In *Muscle diseases* (ed. J. N. Walton, N. Canal, and G. Scarlato) pp. 585–98. Excerpta Medica International Congress Series No. 199, Amsterdam.

Murphy, E. A. (1973). Probabilies in genetic counselling. *Birth defects: Orig. Art. Ser.* **9**(4), 19–33.

—— and Mutalik, G. S. (1969). The application of Bayesian methods in genetic counselling. *Hum. Hered.* **19**, 126–51.

Murphy, E. G. (1985). Personal communication.

—— and Thompson, M. W. (1969). Manifestations of Duchenne muscular dystrophy in carriers. In *Progress in Neurogenetics* (ed. A. Barbeau and J. R Brunette) pp. 162–8. Excerpta Medica, Amsterdam.

——, Corey, P. N. J., and Conen, P. E. (1965). Varying manifestations of Duchenne muscular dystrophy in a family with affected females. In *Muscle* (ed. W. M. Paul, E. E. Daniel, C. M. Kay, and G. Monckton) pp. 529–45. Pergamon Press, New York.

Murray, J. M., Davies, K. E., Harper, P. S., Meredith, L., Mueller, C. R., and Williamson, R. (1982). Linkage relationship of a cloned DNA sequence on the short arm of the X chromosome to Duchenne muscular dystrophy. *Nature* **300**, 69–71.

Musch, B. C., Papapetropoulos, T. A., McQueen, D. A., Hudgson, P., and Weightman, D. (1975). A comparison of the structure of small blood vessels in normal, denervated and dystrophic human muscle. *J. Neurol. Sci.* **26**, 221–34.

Mussini, E., Cornelio, F., Colombo, L., De Ponte, G., Giudici, G., Cotellessa, L., and Marcucci, F. (1984). Increased myofibrillar protein catabolism in Duchenne muscular dystrophy measured by 3-methylhistidine excretion in the urine. *Muscle and Nerve* **7**, 388–91.

Nadas, A. S. (1963). *Pediatric cardiology*, 2nd edn, p. 71. W. B Saunders, Philadelphia.

Namba, T., Aberfeld, D. C., and Grob. D. (1970). Chronic proximal spinal muscular atrophy. *J. Neurol. Sci.* **11**, 401–23.

Narazaki, O., Hanai, T., Ueki, Y., and Mitsudome, A. (1985). Duchenne muscular dystrophy in a female with an X-autosome translocation. (Japanese). *Clin. Neurol.* **25**, 432–6.

Nasse, C. F. (1820). Von einer erblichen Neigung zu tödlichen Blutungen. *Arch. Med. Erfahrung. Geb. Praktischen Med. Staatsarzneikunde*, p. 385.

Nassi, P., Liguri, G., Landi, N., Berti, A., Stefani, M., Pavolini, B., and Ramponi, G. (1985). Acylphosphatase from human skeletal muscle: purification, some properties and levels in normal and myopathic muscles. *Biochem. Med.* **34**, 166–75.

Nayler, W. G. (1980). The pharmacological protection of the ischaemic heart: the use of calcium and beta-adrenoceptor antagonists. *European Heart J.* **1** (Supplement B), 5–13.

Neerunjun, J. S., Allsop, J., and Dubowitz, V. (1979). Hypoxanthine-guanine phosphoribosyltransferase activity of blood and muscle in Duchenne dystrophy. *Muscle and Nerve* **2**, 19–23.

Neligan, G. and Prudham, D. (1969). Norms for four standard developmental milestones by sex, social class and place in family. *Develop. Med. Child. Neurol.* **11**, 413–22.

Neville, H. E. and Harrold, S. (1985). Protein degradation in cultured skeletal muscle from Duchenne muscular dystrophy patients. *Muscle and Nerve* **8**, 253–7.

Nevin, N. C., Hughes, A. E., Calwell, M., and Lim, J. H. K. (1986). Duchenne muscular dystrophy in a female with a translocation involving Xp21. *J. Med. Genet.* **23**, 171–3.

Newberry, P. E. (1893). Beni Hasan, Part II. In *Archaeological survey of Egypt* (ed. F. L. Griffith). Kegan Paul, Trench, Trübner and Co., London.

Newman, R. J., Bore, P. J., Chan, L., Gadian, D. G., Styles, P., Taylor, D., and Radda, G. K. (1982). Nuclear magnetic resonance studies of forearm muscle in Duchenne dystrophy. *Brit. Med. J.* **284**, 1072–4.

Newsom-Davis, J. (1980). The respiratory system in muscular dystrophy. *Brit. Med. Bull.* **36**, 135–8.

Nicholson, G. A., Gardner-Medwin, D., Pennington, R. J. T., and Walton, J. N. (1979). Carrier detection in Duchenne muscular dystrophy: assessment of the effect of age on detection-rate with serum-creatine-kinase-activity. *Lancet* **i**, 692–4.

——, Lane, R. J. M., Gardner-Medwin, D., and Walton, J. N. (1981). Carrier testing in families of isolated cases of Duchenne muscular dystrophy. *J. Neurol. Sci.* **51**, 29–42.

—— and Sugars, J. (1982). An evaluation of lymphocyte capping in Duchenne muscular dystrophy. *J. Neurol. Sci.* **53**, 511–8.

Nicholson, L. V. B. (1981). Serum myoglobin in muscular dystrophy and carrier detection. *J. Neurol. Sci.* **51**, 411–26.

Niebrój-Dobosz, I. (1984). Surface membrane enzymes in human dystrophic muscle. In *Neuromuscular diseases* (ed. G. Serratrice *et al.*) pp. 115–8. Raven Press, New York.

Nigro, G., Comi, L. I., Limongelli, F. M., Giugliano, M. A. M., Politano, L., Petretta, V., Passamano, L., and Stefanelli, S. (1983). Prospective study of X-linked progressive muscular dystrophy in Campania. *Muscle and Nerve* **6**, 253–62.

——, Politano, L., Giugliano, M. A. M., Passamano, L., Porfidia, A., and Storace, R. (1984). Electrocardiographic evaluation of the P-type stage of dystrophic cardiomyopathy. *Cardiomyology* **3**(No. 1), 45–58.

Nowak, T. V., Ionasescu, V., and Anuras, S. (1982). Gastrointestinal manifestations of the muscular dystrophies. *Gastroenterology* **82**, 800–10.

Nutting, D. F., MacPike, A. D., and Meier, H. (1980). The calcium content of various tissues from myodystrophic and dystrophic mice. *J. Heredity* **71**, 15–8.

O'Brien, T., Sibert, I. R., and Harper, P. S. (1983). Implications of diagnostic delay in Duchenne muscular dystrophy. *Brit. Med. J.* **287**, 1106–7.

Oka, S., Igarashi, Y., Takagi, A., Nishida, M., Sato, K., Nakada, K., and Ikeda, K. (1982). Malignant hyperpyrexia and Duchenne muscular dystrophy: a case report. *Can. Anaesth. Soc. J.* **29**, 627–9.

Olson, B. J. and Fenichel, G. M. (1982). Progressive muscle disease in a young woman with family history of Duchenne's muscular dystrophy. *Arch. Neurol.* **39**, 378–80.

Olsson, T., Henriksson, K. G., Klareskog, L., and Forsum, U. (1984). HLA-DR expression, T lymphocyte phenotypes, OKM 1 and OKT 9 reactive cells in inflammatory myopathy. *Acta Neurol. Scand.* **69**, Suppl. 98, 200–1.

Ortaggio, F., Guidetti, D., Motti, L., Marcello, N., Solime, F., and Lucci, B. (1984). Studio longitudinale della funzionalita respiratoria nella distrofia muscolare di Duchenne. *Cardiomyology* **3**(No. 2–3), 73–83.

Oswald, A., Goldblatt, J., Horak, A., and Beighton, P. (1986), Emery–Dreifuss muscular dystrophy in a South African kindred. (In press).

Ott, J. (1974). Estimation of the recombination fraction in human pedigrees: efficient computation of the likelihood for human linkage studies. *Amer. J. Hum. Genet.* **26**, 588-97.

Panayiotopoulos, C. P. (1975). The neural hypothesis. In *Recent advances in myology* (ed. W. G. Bradley, D. Gardner-Medwin, and J. N. Walton) pp. 159-62. Excerpta Medica, Amsterdam.

Parry, R. (1984). Basic counselling techniques. In *Psychological aspects of genetic counselling* (ed. A. E. H. Emery and I. M. Pullen) pp. 11-21. Academic Press, London, New York.

Passos, M. R., Gonzalez, C. H. and Zatz, M. (1985). Creatine-kinase and pyruvate-kinase activities in normal children: implications in Duchenne muscular dystrophy carrier detection. *Amer. J. Med. Genet.* **22**, 255-62.

Patterson, M., Ong, H., and Drake, A. (1964). Intestine absorption in muscular dystrophy patients. *Arch. Intern. Med.* **114**, 67-70.

Paulson, O. B., Engel, A. G., and Gomez, M. R. (1974). Muscle blood flow in Duchenne type muscular dystrophy, limb-girdle dystrophy, polymyositis and in normal controls. *J. Neurol. Neurosurg. Psychiat.* **37**, 685-90.

Pearce, J. and Harriman, D. G. F. (1966). Chronic spinal muscular atrophy. *J. Neurol. Neurosurg. Psychiat.* **29**, 509-20.

Pearn, J. H. (1973). Patients' subjective interpretation of risks offered in genetic counselling. *J. Med. Genet.* **10**, 129-34.

—— (1983). Spinal muscular atrophies. In *Principles and practice of medical genetics* (ed. A. E. H. Emery and D. Rimoin) pp. 414-25. Churchill Livingstone, Edinburgh.

—— and Hudgson, P. (1979). Anterior-horn cell degeneration and gross calf hypertrophy with adolescent onset. *Lancet* **i**, 1059-61.

Pearson, C. M. (1962). Histopathological features of muscle in the preclinical stages of muscular dystrophy. *Brain* **85**, 109-20.

—— and Fowler, W. M. (1963). Hereditary non-progressive muscular dystrophy inducing arthrogryposis syndrome. *Brain* **86**, 75-88.

—— and Wright, S. W. (1963). X-chromosome mosaicism in females with muscular dystrophy. *Proc. Natl. Acad. Sci. (USA)* **50**, 24-31.

Pelham, H. R. B. and Jackson, R. J. (1976). An efficient mRNA-dependent translation system from reticulocyte lysates. *Eur. J. Biochem.* **67**, 247-56.

Pellié, C., Feingold, J., and Démos, J. (1973). Age parental et mutation. A propos d'une enquête sur la myopathie de Duchenne de Boulogne. *J. Génét. Hum.* **21**, 33-41.

Pembrey, M. E., Davies, K. E., Winter, R. M., Elles, R. G., Williamson, R., Fazzone, T. A., and Walker, C. (1984). Clinical use of DNA markers linked to the gene for Duchenne muscular dystrophy. *Arch. Dis. Child.* **59**, 208-16.

Pena, S. D. J., Karpati, G., Carpenter, S., and Fraser, F. C. (1982). The clinical consequences of X-chromosomal inactivation: Duchenne muscular dystrophy in one of monozygotic twins. *Neurology* **32**, A83 (Abstract).

Penn, A. S., Lisak, R. P., and Rowland, L. P. (1970). Muscular dystrophy in young girls. *Neurology* **20**, 147-59.

Pennington, R. J. T. (1962). Some enzyme studies in muscular dystrophy. *Proc. Assoc. Clin. Biochem.* **2**, 17-8.

—— (1977a). Serum enzymes. In *Pathogenesis of human muscular dystrophies* (ed.

L. P. Rowland) pp. 341-9. Excerpta Medica, Amsterdam, Oxford.

—— (1977b). Proteinases of muscle. In *Proteinases in mammalian cells and tissues* (ed. A. J. Barrett) pp. 515-43. Elsevier/North-Holland, Amsterdam.

—— (1980). Clinical biochemistry of muscular dystrophy. *Brit. Med. Bull.* **36**, 123-6.

—— (1987). Biochemical aspects of muscle disease. In *Disorders of voluntary muscle*, 5th edn (ed. J. N. Walton). Churchill Livingstone, Edinburgh. (In press).

Pennington, R. J. and Robinson, J. E. (1968). Cathepsin activity in normal and dystrophic human muscle. *Enzymol. Biol. Clin.* **9**, 175-82.

Penrose, L. S. (1951). Measurement of pleiotropic effects in phenylketonuria. *Ann. Eugen., London* **16**, 134-41.

—— (1955). Parental age and mutation. *Lancet* **ii**, 312-3.

Percy, M. E., Andrews, D. F., and Thompson, M. W. (1982). Serum creatine kinase in the detection of Duchenne muscular dystrophy carriers: effects of season and multiple testing. *Muscle and Nerve* **5**, 58-64.

——, Pichora, G. A., Chang, L. S., Manchester, K. E., and Andrews, D. F. (1984). Serum myoglobin in Duchenne muscular dystrophy carrier detection: a comparison with creatine kinase and hemopexin using logistic discrimination. *Amer. J. Med. Genet.* **18**, 279-87.

Perez Vidal, M. T., Grau, E. S., Viñas, J. P., Bayona, T. V., and Rustein, P. (1983). Distrofia muscular tipo Duchenne en una hembra con una translocación equilibrada X/6. *Rev. Neurol., Barcelona* **XI**, **(51)**, 155-8.

Perloff, J. K., De Leon, A. C., and O'Doherty, D. (1966). The cardiomyopathy of progressive muscular dystrophy. *Circulation* **33**, 625-48.

——, Roberts, W. C., De Leon, A. C., and O'Doherty, D. (1967). The distinctive electrocardiogram of Duchenne's progressive muscular dystrophy. *Amer. J. Med.* **42**, 179-88.

Perry, T. B. and Fraser, F. C. (1973). Variability of serum creatine phosphokinase activity in normal women and carriers of the gene of Duchenne muscular dystrophy. *Neurology* **23**, 1316-23.

Peter, J. B., Worsfold, M., and Pearson, C. M. (1969). Erythrocyte ghost adenosine triphosphatase (ATPase) in Duchenne dystrophy. *J. Lab. Clin. Med.* **74**, 103-8.

Peterson, R., Masurovsky, E. B., Spiro, A. J., Crain, S. M. (1986). Duchenne dystrophic muscle develops lesions in long-term coculture with monse spinal cord. *Muscle and Nerve* **9**, 787-808.

Pickard, N. A., Gruemer, H. D., Verrill, H. L., Isaacs, E. R., Robinow, M., Nance, W. E., Myers, E. C., and Goldsmith, B. (1978). Systemic membrane defect in the proximal muscular dystrophies. *New Engl. J. Med.* **299**, 841-6.

Pöch, H. and Becker, P. E. (1955). Eine Muskeldystrophie auf einem altägyptischen Relief. *Nervenarzt* **26**, 528-30.

Pöche, H. and Schulze, H. (1985). Ribosomal protein synthesis in altered skin fibroblast cells obtained from patients with Duchenne muscular dystrophy. *J. Neurol. Sci.* **70**, 295-304.

Poore, G. V. (1883). *Selections from the clinical works of Dr. Duchenne de Boulogne.* The New Sydenham Society, London.

Porter, I. H., Schulze, J., and McKusick, V. A. (1962). Genetic linkage between the loci for glucose-6-phosphate dehydrogenase deficiency and colour blindness in American Negroes. *Ann. Hum. Genet.* **26**, 107-22.

Proschek, L. and Jasmin, G. (1982). Hereditary polymyopathy and cardiomyopathy in the Syrian hamster. II. Development of heart necrotic changes in relation to defective mitochondrial function. *Muscle and Nerve* 5, 26-32.

Prosser, E. J., Murphy, E. G., and Thompson, M. W. (1969). Intelligence and the gene for Duchenne muscular dystrophy. *Arch. Dis. Child.* 44, 221-30.

Prot, J. (1971). Genetic-epidemiological studies in progressive muscular dystrophy. *J. Med. Genet.* 8, 90-6.

Pullen, I. M. (1984). Physical handicap. In *Psychological aspects of genetic counselling* (ed. A. E. H. Emery and I. M. Pullen) pp. 107-24. Academic Press, London, New York.

Radu, H. and Sarközi, A. (1978). Personal communication to P. Becker, 1980.

——, Migea, S. Török, Z., Bordeianu, L., and Radu, A. (1968). Carrier detection in X-linked Duchenne type muscular dystrophy. A pluridimensional investigation. *J. Neurol. Sci.* 6, 289-300.

Ray, P. N., Belfall, B., Duff, C., Logan, C., Kean, V., Thompson, M. W., Sylvester, J. E., Gorski, J. L., Schmickel, R. D., and Worton, R. G. (1985). Cloning of the breakpoint of an X;21 translocation associated with Duchenne muscular dystrophy. *Nature* 318, 672-5.

Read, A. P., Storrar, L. K., Mountford, R. C., Elles, R. G., and Harris, R. (1986). A register based system for gene tracking in Duchenne muscular dystrophy. *J. Med. Genet.* (In press).

Reddy, B. K., Anandavalli, T. E., and Reddi, O. S. (1984). X-linked Duchenne muscular dystrophy in an unusual family with manifesting carriers. *Hum. Genet.* 67, 460-2.

Renier, W. O., Nabben, F. A. E., Hustinx, T. W. J., Veerkamp, J. H., Otten, B. J., Ter Laak, H. J., Ter Haar, B. G. A., and Gabreels, F. J. M. (1983). Congenital adrenal hypoplasia, progressive muscular dystrophy, and severe mental retardation, in association with glycerol kinase deficiency, in male sibs. *Clin. Genet.* 24, 243-51.

Rennie, M. J., Edwards, R. H. T., Millward, D. L., Wolman, S. L., Halliday, D. H., and Matthews, D. E. (1982). Effects of Duchenne muscular dystrophy on muscle protein synthesis. *Nature* 296, 165-7.

Riad, N. (1955). *La médecine au temps des Pharaons*, p. 242. Librairie Maloine, Paris.

Ribeiro, M. C. M., Melaragno, M. I., Schmidt, B., Brunoni, D., Gabbai, A. A., and Hackel, C. (1986). Duchenne muscular dystrophy in a girl with an (X;15) translocation. *Amer. J. Med. Genet.* 25, 231-6.

Richards, W. C. (1972). Anaesthesia and serum creatine phosphokinase levels in patients with Duchenne's pseudohypertrophic muscular dystrophy. *Anaesth. Intens. Care* 1, 150-3.

Rideau, Y. M. (1979). *Outlines of muscular dystrophy* (edited, revised, and translated from the French). Serem, Poitiers, France.

Rideau, Y., Gatin, G., Bach, J., and Ginies, G. (1983b). Prolongation of life in Duchenne's muscular dystrophy. *Acta Neurol.* (New Series), 5, 118-24.

——, Glorion, B., and Duport, G. (1983a). Prolongation of ambulation in the muscular dystrophies. *Acta Neurol.* (New Series), 5, 390-7.

——, DeLaubier, A., Tarle, O., and Bach, J. (1984). The treatment of scoliosis in Duchenne muscular dystrophy. *Muscle and Nerve* 7, 281-6.

Ringel, S. P., Carroll, J. E., and Schold, S. C. (1977). The spectrum of mild X-linked recessive muscular dystrophy. *Arch. Neurol.* 34, 408-16.

Robert, J. M. and Vignon, E. (1972). Les formes tardives des dystrophies musculaires liées a l'X. *Sciences Medicales* **3**, 397–402.

Robin, G. C. (1976). Scoliosis in Duchenne muscular dystrophy. In *Muscular dystrophy 1976* (ed. G. C. Robin and G. Falewski de Leon) pp. 119–22. Karger, Basel.

—— and Falewski, G. de L. (1963). Acute gastric dilatation in progressive muscular dystrophy. *Lancet* **ii**, 171–2.

Rodeck, C. H. and Morsman, J. M. (1983). First-trimester chorion biopsy. *Brit. Med. Bull.* **39**, 338–42.

Ronan, J. A., Perloff, J. K., Bowen, P. J., and Mann, O. (1972). The vectorcardiogram in Duchenne's progressive muscular dystrophy. *Amer. Heart J.* **84**, 588–96.

Ronzoni, E., Berg, L., and Landau, W. (1960). Enzyme studies in progressive muscular dystrophy. *Res. Publ. Assoc. Res. Nerv. Ment. Dis.* **38**, 721–9.

Ropers, H-H., Wienker, T. F., Grimm, T., Schroetter, K., and Bender, K. (1977). Evidence for preferential X-chromosome inactivation in a family with Fabry disease. *Amer. J. Hum. Genet.* **29**, 361–70.

——, Zuffardi, O., Bianchi, E., and Tiepolo, L. (1982). Agenesis of corpus callosum, ocular and skeletal anomalies (X-linked dominant Aicardi's syndrome) in a girl with balanced X/3 translocation. *Hum. Genet.* **61**, 364–8.

Rosalki, S. B. (1967). An improved procedure for serum creatine phosphokinase determination. *J. Lab. Clin. Med.* **69**, 696–705.

Roses, A. D. and Appel, S. H. (1976). Erythrocyte spectrin peak II phosphorylation in Duchenne muscular dystrophy. *J. Neurol. Sci.* **29**, 185–93.

——, Herbstreith, M. H., and Appel, S. H. (1975). Membrane protein kinase alteration in Duchenne muscular dystrophy. *Nature* **254**, 350–1.

——, Herbstreith, M., Metcalf, B., and Appel, S. H. (1976a). Increased phosphorylated components of erythrocyte membrane spectrin band II with reference to Duchenne dystrophy. *J. Neurol. Sci.* **30**, 167–78.

——, Roses, M. J., Metcalf, B. S., Hull, K. L., Nicholson, G. A., Hartwig, G. B., and Roe, C. R. (1977). Pedigree testing in Duchenne muscular dystrophy. *Ann. Neurol.* **2**, 271–8.

——, Miller, S. F., Hull, K. L., and Appel, S. H. (1976b). Carrier detection in Duchenne muscular dystrophy. *New Engl. J. Med.* **294**, 193–8.

Rosman, N. P. (1970). The cerebral defect and myopathy in Duchenne muscular dystrophy. A comparative clinicopathological study. *Neurology* **20**, 329–35.

—— and Kakulas, B. A. (1966). Mental deficiency associated with muscular dystrophy. A neuropathological study. *Brain* **89**, 769–88.

Rott, H-D. and Rödl, W. (1985). Imaging techniques in muscular dystrophies. *Clin. Genet.* **28**, 179–80.

Rotthauwe, H. W. and Kowalewski, S. (1966). Gutartige recessiv X-chromosomal vererbte Muskeldystrophie. I. Untersuchungen bei Merkmalsträgern. *Humangenetik* **3**, 17–29.

——, Mortier, W., and Beyer, H. (1972). Neuer Typ einer recessiv X-chromosomal vererbten Muskeldystrophie: scapulo-humero-distale Muskeldystrophie mit frühzeitigen Kontrakturen und Herzrhythmusstörungen. *Humangenetik* **16**, 181–200.

Rowe, D., Isenberg, D. A., and Beverley, P. C. L. (1983). Monoclonal antibodies to human leucocyte antigens in polymyositis and muscular dystrophy. *Clin. Exp. Immunol.* **54**, 327–36.

Rowland, L. P. (1976). Pathogenesis of muscular dystrophies. *Arch. Neurol.* **33**, 315–21.

—— (1980). Biochemistry of muscle membranes in Duchenne muscular dystrophy. *Muscle and Nerve* 3, 3–20.

—— (1984). Myoglobinuria, 1984. *Can. J. Neurol. Sci.* 11, 1–13.

——, Fahn, S., Hirschberg, E., and Harter, D. H. (1964) Myoglobinuria. *Arch. Neurol.* 10, 537–62.

——, Fetell, M., Olarte, M., Hays, A., Singh, N., and Wanat, F. E. (1979). Emery–Dreifuss muscular dystrophy. *Ann. Neurol.* 5, 111–7.

Ruitenbeek, W. (1979). Membrane-bound enzymes of erythrocytes in human muscular dystrophy. (Na^+ + K^+)-ATPase, Ca^{2+}-ATPase, K^+-and Ca^{2+}-*p*-Nitrophenylphosphatase. *J. Neurol. Sci.* 41, 71–80.

Russman, B. S. (1984). Comprehensive management of children with muscular disorders. *Pediatr. Ann.* 13, 103–12.

——, Melchreit, R., and Drennan, J. C. (1983). Spinal muscular atrophy: the natural course of disease. *Muscle and Nerve* 6, 179–81.

Saito, F., Goto, J., Kakinuma, H., Nakamura, F., Murayama, S., Nakano, I., and Tonomura, A. (1986). Inherited Xp21 deletion in a boy with complex glycerol kinase deficiency syndrome. *Clin. Genet.* 29, 92–3.

Salih, M. A. M., Omer, M. I. A., Bayoumi, R. A., Karrar, O., and Johnson, M. (1983). Severe autosomal recessive muscular dystrophy in an extended Sudanese kindred. *Develop. Med. Child. Neurol.* 25, 43–52.

Samaha, F. J. and Congedo, C. Z. (1977). Two biochemical types of Duchenne dystrophy: sarcoplasmic reticulum membrane proteins. *Ann. Neurol.* 1, 125–30.

——, Davis, B., and Nagy, B. (1981). Duchenne muscular dystrophy: adenosine triphosphate and creatine phosphate content in muscle. *Neurology* 31, 916–9.

Sanyal, S. K. and Johnson, W. W. (1982). Cardiac conduction abnormalities in children with Duchenne's progressive muscular dystrophy: electrocardiographic features and morphologic correlates. *Circulation* 66, 853–63.

——, Johnson, W. W., Dische, M. R., Pitner, S. E., and Beard, C. (1980). Dystrophic degeneration of papillary muscle and ventricular myocardium. A basis for mitral valve prolapse in Duchenne's muscular dystrophy. *Circulation* 62, 430–8.

Sarfarazi, M. and Williams, H. (1986). A computer programme for estimation of genetic risk in X linked disorders, combining pedigree and DNA probe data with other conditional information. *J. Med. Genet.* 23, 40–5.

Schanne, F. A. X., Kane, A. B., Young, E. E. and Farber, J. L. (1979). Calcium dependence of toxic cell death: a final common pathway. *Science* 206, 700–2.

Schapira, F., Dreyfus, J. C., Schapira, G., and Démos, J. (1960). Étude de l'aldolase et de la créatine kinase du sérum chez les mères de myopathes. *Rev. Franç. Études Clin. Biol.* 5, 990–4.

Schapira, G. and Dreyfus, J. C. (1963). Biochemistry of progressive muscular dystrophy. In *Muscular dystrophy in man and animals* (ed. G. H. Bourne and M. N. Golarz) pp. 48–87. Hafner Publishing Co., New York.

Scheuerbrandt, G. (1984). Personal communication to G. A. Danieli.

——, Hammerschmidt, M., and Mortier, W. (1984). Voluntary CK screening programme for the early detection of Duchenne muscular dystrophy in infants. In *Research into the origin and treatment of muscular dystrophy* (ed. L. P. ten Kate, P. L. Pearson, and A. M. Stadhouders) pp. 73–7. Excerpta Medica, Amsterdam.

——, Lundin, A., Lövgren, T., and Mortier, W. (1986). Screening for Duchenne muscular dystrophy: an improved screening test for creatine kinase and its application in an infant screening program. *Muscle and Nerve* 9,11–23.

Schiaffino, S., Gorza, L., Dones, I., Cornelio, F., and Sartore, S. (1986). Fetal myosin immunoreactivity in human dystrophic muscle. *Muscle and Nerve* 9, 51–8.

Schiffer, D., Bertolotto, A., De Marchi, M., Doriguzzi, C., Mongini, T., Monnier, C., Palmucci, L., and Verzé, L. (1981). Epidemiology of Duchenne muscular dystrophy in the province of Turin. *Ital. J. Neurol. Sci.* 2, 81–4.

——, Doriguzzi, C., Mongini, T., and Palmucci, L. (1984). Quantitative analysis of muscle biopsy. Results in 30 female controls and in 51 Duchenne carriers. *Ital. J. Neurol. Sci.* (Suppl. 3) 175–6.

Schliephake, E. (1929) Der Kardio-intestinale Symptomenkomplex bei der progressiven Muskeldystrophie. II. Graphische Untersuchungen. *Zeit. Kinderheilk.* 47, 85–93.

Schmalbruch, H. (1982). The muscular dystrophies. In *Skeletal muscle pathology* (ed. F. L. Mastaglia and J. N. Walton) pp. 235–65. Churchill Livingstone, Edinburgh.

Schmidt, C. C. (1838). Krankhafte Hypertrophie des Muskelsystems. Mittheilung von den DDr. Coste und Gioja! In *Schmidt's Jahrbücher der in- und ausländischen gesamten Medizin,* 24, 176.

Scholte, H. R. and Busch, H. F. M. (1980). Decreased phosphorylase activity in leucocytes of Duchenne carriers. *Clin. Chim. Acta* 105, 137–9.

Schorer, C. E. (1964). Muscular dystrophy and the mind. *Psychosom. Med.* 26, 5–13.

Schröder, J. M. (1982). *Pathologie der Muskulatur.* Springer-Verlag, Berlin.

Schrödinger, E. (1944). *What is Life?* Cambridge University Press, Cambridge.

Scott, O. M., Hyde, S. A., Goddard, C., Jones, R., and Dubowitz, V. (1981). Effect of exercise in Duchenne muscular dystrophy. *Physiotherapy* 67, 174–6.

——, and Dubowitz, V. (1982). Quantitation of muscle function in children: a prospective study in Duchenne muscular dystrophy. *Muscle and Nerve* 5, 291–301.

Seay, A. R., Ziter, F. A., and Thompson, J. A. (1978). Cardiac arrest during induction of anesthesia in Duchenne muscular dystrophy. *J. Pediat.* 93, 88–90.

Seeger, B. R., Sutherland, A. D. A., and Clark, M. S. (1984). Orthotic management of scoliosis in Duchenne muscular dystrophy. *Arch. Phys. Med. Rehab.* 65, 83–6.

Serratrice, G., Pellissier, J. F., Pouget, J., and Desnuelle, C. (1984). Des formes précoces aux formes tardives des amyotrophies spinales chroniques. A propos de quatre-vingt-quatorze observations. *Sem. Hôp., Paris* 60, 2867–74.

——, Pouget, J., Pellissier, J. F., Gastaut, J. L and Cros, D. (1982). Les atteintes musculaires a transmission récessive liées a l'X avec rétractions musculaires précoces et troubles de le conduction cardiaque. *Rev. Neurol., Paris* 138, 713–24. (*See also* Serratrice, G. and Pouget, J. (1986). *Rev. Neurol. Paris* (In press).)

Shalev, O., Leida, M. N., Hebbel, R. P., Jacob, H. S., and Eaton, J. W. (1981). Abnormal erythrocyte calcium homeostasis in oxidant-induced hemolytic disease. *Blood* 58, 1232–5.

Shapiro, F. and Bresnan, M. J. (1982). Orthopaedic management of childhood neuromuscular disease. Part III. Diseases of muscle. *J. Bone & Joint Surg.* 64(A), 1102–7.

Shaw, R. F. and Dreifuss, F. E. (1969). Mild and severe forms of X-linked muscular dystrophy. *Arch. Neurol.* 20, 451–60.

Sherwin, A. C. and McCully, R. S. (1961). Reactions observed in boys of various ages (10–14) to a crippling progressive and fatal illness (muscular dystrophy). *J. Chronic Dis.* 13, 59–68.

Shoji, S. (1981). Calcium flux of erythrocytes in Duchenne muscular dystrophy.

J. Neurol. Sci. **51**, 427–35.

Shokeir, M. H. K. and Kobrinsky, N. L. (1976). Autosomal recessive muscular dystrophy in Manitoba Hutterites. *Clin. Genet.* **9**, 197–202.

—— and Rozdilsky, B. (1985). Muscular dystrophy in Saskatchewan Hutterites. *Amer. J. Med. Genet.* **22**, 487–93.

Short, J. K. (1963). Congenital muscular dystrophy, a case report with autopsy findings. *Neurology* **13**, 526–30.

Shumate, J. B., Carroll, J. E., Brooke, M. H., and Choksi, R. M. (1982). Palmitate oxidation in human muscle: comparison to CPT and carnitine. *Muscle and Nerve* **5**, 226–31.

Sibert, J. R., Harper, P. S., Thompson, R. J., and Newcombe, R. G. (1979). Carrier detection in Duchenne muscular dystrophy. *Arch. Dis. Child.* **54**, 534–7.

Sibley, J. A. and Lehninger, A. L. (1949). Aldolase in the serum and tissues of tumour-bearing animals. *J. Nat. Cancer Inst.* **9**, 303–9.

Sidler, A. (1944). Beitrag zur Vererbung der progressiven Muskeldystrophie. *Arch. Julius Klaus Stift.* **19**, 213–23.

Siegel, I. M. (1977a). *The clinical management of muscular disease.* Wm. Heineman, London.

Siegel, I. M. (1977b). Fractures of long bones in Duchenne muscular dystrophy. *J. Trauma* **17**, 219–22.

Siegel, I. M. (1978). The management of muscular dystrophy: a clinical review *Muscle and Nerve* **1**, 453–60.

—— (1980). Maintenance of ambulation in Duchenne muscular dystrophy. *Clin. Pediat.* **19**, 383–8.

——, Miller, J. E., and Ray, R. D. (1968). Subcutaneous lower limb tenotomy in the treatment of pseudohypertrophic muscular dystrophy. *J. Bone & Joint Surg.* **50A**, 1437–43.

Silverman, L. M., Mendell, J. R., Sahenk, Z., and Fontana, M. B. (1976). Significance of creatine phosphokinase isoenzymes in Duchenne dystrophy. *Neurology* **26**, 561–4.

Simpson, A. C., Holmes, D., and Pennington, R. J. T. (1979). Dilution effect on serum creatine kinase in carriers of Duchenne muscular dystrophy. *Ann. Clin. Biochem.* **16**, 54–5.

Simpson, J., Zellweger, H., Burmeister, L. F., Christee, R., and Nielsen, M. K. (1974). Effect of oral contraceptive pills on the level of creatine phosphokinase with regard to carrier detection in Duchenne muscular dystrophy. *Clin. Chim. Acta.* **52**, 219–23.

Skinner, R., Emery, A. E. H., Scheuerbrandt, G., and Syme, J. (1982). Feasibility of neonatal screening for Duchenne muscular dystrophy. *J. Med. Genet.* **19**, 1–3.

Skolnick, M., Carmelli, D., and Tyler, F. (1977). A two-locus selection hypothesis for Duchenne muscular dystrophy. *Theoret. Pop. Biol.* **12**, 230–45.

Skyring, A. and McKusick, V. A. (1961). Clinical, genetic and electrocardiographic studies in childhood muscular dystrophy. *Amer. J. Med. Sci.* **242**, 534–47.

Slucka, C. (1968). The electrocardiogram in Duchenne progressive muscular dystrophy. *Circulation* **38**, 933–40.

Smith, C. A. B. and Kilpatrick, S. J. (1958). Estimates of the sex ratio of mutation rates in sex-linked conditions by the method of maximum likelihood. *Ann. Hum. Genet., London* **22**, 244–9.

Smith, I., Elton, R. A., and Thomson, W. H. S. (1979). Carrier detection in

X-linked recessive (Duchenne) muscular dystrophy: serum creatine phosphokinase values in premenarchal, menstruating and postmenopausal and pregnant normal women. *Clin. Chim. Acta.* **98**, 207–16.

Smith, P. E. M., Carty, A., Owen, R., and Edwards, R. H. T. (1986a). Quantitative computerized tomography scanning of psoas and erector spinae in muscular dystrophy. *Muscle & Nerve* **9**, (suppl.), 243 (Abstract).

——, Edwards, R. H. T, Evans, G. A., and Campbell, E. (1986b). Practical considerations of respiratory care of patients with Duchenne muscular dystrophy and related neuromuscular diseases. (In press)

Sollee, N. D., Latham, E. E., Kindlon, D. J. and Bresnan, M. J. (1985). Neuropsychological impairment in Duchenne muscular dystrophy. *J. Clin. Exper. Neuropsychol* **7**, 486–96.

Solti, F., Zádory, E., and Bekény, G. (1963). Electrocardiographic and circulatory changes in progressive muscular dystrophy. *Acta Med. Acad. Sci., Hungary* **19**, 1–10.

Somer, H. (1980). Enzyme release from isolated erythrocytes and lymphocytes in Duchenne muscular dystrophy. *J. Neurol. Sci.* **48**, 445–52.

——, Donner, M., Murros, J., and Konttinen, A. (1973). A serum isozyme study in muscular dystrophy. Particular reference to creatine kinase, aspartate aminotransferase and lactic dehydrogenase isozymes. *Arch. Neurol.* **29**, 343–5.

——, Voutilainen, A., Knuutila, S., Kaitila, I., Rapola, J., and Leinonen, H. (1985). Duchenne-like muscular dystrophy in two sisters with normal karyotypes: evidence for autosomal recessive inheritance. *Clin. Genet.* **28**, 151–6.

——, Willner, J., DeCresce, R. P., Willner, J., and Somer, M. (1980). Duchenne carriers: lactate dehydrogenase isoenzyme 5 in serum and muscle. *Neurology* **30**, 206–9.

Spencer, G. E. and Vignos, P. J. (1962). Bracing for ambulation in childhood progressive muscular dystrophy. *J. Bone & Joint Surg.* **44A**, 234–42.

Spiegler, A. W. J. and Herrmann, F. H. (1983). Erfassung und humangenetische Betreuung von Risikofamilien mit progressiver Muskeldystrophie der Typen Duchenne (DMD) und Becker-Kiener (BMD) im Bezirk Erfurt. *Dt. Gesundh.-Wesen* **38**, 994–9.

Spillane, J. D. (1981). *The doctrine of the nerves – chapters in the history of neurology.* Oxford University Press, Oxford, New York, Toronto.

Spiro, A. J. (1970). Minipolymyoclonus – a neglected sign in childhood spinal muscular atrophy. *Neurology* **20**, 1124–6.

Spowart, G., Buckton, K. E., Skinner, R., and Emery, A. E. H. (1982). X-chromosome in Duchenne muscular dystrophy. *Lancet* **i**, 1251.

Staples, D. (1977). Intellect and psychological problems. In *Severe childhood neuromuscular disease – the management of Duchenne muscular dystrophy and spinal muscular atrophy* (ed. D. H. Bossingham, E. Williams, and P. J. R. Nichols) pp. 30–7. Muscular Dystrophy Group of Great Britain and Northern Ireland, London.

Statham, H. E. and Dubowitz, V. (1979). Duchenne muscular dystrophy: ^{45}Ca exchange in cultured skin fibroblasts and the effect of calcium ionophore A23187. *Clin. Chim. Acta.* **96**, 225–31.

Stephens, F. E. and Tyler, F. H. (1951). Studies in disorders of muscle. V. The inheritance of childhood progressive muscular dystrophy in 33 kindreds. *Amer. J. Hum. Genet.* **3**, 111–25.

Stern, L. M., Caudrey, D. J., Clark, M. S., Perrett, L. V., and Boldt, D. W. (1985). Carrier detection in Duchenne muscular dystrophy using computed tomography. *Clin. Genet.* **27**, 392–7.

Stern, L. Z. (1984). Criteria for therapeutic trials in Duchenne muscular dystrophy. In *Neuromuscular diseases* (ed. G. Serratrice *et al.*) pp. 525–8. Raven Press, New York.

Stern, R. and Eldridge, R. (1975). Attitudes of patients and their relatives to Huntington's disease. *J. Med. Genet.* **12**, 217–23.

——, Godbold, J. H., Chess, Q., and Kagen, L. J. (1984). ECG abnormalities in polymyositis. *Arch. Intern. Med.* **144**, 2185–9.

Stevenson, A. C. (1953). Muscular dystrophy in Northern Ireland. *Ann. Eugen., London* **18**, 50–91.

—— (1958). Muscular dystrophy in Northern Ireland. IV. Some additional data. *Ann. Hum. Genet.* **22**, 231–4.

Sugita, H. (1985). Personal communication.

——, Ishiura, S., and Kohama, K. (1984). Lysosomal and nonlysosomal enzymes and amino acid fluxes in catabolic states. In *Neuromuscular diseases* (ed. G. Serratrice *et al.*) pp. 143–7. Raven Press, New York.

—— and Tyler, F. H. (1963). Pathogenesis of muscular dystrophy. *Trans. Assoc. Amer. Physicians* **76**, 231–43.

Sussman, M. D. (1984). Advantage of early spinal stabilization and fusion in patients with Duchenne muscular dystrophy. *J. Pediat. Orthop.* **4**, 532–7.

—— (1985). Treatment of scoliosis in Duchenne muscular dystrophy. *Develop. Med. Child. Neurol.* **27**, 522–4.

Sutherland, D. H., Olshen, R., Cooper, L., Wyatt, M., Leach, J., Mubarak, S., and Schultz, P. (1981). The pathomechanics of gait in Duchenne muscular dystrophy. *Develop. Med. Child. Neurol.* **23**, 3–22.

Swash, M. and Schwartz, M. S. (1981). *Neuromuscular diseases – a practical approach to Diagnosis and management*. Springer-Verlag, Berlin.

——, Carter, N. D., Heath, R., Leak, M., and Rogers, K. L. (1983). Benign X-linked myopathy with acanthocytes (McLeod syndrome). Its relationship to X-linked muscular dystrophy. *Brain* **106**, 717–33.

Swinyard C. A., Deaver, G. G., and Greenspan, L. (1957) Gradients of functional ability of importance in rehabilitation of patients with progressive muscular and neuromuscular diseases. *Arch. Phys. Med. Rehab.* **38**, 574–9.

Szibor, R., Till, U., Lösche, W., and Steinbicker, V. (1981). Red cell response to A23187 and valinomycine in Duchenne muscular dystrophy. *Acta Biol. Med. Germ.* **40**, 1187–90.

Taft, L. T. (1973). The care and management of the child with muscular dystrophy. *Develop. Med. Child. Neurol.* **15**, 510–8.

Takagi, A. (1984). Sarcoplasmic reticulum of Duchenne muscular dystrophy: a study on skinned muscle fiber. In *Neuromuscular diseases*. (ed. G. Serratrice *et al.*) pp. 123–5. Raven Press, New York.

—— and Nonaka, I. (1981). Duchenne muscular dystrophy: unusual activation of single fibers *in vitro*. *Muscle and Nerve* **4**, 10–5.

——, Shimada, Y., and Mozai, T. (1970). Studies on plasma free fatty acid and ketone bodies in young patients with muscular atrophy. *Neurology* **20**, 904–8.

Takamoto, K., Hirose, K., Uono, M., and Nonaka, I. (1984). A genetic variant of Emery-Dreifuss disease: muscular dystrophy with humeropelvic distribution, early joint contracture, and permanent atrial paralysis. *Arch. Neurol.* **41**, 1292–3.

Tanzer, M. L and Gilvarg, C. (1959). Creatine and creatine kinase measurement. *J. Biol. Chem.* **234**, 3201–4.

Templeton, A. R. and Yokoyama, S. (1980). Effect of reproductive compensation and the desire to have male offspring on the incidence of a sex-linked lethal disease. *Amer. J. Hum. Genet.* **32**, 575–81.

Thomas, A., Bax, M., Coombes, K., Goldson, E., Smyth, D., and Whitmore, K. (1985). The health and social needs of physically handicapped young adults: Are they being met by the statutory services? *Develop. Med. Child. Neurol.* Vol. 27, Suppl. 50, No. 4.

Thomas, N. S. T. Williams, H., Elsas, L. J., Hopkins, L. C., Sarfarazi, M., and Harper, P. S. (1986). Localization of the gene for Emery–Dreifuss muscular dystrophy to the distal long arm of the X-chromosome. *J. Med. Genet.* (In press)

Thomas, P. K., Calne, D. B., and Elliott, C. F. (1972). X-linked scapuloperoneal syndrome. *J. Neurol. Neurosurg. Psychiat.* **35**, 208–15.

——, Schott, G. D., and Morgan-Hughes, J. A. (1975). Adult onset scapuloperoneal myopathy. *J. Neurol. Neurosurg, Psychiat.* **38**, 1008–15.

Thompson, C. E. (1978). Reproduction in Duchenne dystrophy. *Neurology* **28**, 1045–47.

Thompson, M. W. (1984). Genetic management of pregnancies of carriers and possible carriers of Duchenne muscular dystrophy. In *Neuromuscular diseases* (ed. G. Serratrice *et al.*) pp. 21–3. Raven Press, New York.

——, Ludvigsen, B., and Monckton, G. (1962). Some problems in genetics of muscular dystrophy. *Rev. Canad. Biol.* **21**, 543–50.

Thompson, R. G., Nickel, B., Finlayson, S., Meuser, R., Hamerton, J. L., and Wrogemann, K. (1983). 56K fibroblast protein not specific for Duchenne muscular dystrophy but for skin biopsy site. *Nature* **304**, 740–1.

Thompson, W. H. S. (1968). Determination and statistical analyses of the normal ranges for five serum enzymes. *Clin. Chim. Acta* **21**, 469–78.

—— (1971). Serum enzyme studies in acquired disease of skeletal muscle. *Clin. Chim. Acta* **35**, 193–9.

——, Sweetin, J. C., and Elton, R. A (1974). The neurogenic and myogenic hypotheses in human (Duchenne) muscular dystrophy. *Nature* **249**, 151–2.

Tippett, P. A., Dennis, N. R., Machin, D., Price, C. P., and Clayton, B. E. (1982). Creatine kinase activity in the detection of carriers of Duchenne muscular dystrophy: comparison of two methods. *Clin. Chim. Acta* **121**, 345–59.

Tomelleri, G., Orrico, D., De Grandis, D., and Fiaschi, A. (1980). Emery–Dreifuss muscular dystrophy in two brothers. In *Muscular dystrophy research: advances and new trends* (ed. C. Angelini, G. A. Danieli, and D. Fontanari) pp. 307–8. Excerpta Medica, Amsterdam.

Toop, J. (1975). The histochemical development of human skeletal muscle and its motor innervation. In *Recent advances in myology* (ed. W. G. Bradley, D. Gardner-Medwin, and J. N. Walton) pp. 322–9. Excerpta Medica, Amsterdam.

—— and Emery, A. E. H. (1974). Muscle histology in fetuses at risk for Duchenne muscular dystrophy. *Clin. Genet.* **5**, 230–3.

Totsuka, T., Watanabe, K., and Kiyono, S. (1981) Masking of a dystrophic symptom in genotypically dystrophic-dwarf mice. *Proc. Japan Acad. (Ser. B).* **57**, 109–13.

—— and Uramoto, I. (1983). A bone-muscle imbalance hypothesis for the pathogenesis of murine muscular dystrophy. In *Muscular dystrophy: biomedical aspects* (ed. S. Ebashi and E. Ozawa) pp. 29–38. Springer-Verlag, Berlin.

Tyler, F. H. (1950). Studies in disorders of muscle. III. "Pseudohypertrophy" of muscle in progressive muscular dystrophy and other neuromuscular diseases. *Arch. Neurol. Psychiat.* **63**, 425–32.

—— and Wintrobe, M. M. (1950). Studies in disorders of muscle. I. The problems of progressive muscular dystrophy. *Ann. Int. Med.* **32**, 72–9.

Tzvetanova, E. (1971). Aldolase isoenzymes in serum and muscle from patients with progressive muscular dystrophy and from human foetus. *J. Neurol. Sci.* **14**, 483–9.

Usuki, F., Nakazato, O., Osame, M., and Igata, A. (1985). Hyperestrogenemia in Duchenne muscular dystrophy (DMD). *Clin. Neurol.* **25**, 711–5.

Vainzof, M., Zatz, M., and Otto, P. A. (1985). Serum CK–MB activity in progressive muscular dystrophy: Is it of nosologic value? *Amer. J. Med. Genet.* **22**, 81–87.

Vasari G. (1568). *Lives of the artists.* (Translated and reprinted in *Penguin*, London, 1981.)

Vassella, F., Mumenthaler, M., Rossi, E., Moser, H., and Wiesmann, U. (1967). Die kongenitale Muskeldystrophie. *Deutsche Zeit. Nervenheilk.* **190**, 349–74.

Verellen, C., De Meyer, R., Freund, M., Laterre, C., Scholberg, B., and Frédéric, J. (1977). Progressive muscular dystrophy of the Duchenne type in a young girl associated with an aberration of chromosome X. In *Proc. 5th Internat. Congr. Birth Defects* p. 42 (Abstract). Excerpta Medica, Amsterdam.

——, Markovic, V., De Meyer, R., Freund, M., Laterre, C., and Worton, R. (1978). Expression of an X-linked recessive disease in a female due to non-random inactivation of the X chromosome. *Amer. J. Hum. Genet.* **30**, 97A (Abstract).

Verellen-Dumoulin, C. (1986). Personal communication.

——, Freund, M., De Meyer, R., Laterre, C., Frédéric, J., Thompson, M. W., Markovic, V. D., and Worton, R. G. (1984). Expression of an X-linked muscular dystrophy in a female due to a translocation involving Xp21 and non-random inactivation of the normal X chromosome. *Hum. Genet.* **67**, 115–9.

Vignos, P. J. (1977a). Intellectual function and educational achievement in Duchenne muscular dystrophy. In *Muscular dystrophy, 1976* (ed. G. C. Robin and G. Falewski de Leon) pp. 131–8. Karger, Basel.

—— (1977b). Respiratory function and pulmonary infection in Duchenne muscular dystrophy. In *Muscular Dystrophy, 1976* (ed. G. C. Robin and G. Falewski de Leon) pp. 123–30. Karger, Basel.

—— (1979). Rehabilitation in the myopathies. In *Handbook of clinical neurology* (ed. P. J. Vinken and G. W. Bruyn) Vol. 41, pp. 457–500. Elsevier/North-Holland, Amsterdam.

—— and Lefkowitz, M. (1959). A biochemical study of certain skeletal muscle constituents in human progressive muscular dystrophy *J. Clin. Invest.* **38**, 873–81.

——, Spencer, G. E., and Archibald, K. C. (1963) Management of progressive muscular dystrophy of childhood. *Jour. Amer. Med. Assoc.* **184**, 89–96.

—— and Watkins, M. P. (1966). The effect of exercise in muscular dystrophy. *Jour. Amer. Med. Assoc.* **197**, 121–6.

de Visser, M. and Verbeeten, B. (1985a). Computed tomography of the skeletal musculature in Becker-type muscular dystrophy and benign infantile spinal muscular atrophy. *Muscle and Nerve* **8**, 435–44.

—— (1985b). Computed tomographic findings in manifesting carriers of Duchenne muscular dystrophy. *Clin. Genet.* **27**, 269–75.

Vogel, F. (1983). Mutation in man. In *Principles and practice of medical genetics* (ed. A. E. H. Emery and D. Rimoin) pp. 26–48. Churchill Livingstone, Edinburgh.

Wadia, R. S., Wadgaonkar, S. U., Amin, R. B., and Sardesai, H. V. (1976). An unusual family of benign 'X' linked muscular dystrophy with cardiac involvement. *J. Med. Genet.* **13**, 352-6.

Walton, J. N. (1955). On the inheritance of muscular dystrophy. *Ann. Hum. Genet.* **20**, 1-38.

—— (1956). Amyotonia congenita, a follow-up study. *Lancet* **i**, 1023-7.

—— (1957). The inheritance of muscular dystrophy. *Acta Genet., Basel.* **7**, 318-20.

—— (1969). Muscular dystrophies and their management. *Brit. Med. J.* **3**, 639-42.

—— (ed.) (1987). *Disorders of voluntary muscle*, 5th edn. Churchill Livingstone, Edinburgh.

—— and Gardner-Medwin, D. (1981). Progressive muscular dystrophy and the myotonic disorders. In *Disorders of voluntary muscle*, 4th edn (ed. J. N. Walton) pp. 481-524. Churchill Livingstone, Edinburgh, London, New York.

—— and Nattrass, F. J. (1954). On the classification, natural history and treatment of the myopathies. *Brain* **77**, 169-231.

—— and Warrick, C. K. (1954). Osseous changes in myopathy. *Brit. J. Radiology* **27**, 1-15.

Waters, D. D., Nutter, D. O., Hopkins, L. C., and Dorney, E. R. (1975). Cardiac features of an unusual X-linked humeroperoneal neuromuscular disease. *New Engl. J. Med.* **293**, 1017-22.

Watters, G., Karpati, G., and Kaplan, B. (1977). Post-anaesthetic augmentation of muscle damage as a presenting sign in three patients with Duchenne muscular dystrophy. *Canad. J. Neurol. Sci.* **4**, 228 (Abstract).

Weiller, C. (1985). Muskeldystrophie Duchenne. Ein Fallbericht. *Pathologe* **6**, 32-7.

Wharton, B. A. (1965). An unusual variety of muscular dystrophy. *Lancet* **i**, 248-9.

Wiegand, V., Rahlf, G., Meinck, M., and Kreuzer, H. (1984). Kardiomyopathie bei Trägerinnen des Duchenne-Gens. *Zeit. Kardiol.* **73**, 188-91.

Wieme, R. J. and Herpol, J. E. (1962). Origin of the lactate dehydrogenase iso-enzyme pattern found in the serum of patients having primary muscular dystrophy. *Nature* **194**, 287-8.

Wilcox, D. E., Affara, N. A., Yates, J. R. W., Ferguson-Smith, M. A., and Pearson, P. L. (1985). Multipoint linkage analysis of the short arm of the human X chromosome in families with X-linked muscular dystrophy. *Hum. Genet.* **70**, 365-75.

——, Cooke, A., Colgan, J., Boyd, E., Aitken, D. A., Sinclair, L., Glasgow, L., Stephenson, J. B. P., and Ferguson-Smith, M. A. (1986). Duchenne muscular dystrophy due to a familial Xp21 deletion detectable by DNA analysis and flow cytometry. *Hum. Genet.* **73**, 175-80.

Williams, E. A., Read, L., Ellis, A., Galasko, C. S. B., and Morris, P. (1984). The management of equinus deformity in Duchenne muscular dystrophy. *J. Bone & Joint Surg.* **66B**, 546-50.

Williams, W. R., Thompson, M. W., and Morton, N. E. (1983). Complex segregation analysis and computer-assisted genetic risk assessment for Duchenne muscular dystrophy. *Amer. J. Med. Genet.* **14**, 315-33.

Winter, R. M. (1980). Estimation of male to female ratio of mutation rates from carrier-detection tests in X-linked disorders. *Amer. J. Hum. Genet.* **32**, 582-8.

—— and Pembrey, M. E. (1982). Does unequal crossing over contribute to the mutation rate in Duchenne muscular dystrophy? *Amer. J. Med. Genet.* **12**, 437–41.

Witkowski, J. A. (1986a). Tissue culture studies of muscle disorders: Part 1. Techniques, cell growth, morphology, cell surface. *Muscle and Nerve* **9**, 191–207.

—— (1986b). Tissue culture studies of muscle disorders: Part 2. *Muscle and Nerve* **9**, 283–98.

—— and Dubowitz, V. (1985). Duchenne muscular dystrophy: studies of cell motility *in vitro. J. Cell Sci.* **76**, 225–34.

Wohlfart, G., Fex, J., and Eliasson, S. (1955). Hereditary proximal spinal muscular atrophy – a clinical entity simulating progressive muscular dystrophy. *Acta Psychiat. Neurol. (Kbh)* **30**, 395–406.

Wood, D. S. (1984). Excitation-contraction coupling in Duchenne muscular dystrophy. In *Neuromuscular diseases* (ed. G. Serratrice *et al.*) pp. 185–90. Raven Press, New York.

Worden, D. K. and Vignos, P. J. (1962). Intellectual function in childhood progressive muscular dystrophy. *Pediatrics* **29**, 968–77.

Worton, R. G., Duff, C., Sylvester, J. E., Schmickel, R. D. and Willard, H. F. (1984). Duchenne muscular dystrophy involving translocation of the *dmd* gene next to ribosomal RNA genes. *Science* **224**, 1447–9.

Wrogemann, K. and Pena, S. D. J. (1976). Mitochondrial calcium overload: a general mechanism for cell-necrosis in muscle diseases. *Lancet* **i**, 672–4.

Yasin, R., Walsh, F. S., Landon, D. N., and Thompson, E. J. (1983). New approaches to the study of human dystrophic muscle cells in culture. *J. Neurol. Sci.* **58**, 315–34.

Yasuda, N. and Kondo, K. (1980). No sex difference in mutation rates of Duchenne muscular dystrophy. *J. Med. Genet.* **17**, 106–11.

—— (1982). The effect of parental age on rate of mutation for Duchenne muscular dystrophy. *Amer. J. Med. Genet.* **13**, 91–9.

Yates, J. R. W. and Emery, A. E. H. (1985). A population study of adult onset limb-girdle muscular dystrophy. *J. Med. Genet.* **22**, 250–57.

Yoshioka, M., Itagaki, Y., Saida, K., and Nishitani, Y. (1986). Clinical and genetic studies of muscular dystrophy in young girls. *Clin Genet.* **29**, 137–42.

——, Okuno, T., Honda, Y., and Nakano, Y. (1980) Central nervous system involvement in progressive muscular dystrophy. *Arch. Dis. Child.* **55**, 589–94.

Young, A., Johnson, D., O'Gorman, E., Macmillan, T., and Chase, A. P. (1984). A new spinal brace for use in Duchenne muscular dystrophy. *Develop. Med. Child. Neurol.* **26**, 808–13.

Yu, Y. L. and Murray, N. M. F. (1984). A comparison of concentric needle electromyography, quantitative EMG and single fibre EMG in the diagnosis of neuromuscular diseases. *Electroencephalogr. Clin. Neurophysiol.* **58**, 220–5.

Zalman, F., Perloff, J. K., Durant, N. N., and Campion, D. S. (1983). Acute respiratory failure following intravenous verapamil in Duchenne's muscular dystrophy. *Amer. Heart J.* **105**, 510–11.

Zatz, M. (1983). Effects of genetic counseling on Duchenne muscular dystrophy families in Brazil. *Amer. J. Med. Genet.* **15**, 483–90.

—— (1986). Personal communication.

——, Betti, R. T. B., and Frota-Pessoa, O. (1986). Treatment of Duchenne muscular dystrophy with growth hormone inhibitors. *Amer. J. Med. Genet.* **24**, 549–66.

—— and Levy, J. A. (1981b). Benign Duchenne muscular dystrophy in a patient with growth hormone deficiency. *Amer. J. Med. Genet.* **10**, 301–4 (and also *Amer. J. Med. Genet.* **24**, 567–72 (1986)).

—— and Frota-Pessoa, O. (1981). Suggestion for a possible mitigating treatment of Duchenne muscular dystrophy. *Amer. J. Med. Genet.* **10**, 305–7.

——, Levy, J. A. and Peres, C. A. (1976). Creatine phosphokinase (CPK) activity in relatives of patients with X-linked muscular dystrophies. A Brazilian study. *J. Génét. Hum.* **24**, 153–168.

——, Itskan, S. B., Sanger, R., Frota-Pessoa, O., and Saldanha, P. H. (1974). New linkage data for the X-linked types of muscular dystrophy and G6PD variants, colour blindness and Xg blood groups. *J. Med. Genet.* **11**, 321–7.

——, Shapiro, L. J., Campion, D. S., Oda, E., and Kaback, M. M. (1978). Serum pyruvate kinase (PK) and creatine phosphokinase (CPK) in progressive muscular dystrophies. *J. Neurol. Sci.* **36**, 349–62.

——, Vianna-Morgante, A. M., Campos, P., and Diament, A. J. (1981a) Translocation (X;6) in a female with Duchenne muscular dystrophy: implications for the localisation of the DMD locus. *J. Med. Genet.* **18**, 442–7.

Zellweger, H. (1975). Family counselling in Duchenne muscular dystrophy. In *Recent advances in myology* (ed. W. G. Bradley, D. Gardner-Medwin, and J. N. Walton) pp. 469–71. Excerpta Medica, Amsterdam.

——, Afifi, A., McCormick, W. F. and Mergner, W. (1967). Severe congenital muscular dystrophy. *Amer. J. Dis. Child.* **114**, 591–602.

—— and Antonik, A. (1975). Newborn screening for Duchenne muscular dystrophy. *Pediatrics* **55**, 30–4.

—— and Hanson, J. W. (1967a). Slowly progressive X-linked recessive muscular dystrophy (Type IIIb). *Arch. Int. Med.* **120**, 525–35.

—— (1967b). Psychometric studies in muscular dystrophy type IIIa (Duchenne). *Develop. Med. Child. Neurol.* **9**, 576–81.

—— and Markowitz, E. (1970). Age- and sex-dependent differences of serum enzymes in normal controls. In *Muscle diseases* (ed. J. N. Walton, N. Canal, and G. Scarlato) pp. 445–9. Excerpta Medica, Internat. Congr. Ser. No. 199, Amsterdam.

——, Ionasescu, V., and Simpson, J. (1980). Sporadic Duchenne muscular dystrophy in females; genetic counseling of women with pelvifemoral muscular dystrophy. *Helv. Paediat. Acta* **35**, 343–8.

——, Waziri, M., and Antonik. A. (1975). Screening of the newborn for Duchenne muscular dystrophy. *Brit. Med. J.* **3**, 767.

—— and Niedermeyer, E. (1965). Central nervous system manifestations in childhood muscular dystrophy. I. Psychometric and electroencephalographic findings. *Ann. Paediat.* **205**, 25–42.

Ziter, F. A., Allsop, K. G. and Tyler, F. H. (1977). Assessment of muscle strength in Duchenne muscular dystrophy. *Neurology* **27**, 981–4.

Index